Suzanne Brown CRNA

ATLAS OF PROCEDURES
IN ANESTHESIA
AND CRITICAL CARE

Foreword

The concept and fulfillment of an *Atlas of Procedures in Anesthesia and Critical Care* amply depict the burgeoning of technology in anesthesia over recent decades and the overlapping of interests with critical care medicine. After all, of what does anesthesia consist but the intimate critical care of surgical patients often quite ill, where the balance between survival and death may be influenced by the physiologic effects of anesthetics.

John Butterworth in his unitary approach to this subject has resorted to a venerable medium wherein the use of a commonality of illustrations and minimal text is the strategy. Andreas Vesalius, to be sure, was the progenitor of this approach. As part of a series of surgical lectures given at the University of Padua in 1537, Vesalius had prepared a large illustration of the veins. The detail and quality of this drawing represented such a novel and pedagogical device, "that the professors and students of medicine urged me to make similar illustrations of the arteries and nerves." These would become a part of the *Tabulae anatomicae* so ably executed in wood engravings by Jan Stephan van Calcar.

In this text, management of the airway is appropriately heralded, perhaps in greater detail than can be found in more general works; essentially we are provided with a manual within an atlas. And so it goes with current monitoring techniques, both invasive and noninvasive. While relevant to anesthesia, the chapters on regional anesthesia may also intrigue the intensivist. Some of the nerve blocks may also apply to emergent surgical procedures that need to be performed in the intensive care unit. In a concluding chapter, Butterworth suggests that few physicians, with the exception of anesthesiologists, are aware of the problems inherent in careful positioning of patients whereby the physiologic stresses may be great indeed.

I take pride in offering these prefatory remarks on the *Atlas* because I have long been aware of John Butterworth's abilities as an anesthesiologist and his incisive approach to all manner of problems. He has succeeded in compiling an important work of a conceptual nature nicely tied together by a series of illustrations done by the one medical illustrator.

LEROY D. VANDAM, MD
Boston, Massachusetts
September, 1991

ATLAS OF PROCEDURES IN ANESTHESIA AND CRITICAL CARE

John F. Butterworth IV, MD

Associate Professor
Department of Anesthesia
The Bowman Gray School of Medicine
Wake Forest University
Winston-Salem, North Carolina

Illustrated by Greg Marlow

W. B. SAUNDERS COMPANY
Harcourt Brace Jovanovich, Inc.

Philadelphia   London   Toronto   Montreal   Sydney   Tokyo

W. B. SAUNDERS COMPANY
Harcourt Brace Jovanovich, Inc.

The Curtis Center
Independence Square West
Philadelphia, PA 19106

> **Library of Congress Cataloging-in-Publication Data**
>
> Butterworth, John F.
>   Atlas of procedures in anesthesia and critical care/John F. Butterworth IV; illustrated by Greg Marlow.
>   p. cm.
>   ISBN 0-7216-2916-4
>   1. Anesthesia—Atlases.   2. Critical care medicine—Atlases. I. Title.
>   [DNLM: 1. Anesthesia—methods—atlases. 2. Critical Care—methods—atlases.   WO 517 B988a]
>   RD81.B84   1992
>   617.9'6—dc20
>   DNLM/DLC   91—18528

Editor: Richard Zorab
Designer: Bill Donnelly
Production Manager: Ken Neimeister
Manuscript Editors: Jeanne M. Carper and Tina Rebane
Illustrator: Greg Marlow
Illustration Coordinator: Cecelia Roberts
Indexer: Helene Taylor
Cover Designer: Anita Curry

ATLAS OF PROCEDURES IN ANESTHESIA
AND CRITICAL CARE   ISBN 0-7216-2916-4

Copyright © 1992 by W. B. Saunders Company.

All rights reserved.   No part of this publication may be reproduced or transmitted in any form or by any means, electronic or mechanical, including photocopy, recording, or any information storage and retrieval system, without permission in writing from the publisher.

Printed in MEXICO.

Last digit is the print number: 9   8   7   6   5   4   3   2   1

Preface

The practice of anesthesia and critical care medicine includes aspects of both the "cognitive" and the "procedural" sides of medicine. As with other specialties, the "cognitive" side is usually emphasized in the standard textbooks, leaving instruction in the more "mundane" manual skills of the specialty to colleagues and to scattered subspecialty texts. An atlas that would illustrate the more representative regional anesthetic, airway management, invasive monitoring, and positioning techniques in one volume is clearly warranted.

The list of procedures detailed in this volume is not all-inclusive. The block techniques include only those that have formed part of the day-to-day practice of the hospitals in which I have worked. Thus, cervical epidural block, a common procedure in the pain management clinic but rarely used for surgical anesthesia, is not included. On the other hand, transtracheal jet ventilation is rarely used but is often lifesaving. Because I believe it should be part of the armamentarium of all who may need to intubate an apneic patient with abnormal airway anatomy, the technique is illustrated and described in detail. In short, I have tried to limit the book to essentials, but I recognize that my selection represents personal and institutional biases.

I would like to acknowledge the invaluable assistance of my illustrator, Greg Marlow. In addition to his obvious skills as an illustrator, Greg has also served as a reviewer of the text. I would also like to thank Faith McLellan for critically reading and rereading all the chapters for style and grammar. I thank the numerous colleagues who have made suggestions about the illustrations and text. I thank Leroy Vandam for forwarding and recommending my embryonic idea for a book to Lewis Reines, president of the W. B. Saunders Company. Finally, I thank my family for their support.

JOHN F. BUTTERWORTH IV, MD

A Note About Monitoring and Resuscitation Standards

Throughout the text I have referred to "usual monitoring devices" and "resuscitation drugs and equipment." Monitoring standards for anesthesia practice were adopted by a vote of the House of Delegates of the American Society of Anesthesiologists (ASA) and are summarized in Table I–1. Note that *continuous* means

TABLE I–1

MONITORING STANDARDS FOR ANESTHESIA PRACTICE

Required during *Every* Anesthetic Procedure
- Continuous presence of a qualified anesthesia provider
- Continual evaluation of the patient
  Oxygenation
  1. Measurement of oxygen in inspired gas (including a low-oxygen concentration limit alarm)
  2. Quantitative assessment of blood oxygenation (e.g., pulse oximetry)

  Ventilation
  1. Continual assessment of adequacy of ventilation with (at least) clinical observation and auscultation of breath sounds (capnography is recommended)
  2. Verification of correct positioning of endotracheal tubes by clinical assessment and by identification of carbon dioxide in expired gas
  3. A disconnection alarm shall be used during mechanical ventilation

  Circulation
  1. The electrocardiogram shall be continuously displayed during anesthetics
  2. Arterial blood pressure and heart rate shall be determined at least every 5 minutes
  3. During *general anesthesia* at least one of the following will be used continually
     Palpation of a peripheral pulse
     Auscultation of heart sounds
     Monitoring of intraarterial pressures
     Ultrasound peripheral pulse monitoring
     Pulse plethysmography
     Pulse oximetry

  Body Temperature
  Body temperature shall be measured continuously when changes in body temperature are intended, anticipated, or suspected

TABLE I–2

DRUGS AND EQUIPMENT ESSENTIAL FOR RESUSCITATION

Drugs
- Oxygen
- Atropine
- Epinephrine
- Lidocaine
- Procainamide
- Bretylium
- Adenosine
- Verapamil
- Esmolol
- Calcium chloride or calcium glutamate (controversial)
- Sodium bicarbonate (controversial)
- Thiopental
- Succinylcholine
- Phenylephrine (or ephedrine or other vasoconstrictor)

Equipment
- Bag–valve–mask ventilation system
- Oropharyngeal and nasopharyngeal airways
- Laryngoscope and blades
- Tracheal tubes
- Defibrillator
- Suction equipment
- Intravenous supplies (including syringes and needles)

uninterrupted, whereas *continual* means repeated regularly and frequently. Standards of practice evolve with time, and thus capnography may one day be mandated by the ASA.

Resuscitation drugs and equipment and their use are described in the American Heart Association's *Textbook of Advanced Cardiac Life Support*. Those drugs essential for resuscitation are contained on most hospital "crash carts." Clearly, all those drugs and items of equipment necessary to perform basic and advanced cardiac life support must be available in the operating room, postanesthesia care unit, nerve block room, and intensive care unit, just as they are in other areas of the hospital. In addition, drugs (e.g., oxygen, thiopental, succinylcholine) and equipment (e.g., ventilation and intubation supplies) for management of local anesthetic toxic side effects must also be readily available during regional anesthesia. These items are summarized in Table I–2. The availability of resuscitation drugs and equipment is essential, but I do not mean to imply that an epinephrine infusion must be mixed prior to performing a median nerve block at the wrist; rather I hope to emphasize that the practitioner always be certain that the resuscitation drugs and equipment that may be required are accessible before the need for them actually arises.

References

American Heart Association: Textbook of Advanced Cardiac Life Support. Dallas, American Heart Association, 1987

Standards for Basic Intraoperative Monitoring. ASA Newsletter, vol 54, pp 17–18. Park Ridge, IL, American Society of Anesthesiologists, 1990

Contents

I
AIRWAY MANAGEMENT

1. Ventilation with Bag and Mask 3
2. Laryngeal Anesthesia 7
3. Orotracheal Intubation 11
4. Nasotracheal Intubation 21
5. Failed Intubation 27
6. Fiberoptic Laryngoscopy 31
7. Transtracheal Jet Ventilation 37
8. Cricothyroidotomy 41
9. Retrograde Intubation 45
10. Intubation with Lighted Stylet 49
11. Intubation with Double-Lumen Endobronchial Tubes 53
12. Replacement of an Endotracheal Tube 63
13. Emergency Needle Thoracentesis 67

II
INTRAVASCULAR CANNULATION

14. Intravenous Cannulation 71
15. Central Venous Cannulation 75
16. Intravascular Electrocardiography 101

17	Pulmonary Artery Catheterization	105
18	Arterial Cannulation	115
19	Suture Techniques	125

III
REGIONAL ANESTHESIA

20	Local Infiltration of Anesthetic	135
21	Intravenous Regional Anesthesia	137
22	Digital Nerve Block	143
23	Upper Extremity Nerve Blocks	145
24	Lower Extremity Nerve Blocks	167
25	Spinal Anesthesia	179
26	Epidural Anesthesia	191
27	Intercostal Nerve Blocks	209
28	Cervical Plexus Block	213
29	Use of the Electrical Nerve Stimulator for Regional Anesthesia	217

IV
POSITIONING THE PATIENT ON THE OPERATING ROOM TABLE

30	Operation of the Surgical Table	221
31	Patient Positions	227
	Index	235

AIRWAY MANAGEMENT

1

Ventilation with Bag and Mask

Although nearly all patients undergoing general anesthesia also undergo tracheal intubation, an anesthetist's ability to maintain an unobstructed airway with bag and mask is no less important now than it was in the past. Brief general anesthetic procedures (e.g., for electroconvulsive therapy) are still most commonly performed without intubation. All patients who will be intubated are managed initially with bag and mask. And, despite the best intentions of the anesthetist, not every patient will be intubated on the first attempt.

Masks and Mask "Fit"

When a bag and mask system is used to provide unobstructed ventilation, the mask must be of an appropriate size so that it will form a seal with the skin of the face. Obtaining a seal with the mask is often difficult in bearded or edentulous patients. Transparent masks permit early visual detection of hypoxemia (by checking the color of the lips) and regurgitation.

If a mask of proper size has been applied to the patient's face, *spontaneous* (the patient inspires spontaneously without assistance), *assisted* (the anesthetist provides a positive-pressure breath as the patient inspires spontaneously), or *controlled* (the anesthetist provides positive-pressure breaths without contribution from the patient) ventilation can be provided. For any of these techniques it is vital that the flow of inspired and expired gases not be obstructed by the tongue. Unconscious and semiconscious patients lack sufficient voluntary motor tone to elevate the tongue out of the oropharynx. If the airway is wholly or partially obstructed, positive-pressure mask ventilation may result only in distention of the stomach with gas. Usually the obstruction can be overcome by lifting the patient's mandible with the third, fourth, and fifth fingers while holding the mask in place with the thumb and index finger of the left hand (Fig. 1–1). It is important to lift the mandible, not the soft tissues adjacent to the mandible, with the fingers of the left hand.

Oropharyngeal and Nasopharyngeal Airways

When gas exchange remains obstructed despite elevation of the mandible, several options remain. An oropharyngeal or nasopharyngeal airway can be placed to provide a conduit for inspired and expired gases to pass around the obstructing

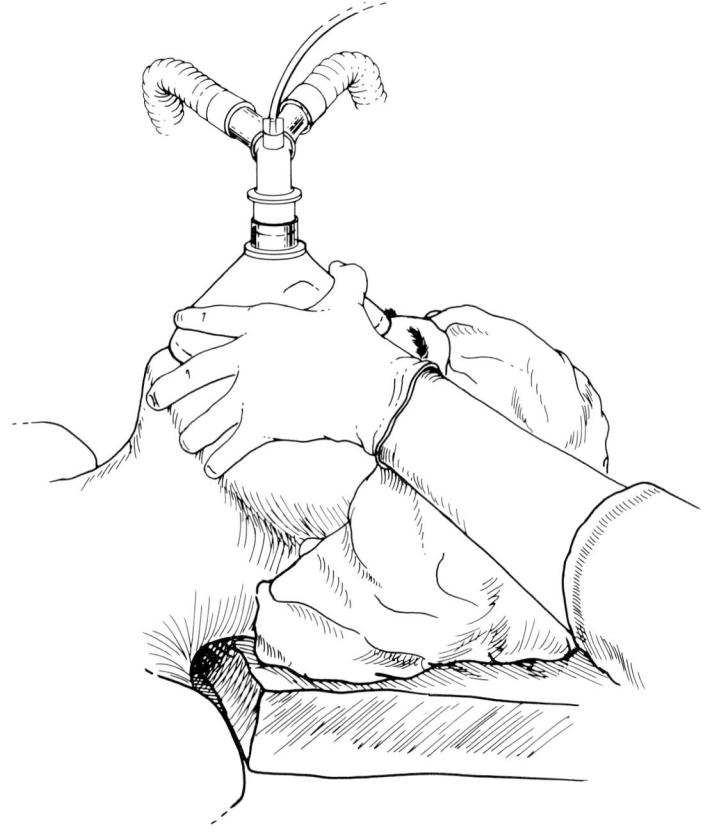

FIGURE 1–1

tongue. To insert an oropharyngeal airway, scissor the mouth open with the index (or middle) finger and thumb of the gloved right hand (Fig. 1–2). Lift the tongue with a tongue depressor (held with the left hand), and insert the oropharyngeal airway (with the right hand) (Fig. 1–3). The curve of the oropharyngeal airway should follow the natural curvature of the oropharynx (Fig. 1–4). If a nasopharyngeal airway is selected, lubricate it before gently advancing it through either nostril (Fig. 1–5). The tips of the oropharyngeal and nasopharyngeal airways will normally rest in the posterior oropharynx when seated to their entire length.

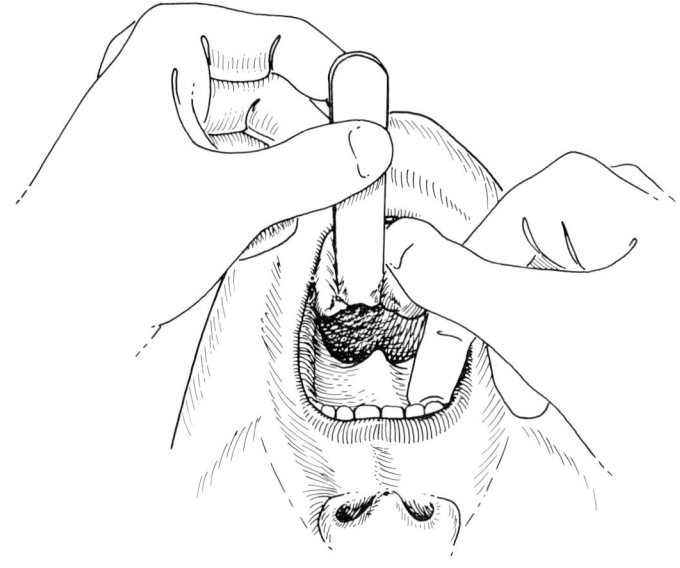

FIGURE 1–2

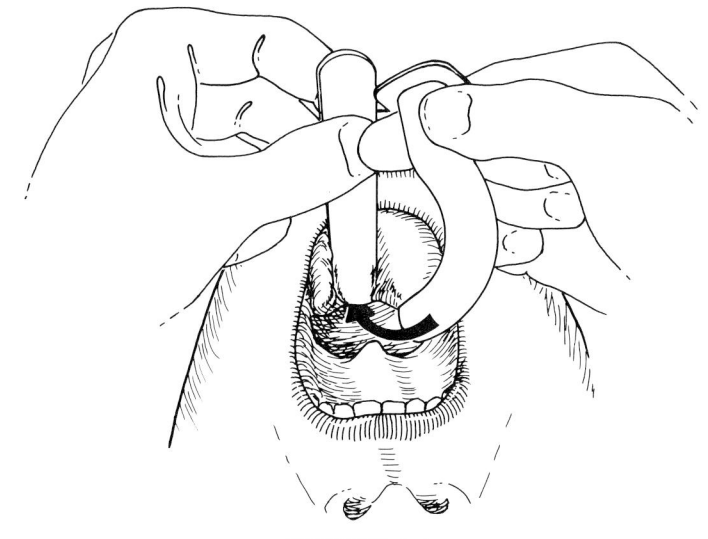

FIGURE 1–3

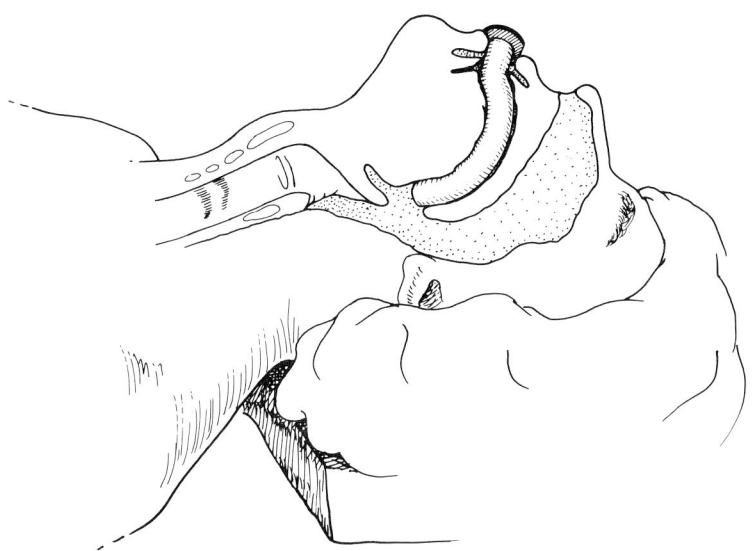

FIGURE 1–4

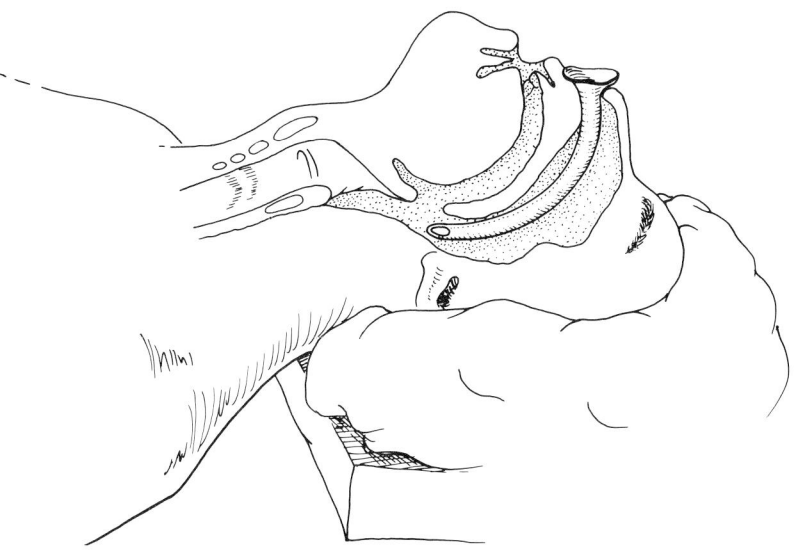

FIGURE 1–5

Patients who are partially anesthetized (i.e., in stage II of general anesthesia) may respond to placement of either oral or nasopharyngeal airways with bouts of coughing or with laryngospasm. Thus, the anesthetist must weigh these risks against the benefits of placing an airway during the onset or offset of inhalational anesthesia. Airway patency often improves as the patient becomes more deeply anesthetized or emerges from anesthesia. If oropharyngeal and nasopharyngeal airways prove unsuccessful in providing an unobstructed airway, tracheal intubation may be required.

Adjunct Maneuvers

In those instances in which anesthesia will be administered by mask for more than 15 minutes, the anesthetist can reduce the work load of his left hand by using elastic straps to help hold the mask in place and/or by placing a folded blanket behind the patient's shoulders (Fig. 1–6). The straps do not substitute for the anesthetist's left hand. Likewise, while the blanket may assist in maintaining airway patency by extending the head on the neck, it usually will not eliminate the need for the anesthetist to lift the patient's mandible with the fingers of his left hand.

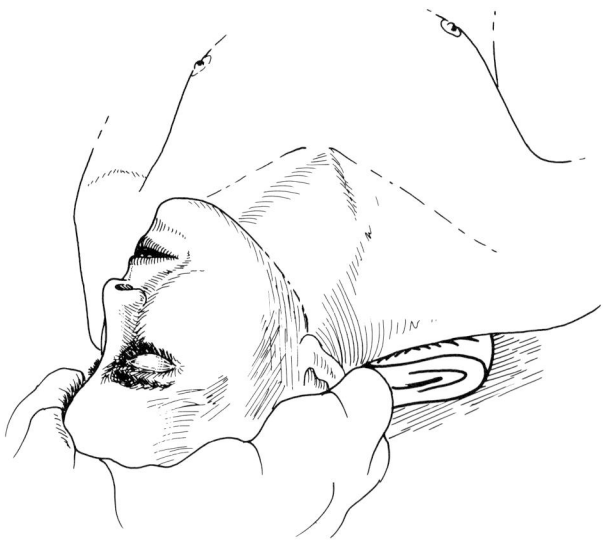

FIGURE 1–6

Adequacy of Ventilation

Assessment of the adequacy of ventilation is no less important during mask ventilation than following tracheal intubation. Observation of chest movements, continuous auscultation of breath and cardiac sounds, capnometry, and finger pulse oximetry are mandatory.

References

Boidin MP: Airway patency in the unconscious patient. Br J Anaesth 57:306–310, 1965

Guedel AE: Inhalation Anesthesia: A Fundamental Guide, ed 2, pp 10–52, 113–117. New York, Macmillan, 1951

Guildner CW: Resuscitation: Opening the airway: A comparative study of techniques for opening an airway obstructed by the tongue. J Am Coll Emerg Physicians 5:588–590, 1976

Morikawa S, Safar P, DeCurlo J: Influence of head position upon upper airway patency. Anesthesiology 22:265–270, 1961

2

Laryngeal Anesthesia

The larynx is innervated by the superior and recurrent laryngeal nerves, both of which are branches of the vagus nerve. The superior laryngeal nerve branches into the external laryngeal nerve (which provides motor innervation to the cricothyroid and inferior constrictor muscles) and the internal laryngeal nerve (which provides sensory innervation to the superior surface of the true vocal cords). The recurrent laryngeal nerve innervates all laryngeal muscles except the cricothyroid and provides sensory innervation to the larynx below the vocal cords. Complete laryngeal anesthesia can be provided prior to awake endoscopy or awake intubation by a combination of bilateral superior laryngeal nerve blocks and transtracheal anesthesia.

Transtracheal anesthesia will anesthetize the upper portion of the trachea up to the vocal cords and, depending on the amount of anesthetic that is coughed beyond the vocal cords, may anesthetize the superior surface of the vocal cords as well. Transtracheal anesthesia does not obviate the need for superior laryngeal nerve block during awake endoscopy.

Technique of Superior Laryngeal Nerve Block

EQUIPMENT NEEDED

Sterile gloves
Antiseptic solution
2 3-ml syringes
2 22-gauge needles
6 ml lidocaine 1%
Usual monitoring devices
Resuscitation drugs and equipment

PROCEDURE

Insert an intravenous cannula in the patient (if one is not already present) and attach it to a crystalloid infusion set. Cleanse the skin of the neck with antiseptic solution. Insert a 22-gauge needle 0.5 cm caudad and medial to the greater cornu of the hyoid bone, and advance it 0.5 cm beneath the skin surface (Fig. 2–1). After aspiration, to ensure that the needle has not entered the external carotid artery, inject 3 ml of 1% lidocaine in a fanwise fashion and withdraw the needle. Repeat the procedure on the opposite side of the neck.

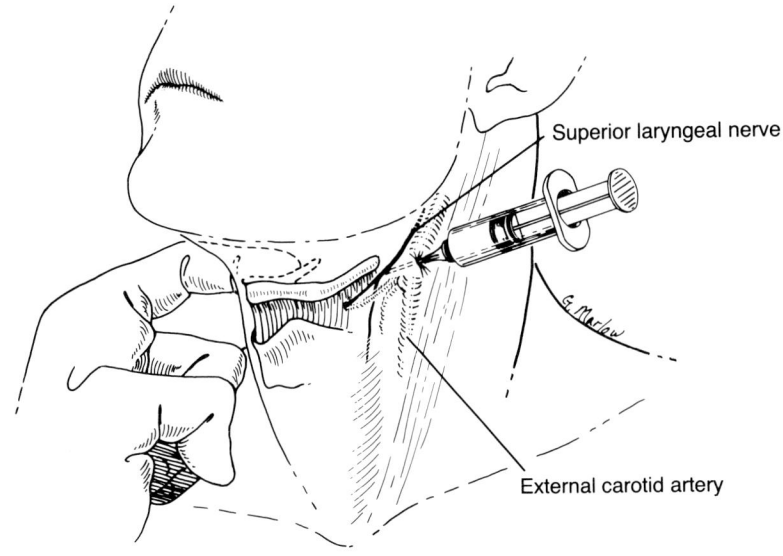

FIGURE 2–1

Technique of Transtracheal (Translaryngeal) Anesthesia

EQUIPMENT NEEDED

Sterile gloves
Antiseptic solution
5-ml syringe
22-gauge needle
4 ml lidocaine 4%
Usual monitoring devices
Resuscitation drugs and equipment

PROCEDURE

Cleanse the skin overlying the cricothyroid membrane with antiseptic solution. Instruct the patient to exhale fully. Insert a 22-gauge needle through the skin and the cricothyroid membrane. A correctly placed needle will permit free aspiration of air through the needle (Figs. 2–2 and 2–3). Inject 4 ml of 4% lidocaine, and then quickly withdraw the needle. The anesthetic will nearly always produce a bout of coughing by the patient.

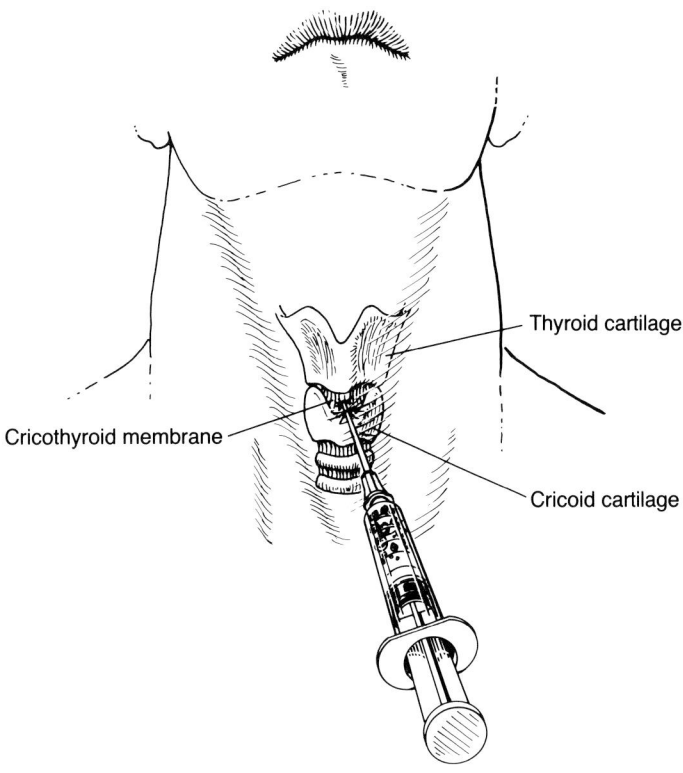

FIGURE 2–2

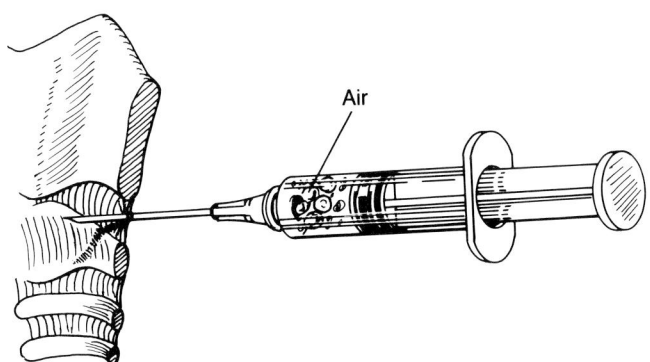

FIGURE 2–3

References

Adriani J: Labat's Regional Anesthesia Techniques and Clinical Applications, pp 187–192. St. Louis, Warren H. Green, 1985

Anderson JE: Grant's Atlas of Anatomy, pp 9–43. Baltimore, Williams & Wilkins, 1983

Applebaum EL, Bruce DL: Tracheal Intubation, pp 38–39. Philadelphia, WB Saunders, 1976

Gejrot T: Anesthesia for ear, nose and throat surgery. In Eriksson E (ed): Illustrated Handbook in Local Anaesthesia, pp 33–42. London, Edward Arnold, 1979

Neill RS: Head, neck and airway. In Wildsmith JAW, Armitage EN (eds): Principles and Practice of Regional Anaesthesia, pp 174–175. Edinburgh, Churchill Livingstone, 1987

Roberts JT: Fundamentals of Tracheal Intubation, pp 12–25, 66. New York, Grune & Stratton, 1983

Tucker HM: The Larynx, pp 17–19. New York, Thieme Medical Publishers, 1987

3

Orotracheal Intubation

Orotracheal intubation is a technique so central to the administration of general anesthesia that all anesthetists must be expert in it. This was not always the case. As late as the 1950s, general anesthesia was virtually synonymous with inhalational anesthesia (usually diethyl ether in North America), which was nearly always accomplished without intubation in a spontaneously breathing patient. With the introduction of neuromuscular paralysis, practitioners became increasingly comfortable with the use of tracheal intubation. At the same time, tracheal intubation, paralysis, and controlled ventilation during general anesthesia permitted neurosurgery, cardiac surgery, and thoracic surgery to flourish. Currently, mask inhalational anesthesia, rather than endotracheal anesthesia, is the rarer technique.

Laryngoscope Blades

I suspect that the vast majority of anesthetists prefer to use one of two laryngoscope designs routinely for their elective orotracheal intubations—the curved MacIntosh blade or the straight Miller blade. Although there are numerous other laryngoscope designs (most of which are variations on either the curved or the straight blade theme), only the intubation technique for the MacIntosh and Miller blades is discussed here (Fig. 3–1).

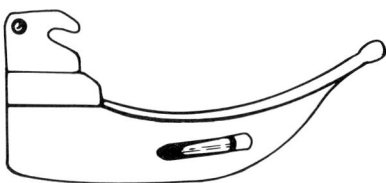

MacIntosh blade

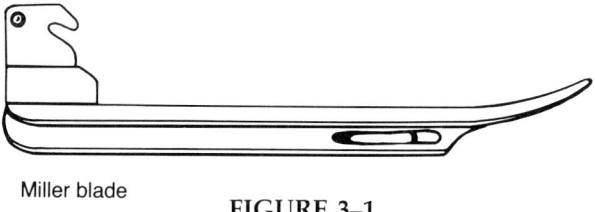

Miller blade

FIGURE 3–1

Awake vs. "Anesthetized" Intubation

As is true for nasotracheal intubation, orotracheal intubation can be accomplished in either awake or anesthetized patients. The anesthetist should be comfortable with either situation and should choose between them based on the needs of a particular patient, rather than on personal insecurity or lack of training. The approach described here emphasizes the anatomy and maneuvers required to accomplish intubation, whether in an awake or an anesthetized patient.

I find awake oral intubation useful in the critically ill patient who requires urgent or emergent intubation for airway protection, for positive-pressure ventilation (with or without positive end-expiratory pressure), or to provide high concentrations of oxygen. I also find it useful to intubate awake patients who require elective endotracheal anesthesia but appear to represent "difficult intubations" or who present with a "full stomach" (particularly those with intestinal obstruction) and a relative contraindication to rapid sequence induction (e.g., those with an airway abnormality).

In the operating room, orotracheal intubation can usually be accomplished with optimal instrumentation and under optimal conditions. The patient has usually been anesthetized and paralyzed, allowing time during laryngoscopy for inspection of the upper airway and glottis for anatomic abnormalities. In contrast, tracheal intubation of the awake patient in the emergency department or intensive care unit is rarely an elegant procedure. Usually it is remarkable because of the desperate situation of the patient and for the skill required on the part of the anesthetist to make the intubation tolerable, safe, and swift.

Technique of Elective Awake Orotracheal Intubation

EQUIPMENT NEEDED

Gloves
Suction device and Yankauer suction tip
Oral and nasal airways
Selection of endotracheal tubes (7.0–8.0 mm for women and 8.0–9.0 mm for men)
Stylet for endotracheal tube
Laryngoscope handle and selection of appropriate-sized blades (for adults, MacIntosh 3 and Miller 2 or 3 blades)
Lidocaine paste
Means for delivering positive-pressure ventilation with bag and mask (e.g., anesthesia machine)
Magill forceps
Stethoscope
Usual monitoring devices
Resuscitation drugs (including neuromuscular blocking drugs) and equipment

PREPARATION AND POSITIONING

Start an intravenous infusion if one is not present (unless intubation is a lifesaving maneuver) for administration of sedative medication and/or neuromuscular blocking agents. Attach the electrocardiographic leads, blood pressure cuff, and pulse oximeter probe for monitoring during the procedure. Administer oxygen by face mask as guided by blood gas analysis or finger pulse oximetry. Confirm that the laryngoscope handle, blades, and light bulbs all function properly. Make certain that suction is readily available.

Position the patient supine on the operating room table. Extend the head at the atlanto-occipital joint into the so-called "sniffing" position by elevating the patient's head approximately 10 cm above the table on a folded towel or blanket (Fig. 3–2). Resist the temptation to elevate the patient's chin excessively, hyperextending the head on the neck. Do not alter the head or neck position of patients with known or suspected instability of the cervical spine (e.g., multiple trauma patients) without the assistance of a neurosurgeon.

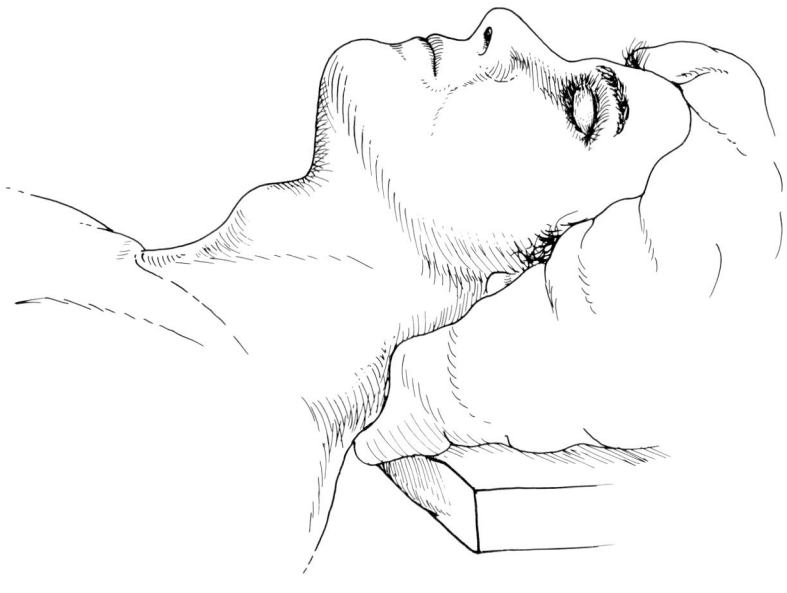

FIGURE 3–2

SEDATION

Sedate the patient with incremental doses of intravenous medication if the patient's clinical condition will permit the use of sedation. I recommend midazolam in 0.015-mg/kg doses, up to a total dose (rarely necessary) of 0.15 mg/kg. With appropriate *small* doses of midazolam and careful application of local anesthetic, awake oral intubation can be rendered relatively comfortable for most patients. Following sedation with midazolam, many patients will not remember the intubation.

ANESTHESIA OF PHARYNX AND LARYNX

Have the patient gargle with viscous lidocaine to anesthetize the oropharynx and tongue and repeat the procedure at least once. Suction the excess local anesthetic and oropharyngeal secretions from the patient's mouth. Use a tongue blade and an atomizer to apply local anesthetic on the tongue and pharynx (Fig. 3–3).

As the tongue and the anterior part of the oropharynx become anesthetized, insert the laryngoscope to expose progressively deeper structures within the oropharynx and spray them with the local anesthetic.

If there is no contraindication, transtracheal anesthesia and superior laryngeal nerve blocks should be performed (see Chapter 2).

EXPOSURE OF GLOTTIS

Advance the laryngoscope farther into the oropharynx and visualize the glottic opening. Spray topical lidocaine on and between the vocal cords in final preparation for intubation (unless the patient has a "full stomach" and is at risk for aspiration of gastric contents, in which case all glottic anesthesia must be omitted) (Fig. 3–4).

14
Airway Management

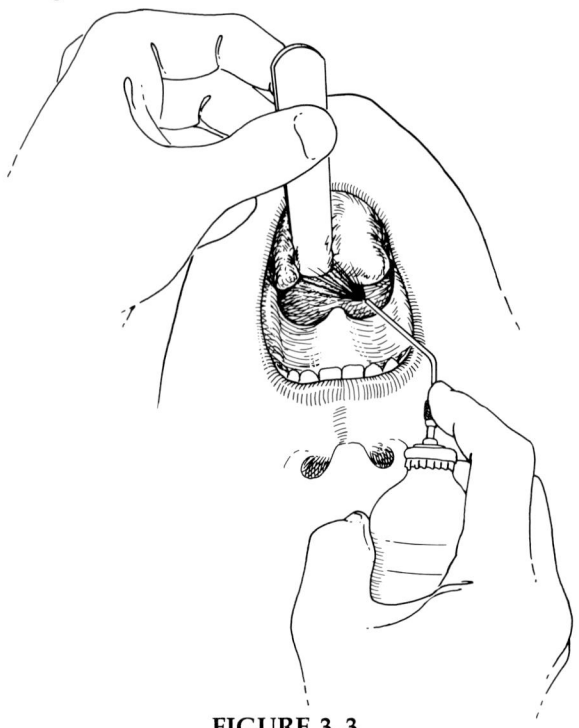

FIGURE 3–3

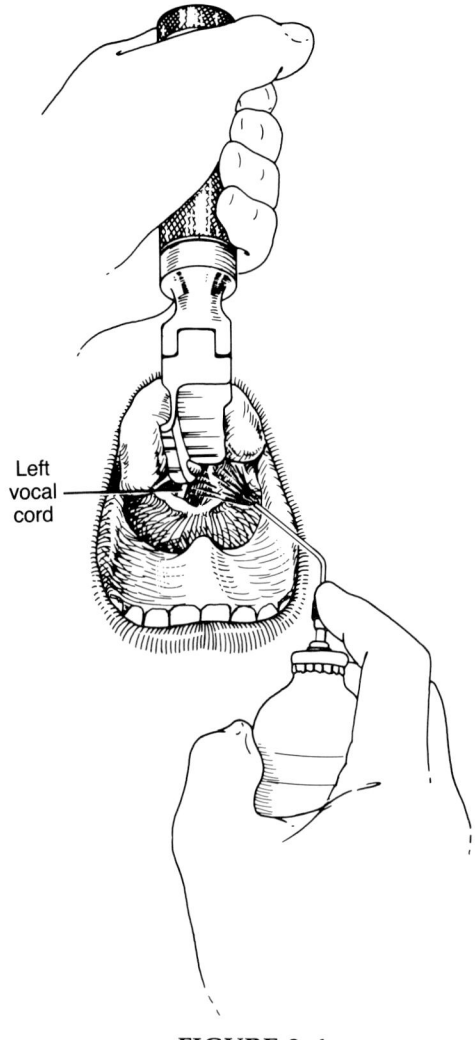

Left vocal cord

FIGURE 3–4

Expose and elevate the glottis, pass the tracheal tube between the vocal cords, and inflate the cuff (Fig. 3–5). Confirm the proper positioning of the tube with auscultation, capnography, and finger pulse oximetry, or with a chest radiograph and blood gas analysis. Secure the tube with adhesive tape or with an umbilical tape passed around the neck and tied securely to the tube (this is especially helpful in bearded persons) (Fig. 3–6).

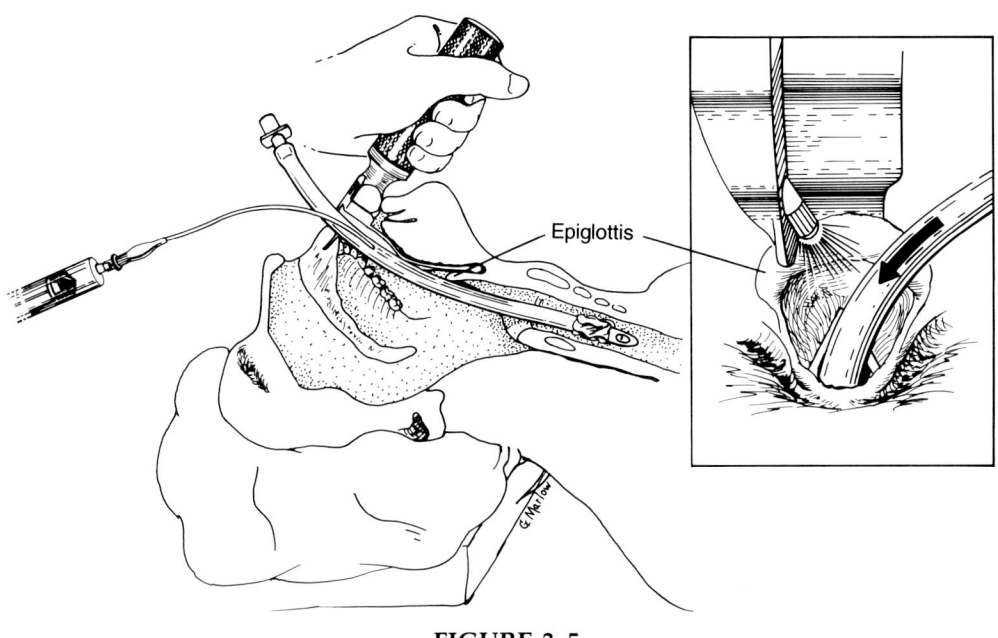

FIGURE 3–5

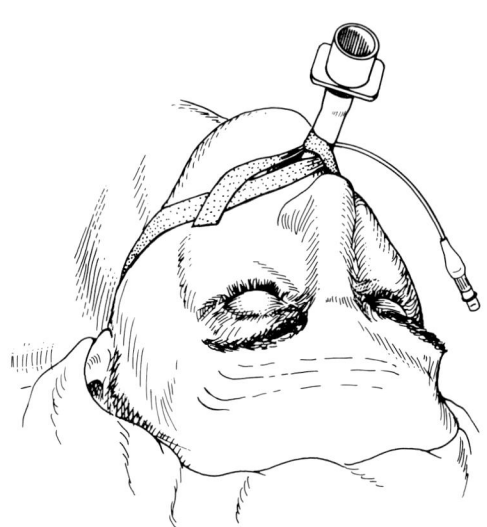

FIGURE 3–6

Mechanics of Using Curved and Straight Laryngoscope Blades

CURVED BLADE (MACINTOSH) TECHNIQUE

Position the patient in the "sniffing" position (see Fig. 3–2). Scissor the mouth open with index finger and thumb of the gloved right hand (Fig. 3–7). With the gloved left hand, insert the laryngoscope blade into the mouth, starting on the far right side of the patient's mouth and tongue. Lift the tongue and sweep it over to the left side of the mouth (Fig. 3–8). Do not "lever" back with the laryngoscope; the laryngoscope should be lifted directly up and away from the floor. The flange on

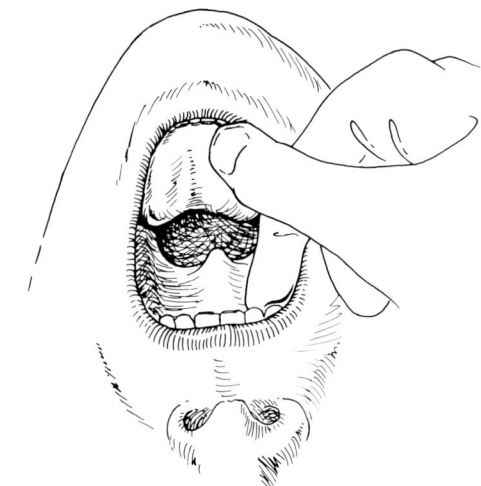

FIGURE 3–7

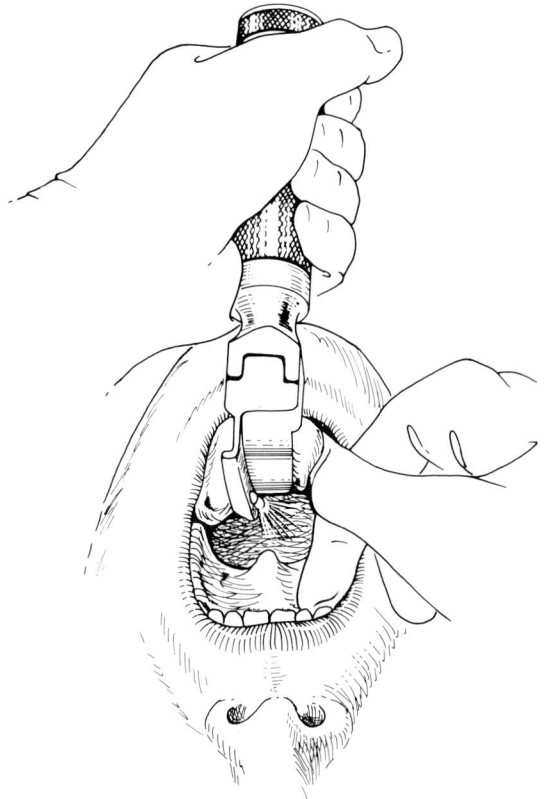

FIGURE 3–8

the MacIntosh blade is designed to prevent the tongue from folding in over the blade and obscuring the view. Ensure that the flange on the blade and the blade itself do not make contact with the teeth (particularly the upper incisors).

Look past the tip of the blade to be sure that it is located in the vallecula (between the epiglottis and the anterior wall of the pharynx) and not within the glottic opening or esophagus. Quickly inspect the oral cavity and the glottis for lesions such as vocal cord polyps, reddened areas on the vocal cords, "white" lesions on the mucosal surfaces, or soft tissue swellings.

Pass the tracheal tube through and beyond the vocal cords, far enough that the cuff will not touch the cords when inflated (see Fig. 3–5). Carefully remove the laryngoscope blade from the mouth. I suspect that dental damage may occur at least as commonly during removal of the laryngoscope blade, when the excitement of intubation has passed, as during insertion of the blade and glottic exposure. Confirm the position of the tube and tape it in place as previously described.

STRAIGHT BLADE (MILLER) TECHNIQUE

Position the patient supine on the operating room table in the "sniffing" position (see Fig. 3–2). Scissor the mouth open with the index finger and thumb of the gloved right hand (see Fig. 3–7). Insert the laryngoscope blade on the right side of the patient's mouth and tongue, sweeping the tongue to the left side (Fig. 3–9).

Advance the tip of the laryngoscope blade (under direct vision) into the glottic opening. When using straight laryngoscope blades, beginners typically advance the blade too far, usually into the esophagus. If bilaterally symmetric, pearly-white vocal cords are not visible, it is a safe bet that the opening under inspection does not lead to the lungs (Fig. 3–10)!

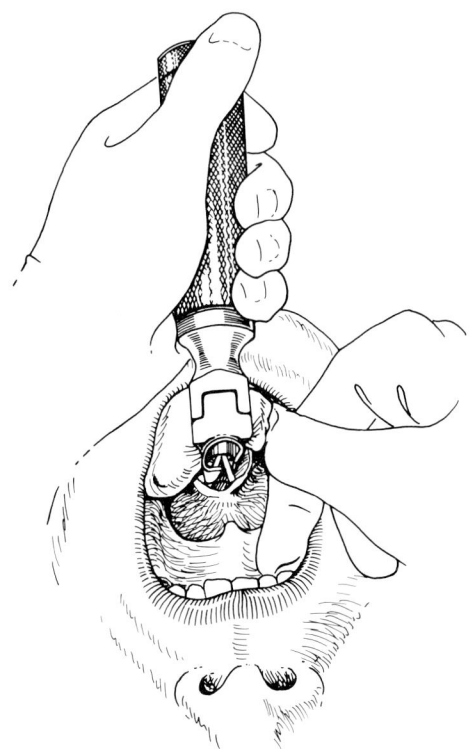

FIGURE 3–9

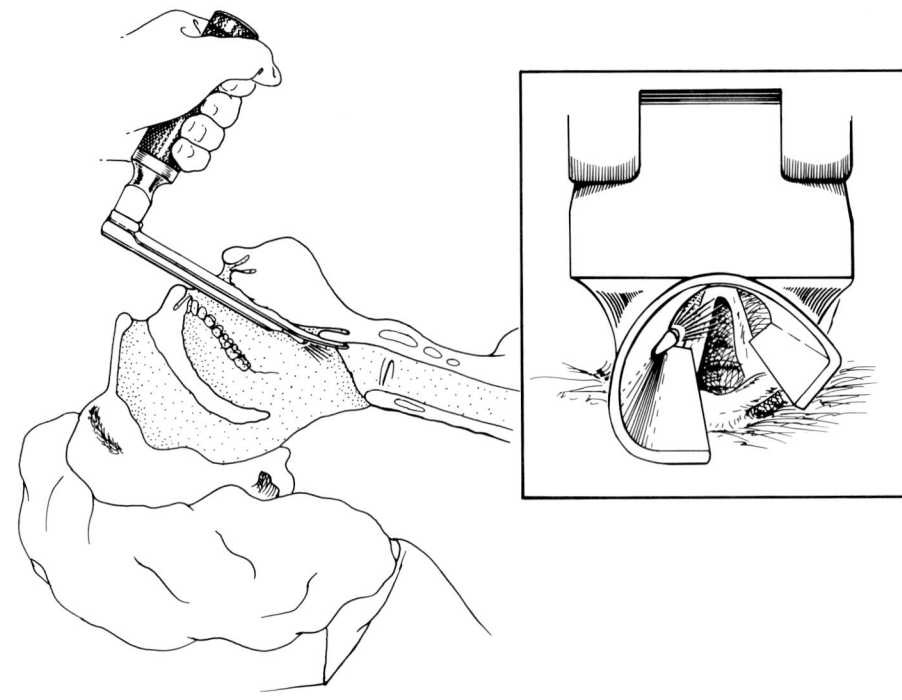

FIGURE 3–10

With the tip of the laryngoscope blade, lift the epiglottis out of the way and expose the vocal cords. A laryngoscope handle or blade should be *elevated*, not "levered." Advance the tracheal tube cuff beyond the vocal cords. Carefully remove the laryngoscope from the mouth and inflate the cuff on the tracheal tube. Confirm the position of the tube and tape it in place as previously described.

Intubation of Infants and Children

ANATOMIC CONCERNS

Intubation of children 8 years of age and older is not much different from intubation of adults, save for differences in the size of the appropriate tube and laryngoscope blade. Intubation of younger children, and especially infants, presents more of a challenge. The infant or young child has a relatively narrow and short (often referred to as "floppy") epiglottis. Unlike the case in adults, in which the epiglottis is parallel to the axis of the trachea, in infants the epiglottis is angled posterior to the axis of the trachea (Fig. 3–11). For this reason, many anesthetists prefer straight laryngoscope blades for infants and small children to lift the epiglottis out of the way during intubation.

In adults, the narrowest portion of the upper airway occurs at the level of the vocal cords, whereas the infant larynx is narrowest below the cords at the level of the cricoid cartilage. Thus, a tube may appear to pass between the vocal cords with ease but be too large for an infant. The key test for proper size of an infant's tracheal tube is to hear gas leak around the endotracheal tube at an airway pressure (measured on an in-line manometer) less than 25 cm H_2O. A tube too large to permit air leak predisposes the child to postextubation croup and should be replaced with a smaller one.

Right mainstem bronchial intubation is very common in infants. Pulse oximetry may not always show desaturation, even when only one lung field is ventilated.

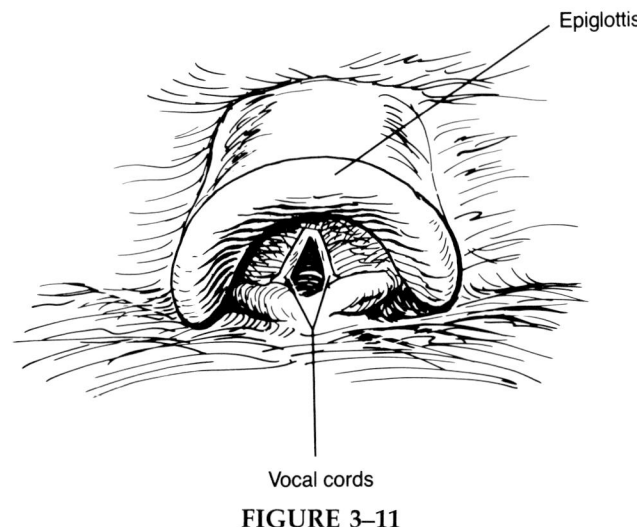

FIGURE 3–11

Auscultation (in both axillae) after intubation is therefore doubly important for infants. Some anesthetists routinely advance endotracheal tubes until only one lung is ventilated and then carefully withdraw the tube (while listening to breath sounds in the axillae) to determine the optimal position. Changes in head position are potentially hazardous to intubated infants. Each time a child's head position is changed, the anesthetist must confirm that the tube has not become malpositioned.

SELECTION AND INSERTION OF A TUBE

There are a number of formulas by which the more mathematically inclined predict the appropriate (uncuffed) tube size for an individual patient; however, I recommend a simpler approach. Full-term newborns generally require a 3.0- or 3.5-mm tube (I use a Miller 0 laryngoscope), 2-year-olds require a 4.0-mm tube (I use a Miller 1 laryngoscope), 5-year-olds require a 5.0-mm tube (I use a MacIntosh or Miller 2 laryngoscope), and 7-year-olds require a 6.0-mm tube. Children of other ages require the tube sizes in between! A properly sized tube will usually approximate the size of the patient's fifth (little) finger. If a formula must be used, (16 + age in years) ÷ 4 will approximate the appropriate size. Always ensure that a selection of tubes is available (usually a size smaller and a size larger than the one that is anticipated to be the correct size).

I generally do not use a cuffed tube until the child has reached school age. I intubate children 8 to 9 years old with a cuffed 5.0-mm tube and inflate the cuff if the air leak is too great. Older children (up to age 13) can be intubated with a cuffed 6.0-mm tube. I treat teenagers as small adults and use 7.0- or 8.0-mm tubes depending on body habitus.

Infants desaturate rapidly even after inhaling 100% oxygen for prolonged periods of time. Thus, intubation of infants should proceed speedily. (A specially modified Miller laryngoscope blade is available with a channel through which oxygen may be insufflated during laryngoscopy). Carefully observe the endotracheal tube passing between the infant's vocal cords. It need enter only as far as the second mark on its tip. Usually the tube will be properly positioned if it is inserted 30 times its internal diameter (in mm) from the teeth. Avoid the natural tendency to "push it in to his toes."

References

Applebaum EL, Bruce DL: Tracheal Intubation. Philadelphia, WB Saunders, 1976

Blanc VF, Trembly NAG: The complications of tracheal intubation: A new classification with a review of the literature. Anesth Analg 53:202–213, 1974

Coté CJ, Todres ID: The pediatric airway. In Ryan SF, Todres ID, Coté CJ, Goudsouzian NG (eds): A Practice of Anesthesia for Infants and Children, pp 35–57. Orlando, FL, Grune & Stratton, 1986

Gillespie NA: Endotracheal Anaesthesia, pp 83–129. Madison, University of Wisconsin Press, 1950

Harmer M: Complications of tracheal intubation. In Latto IP, Rosen M (eds): Difficulties in Tracheal Intubation, pp 36–47. Philadelphia, Baillière Tindall, 1984

Kingston HGG: Airway problems in pediatric patients. In Lynn AM (ed): Problems in Anesthesia, vol 2, pp 545–565. Philadelphia, JB Lippincott, 1990

Koka BV, Jeon IS, Andre JM, Mackay I, Smith RM: Post-intubation croup in children. Anesth Analg 56:501–505, 1977

Marrin KR: Awake intubation. In Latto IP, Rosen M (eds): Difficulties in Tracheal Intubation, pp 90–98. Philadelphia, Baillière Tindall, 1984

Roberts JT: Fundamentals of Tracheal Intubation. New York, Grune & Stratton, 1983

Tucker HM: The Larynx, pp 1–32, 163–179, 181–183. New York, Thieme Medical Publishers, 1987

4

Nasotracheal Intubation

Nasotracheal intubation is commonly used during surgery of the face and mouth, for intubation of patients with respiratory failure, and in those situations in which tracheal intubation is required but oral laryngoscopy presents technical difficulties or might cause the patient harm. When tracheal intubation will be required for more than a day, especially in small children, nasotracheal intubation is preferred. Nasotracheal tubes are more easily secured with tape to the face and are less bothersome to awake patients than orotracheal tubes, but they carry the risks of epistaxis, sinusitis, and bacteremia.

Blind vs. Endoscopic Intubation

Whenever nasotracheal intubation is indicated, the operator may perform the technique "blind" or while visualizing the airway either with a conventional oral laryngoscope or with a fiberoptic endoscope (see Chapter 6) passed through the tracheal tube. If nasal intubation has been selected because oral laryngoscopy must *not* be performed (e.g., in a patient with an unstable neck fracture), nasal intubation can be performed under direct vision with the fiberoptic endoscope.

Requirements of Awake and Anesthetized Patients

Of key importance in determining the local anesthetic requirements for nasotracheal intubation is the state of consciousness of the patient. When the patient will be given general anesthesia prior to nasotracheal intubation, the only additional requirement is that a vasoconstrictor (e.g., tolazoline spray, phenylephrine nose drops, lidocaine with 1:400,000 epinephrine, or topical cocaine) be used to prevent epistaxis. When nasotracheal intubation is to be accomplished in an awake patient, the anesthetist must provide for the patient's comfort during the procedure as well as prevent epistaxis. Often this will require topical anesthesia of the nasal passage and oropharynx, transtracheal local anesthesia of the trachea and glottis, superior laryngeal nerve blocks (see Chapter 2), and careful titration of sedative medication to provide for patient comfort during the procedure.

Technique of Blind Nasal Intubation

EQUIPMENT NEEDED

Gloves
Topical vasoconstrictor (topical tolazoline spray or lidocaine 1% with 1:400,000 epinephrine)
Topical anesthesia spray (lidocaine 4%–10% and an atomizer)
Viscous lidocaine gargle
Lidocaine paste
Nasal (trumpet) airways (small, medium, and large)
Suction apparatus
Means for administering oxygen and positive-pressure ventilation (bag and mask)
Selection of endotracheal tubes (for nasal intubation of adults, size 6.0 or 7.0 mm)
Means for confirming correct tube placement (stethoscope, capnograph, and pulse oximeter are preferred)
Usual monitoring devices
Resuscitation drugs and equipment

PREPARATION

Insert an intravenous cannula in the patient (if one is not already present) and attach it to a crystalloid infusion set. Attach the electrocardiographic leads, blood pressure cuff, and pulse oximeter probe to the patient for monitoring during intubation. Sedate the patient with small doses of intravenous midazolam (1 to 5 mg in the average adult patient). Adequate local anesthesia is a better choice than intravenous narcotics, which tend to cause respiratory depression. Thus, I rarely administer more than 1 to 2 µg/kg of fentanyl (or the equivalent) and often give no narcotic at all. Administer intravenous glycopyrrolate 3 µg/kg if an anticholinergic has not been given with the premedication.

TOPICAL ANESTHESIA OF THE NOSTRIL

Determine which nostril is to be intubated. Ask the patient to breathe selectively through each nostril to determine which side appears to be more widely patent.

Apply vasoconstrictor (either topical tolazoline spray or lidocaine 1% with 1:400,000 epinephrine) to shrink and (if lidocaine is used) anesthetize the nasal mucosa. Vasoconstrictor may be sprayed directly on the mucosa or applied with swabs. Swabs should be placed in the anterior part of the nose first, then moved farther back along the turbinates until the entire nostril has been anesthetized and vasoconstricted (Fig. 4–1). Gently pass lubricated nasal airways of increasing size into the nostril to dilate it (Fig. 4–2).

ANESTHESIA OF PHARYNX AND LARYNX

Spray local anesthetic (lidocaine 4%, 1 to 2 ml total dose) in the back of the patient's mouth (use several applications) (see Fig. 3–4). Ask the patient to gargle with the local anesthetic to produce topical anesthesia of the oropharynx. Suction excess local anesthetic and secretions from the mouth. If there is no contraindication, transtracheal anesthesia and superior laryngeal nerve blocks should be performed (see Chapter 2).

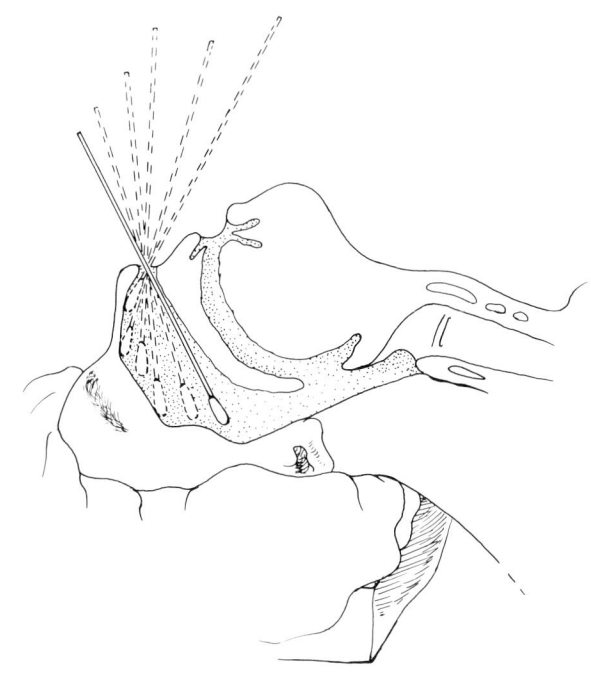

FIGURE 4–1

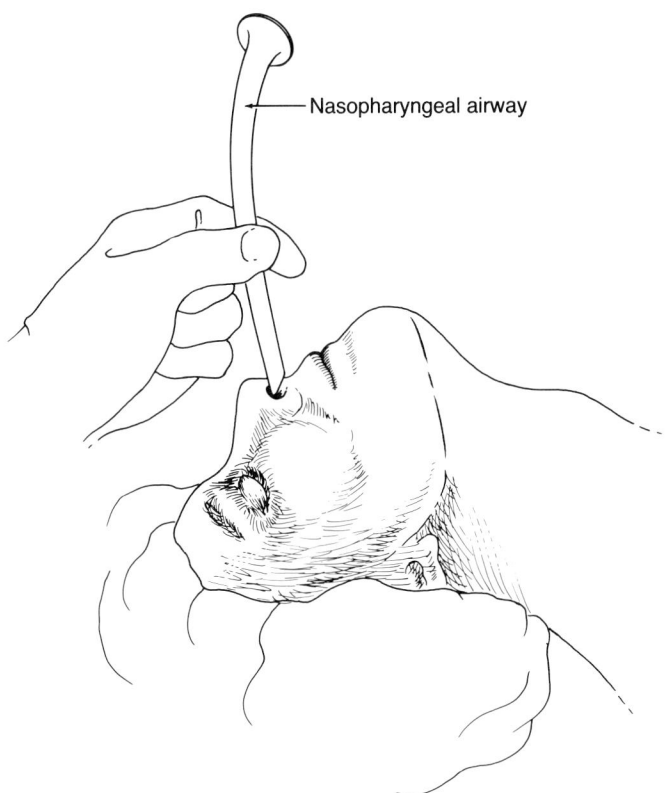

FIGURE 4–2

POSITIONING

Position the patient in a "sniffing" position much as is used during orotracheal intubation, with the head extended at the atlanto-occipital joint and elevated on a folded sheet or foam headrest (Fig. 4–3).

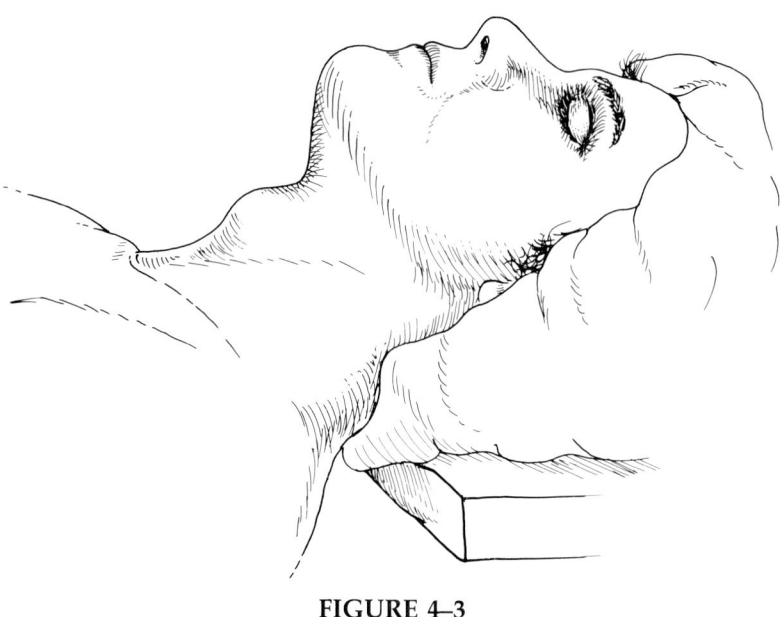

FIGURE 4–3

TUBE INSERTION

Insert a lubricated cuffed plastic endotracheal tube of appropriate size (usually 7.0 mm) gently and slowly through the nostril and into the back of the throat. Warm water can be run over the tube to soften it before inserting it into the patient so that its passage through the nose and pharynx will be less traumatic.

Listen to the character of the breath sounds transmitted through the endotracheal tube, and advance the tube in the direction of the loudest breath sounds (Fig. 4–4). This maneuver is easier than it sounds. Attempt to pass the tube through the vocal cords during a deep inspiration when the vocal cords are widely separated, rather than during expiration when the vocal cords approximate.

If the first few intubation attempts are unsuccessful, and the breath sounds become muffled as the tube is advanced, the tube may be either passing off the midline or into the esophagus. When the former occurs, a "bulge" is often visible on the patient's neck where the tip of the tube is pressing. If so, the tube should be gently rotated toward the opposite side to restore its path to the midline. If the tube appears to be in the midline but is nonetheless not entering the trachea, extend the patient's head at the neck (so that the chin is farther away from the chest) to reorient the tip of the tube into the glottis. Rarely, flexing the patient's head (so that the chin is closer to the chest) may be helpful.

USE OF LARYNGOSCOPY

If these several maneuvers are unsuccessful, and nasal intubation is required, use either peroral endoscopy with a standard laryngoscope or fiberoptic endoscopy through the tube.

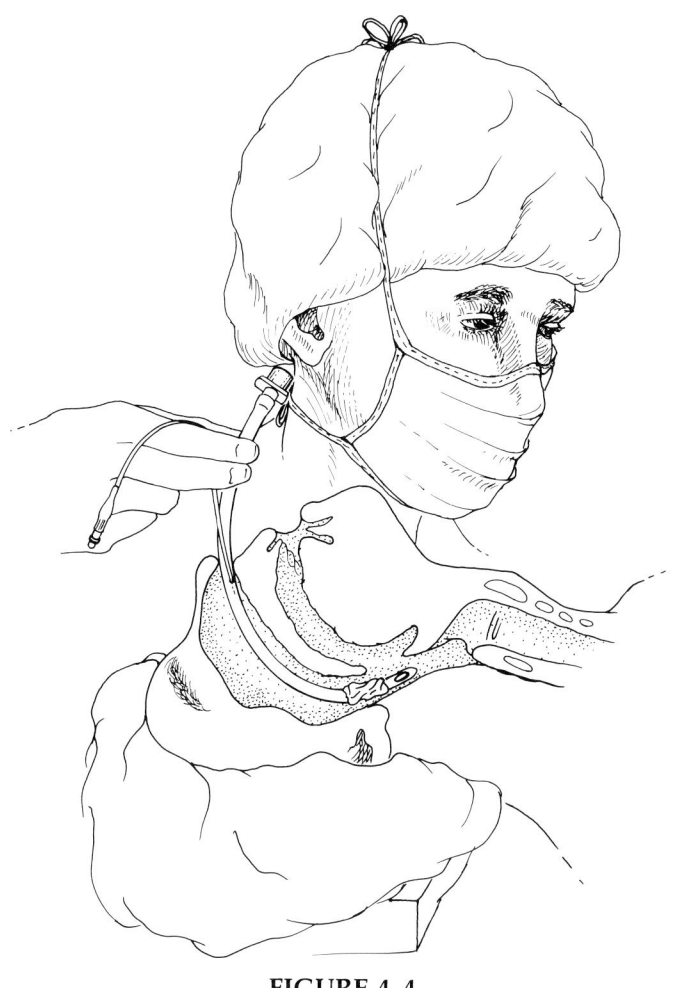

FIGURE 4-4

After exposing the glottis with the laryngoscope, direct the tube between the vocal cords with Magill forceps (as an assistant advances the tube through the nose) (Fig. 4–5). It is nearly impossible both to advance and to aim a nasotracheal tube with Magill forceps. Do not grab the endotracheal tube cuff with Magill forceps, since this may rupture the cuff and necessitate replacing the tube. Fiberoptic intubation and endoscopy are described in Chapter 6.

NASAL INTUBATION AFTER INDUCTION OF GENERAL ANESTHESIA

Nasotracheal intubation is often used in patients undergoing general anesthesia for surgery in the mouth or on the face. In these cases, shrink the nasal mucosa with topical vasoconstrictors and position the patient's head in a "sniffing" position before inducing general anesthesia. If there are no contraindications (e.g., evidence of a difficult intubation), induce general anesthesia with neuromuscular paralysis as for oral intubation. Advance the warmed, lubricated endotracheal tube through the nostril and oropharynx. Nasotracheal intubation often can be accomplished blindly on the first or second attempt. Alternatively, expose the glottis with the laryngoscope (or the fiberoptic endoscope, see Chapter 6), grasp the tip of the endotracheal tube with a Magill forceps, and direct the tube between the vocal cords as the assistant advances the tube into the patient's nostril.

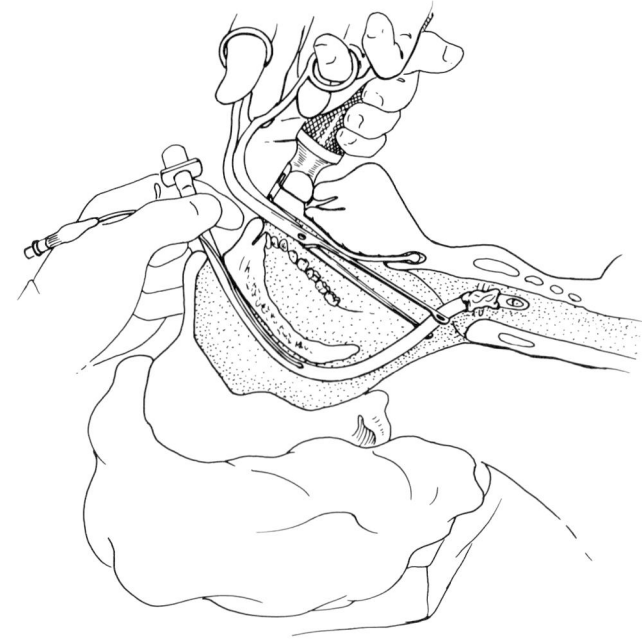

FIGURE 4–5

Confirm that the tube is in proper position in the trachea with auscultation of both axillae, capnometry, and pulse oximetry or with a chest radiograph and blood gas analysis. Secure the tube to the nose with tincture of benzoin and adhesive tape.

References

Applebaum EL, Bruce DL: Tracheal Intubation. Philadelphia, WB Saunders, 1976
Arens JF, LeJeune FE, Webre DR: Maxillary sinusitis, a complication of nasotracheal intubation. Anesthesiology 40:415–416, 1974
Blanc VF, Trembly NAG: The complications of tracheal intubation: A new classification with a review of the literature. Anesth Analg 53:202–213, 1974
Gillespie N: Endotracheal Anesthesia, pp 101–117. Madison, University of Wisconsin Press, 1950
Gold MI, Buechel DR: A method of blind nasal intubation for the conscious patient. Anesth Analg 39:257–263, 1960
Latto IP: Management of difficult intubation. In Latto IP, Rosen M (eds): Difficulties in Tracheal Intubation, pp 116–119. Philadelphia, Baillière Tindall, 1984
Pederson B: Blind nasotracheal intubation: A review and a new guided technique. Acta Anaesthesiol Scand 15:107–124, 1971
Roberts JT: Fundamentals of Tracheal Intubation, pp 93–104. New York, Grune & Stratton, 1983

5
Failed Intubation

Most elective tracheal intubations are successful on the first attempt. Unfortunately, even the most experienced laryngoscopist will have occasional difficulty passing a tracheal tube. The guiding principle in the face of an unexpectedly difficult intubation is *first do no harm*. Provision of adequate ventilation and oxygen delivery to the patient, not successful tracheal intubation, is the primary goal.

With each succeeding intubation attempt, I always try a different technique or intubating instrument. For example, in large patients, a MacIntosh 4 blade may more effectively lift the tongue and provide better glottic exposure than a MacIntosh 3 blade. Smaller tracheal tubes may sometimes be passed successfully when passage of a larger tube has failed. Patients who for anatomic reasons (e.g., an "anteriorly" placed glottis) are difficult to intubate orally are often more easily intubated by the nasal route (see Chapter 4). Nonetheless, I am amazed at how often I have observed a laryngoscopist repeat an unsuccessful maneuver again and again without trying something new.

All anesthetists should have an organized plan for failed intubation, the sequence of which is determined by whether adequate airway support can be provided with bag and mask and by whether the patient is at high risk for pulmonary aspiration of gastric contents.

Etiology and Demographics

Unexpected failed intubation should be a relatively rare event. Sometimes apparently "difficult" intubations result from improper positioning or inadequate paralysis (the latter is a consequence of attempting intubation too soon after administering a neuromuscular blocking agent). Thus, I always check the extent of paralysis and the head position before initiating my "difficult intubation protocol." Difficult intubation can often be anticipated. Patients with anomalies, trauma, or neoplasms of the face, oropharyngeal cavity, or trachea should be treated as if they may be impossible to intubate with direct oral laryngoscopy. Those who cannot extend their necks (at the atlanto-occipital joint) into the "sniffing" position owing to trauma or rheumatic disease; those with disproportionately large tongues, short necks, prominent incisors, or receding mandibles; and those with temporomandibular joint disorders are also often difficult to intubate.

Retrospective studies indicate that failed intubation is more likely to occur in pregnant than in nonpregnant patients. Among the many physiologic changes of pregnancy are engorgement and swelling of the mucosa of the upper airway and mammary enlargement, both of which may interfere with glottic exposure during direct laryngoscopy. Perhaps even more important may be anatomic problems related to left uterine displacement (to prevent aortocaval compression by the gravid uterus), surgical drapes (often placed prior to induction of general anesthesia for cesarean delivery), cricoid pressure (Sellick maneuver), or poor head positioning prior to laryngoscopy.

When I anticipate that tracheal intubation may be difficult or impossible, I tend to select regional over general anesthesia, provided that the proposed surgery can be accomplished with a regional anesthetic technique. Nonetheless, the use of regional anesthesia does not eliminate the possibility that emergency tracheal intubation may be required if, for example, the dermatomal level of spinal anesthesia rises too craniad or local anesthetic is accidentally administered as an intravenous bolus.

Alternatives to Tracheal Intubation and Ventilation by Mask

Whenever intubation cannot be accomplished, the operator must make several assessments, the results of which will determine the subsequent plan (Fig. 5–1). First, the operator must determine whether he can provide adequate ventilation with bag and mask. If he is unable either to intubate or to ventilate the patient with bag and mask, then the remaining options (in an apneic patient) are laryngeal mask ventilation, transtracheal jet ventilation, cricothyroidotomy, or emergency tracheostomy. Although the laryngeal mask shows promise, it has not yet been widely used in North America. Of the remaining three options, I believe the easiest, safest, and fastest is transtracheal jet ventilation.

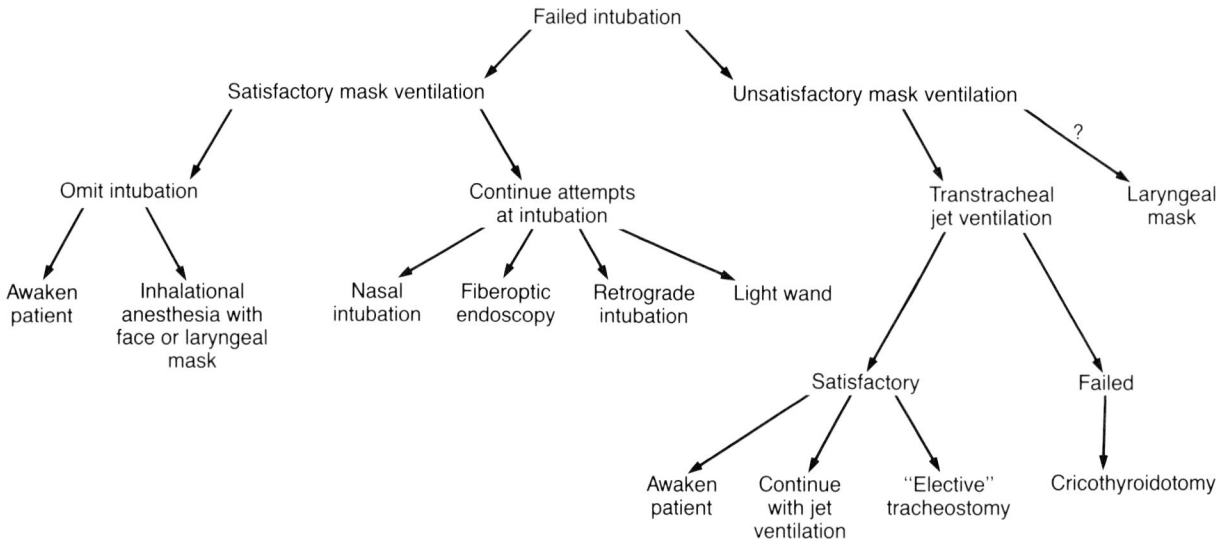

FIGURE 5–1

Difficult Intubation but Easy Mask Ventilation

When a patient cannot be intubated but can be adequately ventilated with bag and mask, the operator has several options. If the patient has undergone induction of general anesthesia and is not at risk for aspiration of gastric contents, the anesthetic may be continued without intubation if the surgical procedure is amenable to inhalational anesthesia by face mask or laryngeal mask. If intubation is required for the surgical procedure, the anesthetist may allow the patient to awaken from general anesthesia before making additional attempts at intubation (e.g., using fiberoptic endoscopy or a retrograde technique). This is a conservative approach that permits the patient and surgeon to reassess the advisability of proceeding with surgery in the face of significant airway difficulties and is particularly appropriate for patients at risk for aspiration of gastric contents. Alternatively, general anesthesia can be maintained while additional attempts at intubation are made.

References

Brain AIJ: Three cases of difficult intubation overcome by the laryngeal mask airway. Anaesthesia 40:353–355, 1985

King TA, Adams AP: Failed tracheal intubation. Br J Anaesth 65:400–414, 1990

Latto IP, Rosen M (eds): Difficulties in Tracheal Intubation. Philadelphia, Baillière Tindall, 1984

Roberts J: Fundamentals of Tracheal Intubation. New York, Grune & Stratton, 1983

Tunstall ME: Failed intubation drill. Anaesthesia 31:850, 1976

6

Fiberoptic Laryngoscopy

The fiberoptic bronchoscope is a valuable aid to nasotracheal and orotracheal intubation, particularly when airway abnormalities are present or when the position of the patient's head and neck must be maintained constant (e.g., with unstable neck fractures).

Intravenous Adjuvants

The anesthetist can make endoscopic intubation easier by adhering to a few simple guidelines. First, endoscopy is always easier when there are few airway secretions. I recommend administration of glycopyrrolate 3 µg/kg intravenously or intramuscularly 30 minutes or more before attempts at instrumentation of the airway begin. Second, during awake endoscopy, a little sedation is good; too much sedation is tragic. I recommend that small incremental doses of intravenous midazolam (0.015 mg/kg) be given up to (in rare instances) a total dose of 0.15 mg/kg. Narcotics provide little benefit and produce respiratory depression, whereas benzodiazepines calm patients and often render them amnestic for the intubation.

Topical Anesthetics and Vasoconstrictors

If intubation is to be accomplished with the patient awake, topical application of anesthesia and vasoconstrictor should proceed as previously described for either oral or nasotracheal intubation (see Chapters 3 and 4), depending on the route of intubation selected. I prefer the nasal route for fiberoptic intubations. When endoscopic nasal intubation will be performed in an anesthetized patient, only a topical vasoconstrictor needs to be applied to the nasal mucosa prior to instrumentation.

Technique

EQUIPMENT NEEDED

Gloves
Bronchoscope
Light source
Suction device

Topical anesthesia spray with vasoconstrictor
Lidocaine paste
2 3-ml syringes (for superior laryngeal blocks and transtracheal injection)
2 22-gauge needles
Endotracheal tube
Silicone lubricant
Nasal airways
Endoscopic mask
Oral airway intubator (or modified Guedel oral airway)
Usual monitoring devices
Resuscitation drugs and equipment

PREPARATION OF INSTRUMENT

Connect the light source to a power outlet and the endoscope to the light source. Adjust the light source to its maximal intensity. Ensure that the suction port of the endoscope is clear and functional. Spray the surface of the endoscope and the inner surface of the endotracheal tube with silicone lubricant. Become familiar with the control knob for directing the tip of the endoscope. Examine a piece of cloth or the back of the hand with the endoscope to be sure that the optics are functional.

PREPARATION AND POSITIONING OF PATIENT

Start an intravenous infusion if one is not already present. Attach electrocardiographic leads, blood pressure cuff, and pulse oximeter probe for monitoring during endoscopy. Move the patient to a semi-sitting position so that gravity will help to direct the tip of the endoscope into the glottis and away from pools of airway secretions. If difficulty is encountered during the endoscopy, it may be helpful to have the patient sit fully upright.

Determine which nostril is to be intubated. Ask the patient to breathe selectively through each nostril to determine which side appears to be more widely patent. Some patients will know this information beforehand. After shrinking and anesthetizing the nasal mucosa with local anesthetic and vasoconstrictor, and anesthetizing the oropharynx and glottis (with topical anesthesia, transtracheal local anesthetic, and superior laryngeal nerve blocks) (see Chapter 2 for techniques), advance a soft nasal airway lubricated with lidocaine paste through the larger naris into the posterior oropharynx to gauge the size and direction of the nasal passage (Fig. 6–1). Next, replace the nasal airway with an endotracheal tube. *Do not advance the tube close to the vocal cords.* Unnecessary manipulation of the endotracheal tube increases production of secretions and increases the likelihood of hemorrhage and laryngospasm.

If intubation through the mouth is preferred over the nasal route, an oropharyngeal airway through which the flexible fiberoptic endoscope will pass has been developed; however, I normally use the partially inserted endotracheal tube as both a bite block and a "conduit" for passage of the endoscope. Alternatively, the rigid fiberoptic laryngoscope could be used for peroral intubations.

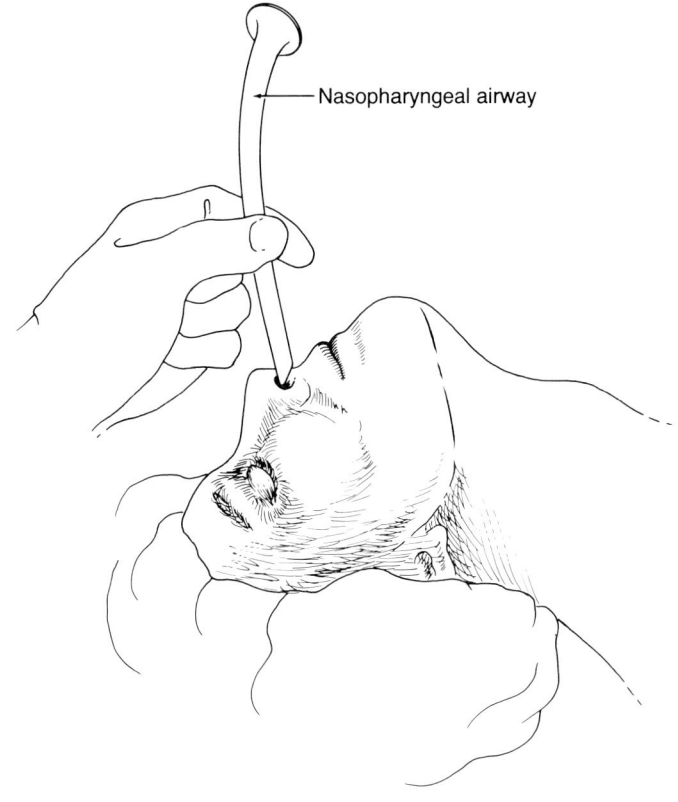

FIGURE 6–1

INSERTION OF ENDOSCOPE

Advance the endoscope through the endotracheal tube and out the distal end. Slowly advance the endoscope while continuously viewing the structures passing before its tip (Fig. 6–2). Insufflate oxygen through the suction port of the endoscope (I have found the suction port ineffective for suctioning). Direct the endoscope into and past the glottic opening (Fig. 6–3). Periodic suctioning (with a Yankauer suction cannula inserted through the mouth) may be necessary, especially if the patient is lying supine during the endoscopy.

Confirm the position of the endoscope within the trachea by observing the tracheal rings (and, if you wish, observing the more distal structures).

INSERTION OF ENDOTRACHEAL TUBE

Pass the endotracheal tube over the endoscope into the trachea (Fig. 6–4). Remove the endoscope. Confirm the proper positioning of the tube with auscultation, capnography (or a carbon dioxide detector), and pulse oximetry, or with a chest radiograph and arterial blood gas analysis.

CLEANING OF INSTRUMENT

After using the fiberoptic instrument, clean its tip with soap and water and flush its suction channel with water. Finally, clean and sterilize the whole instrument as per the manufacturer's instructions. Do not allow secretions, blood, or other material to dry on or within the instrument.

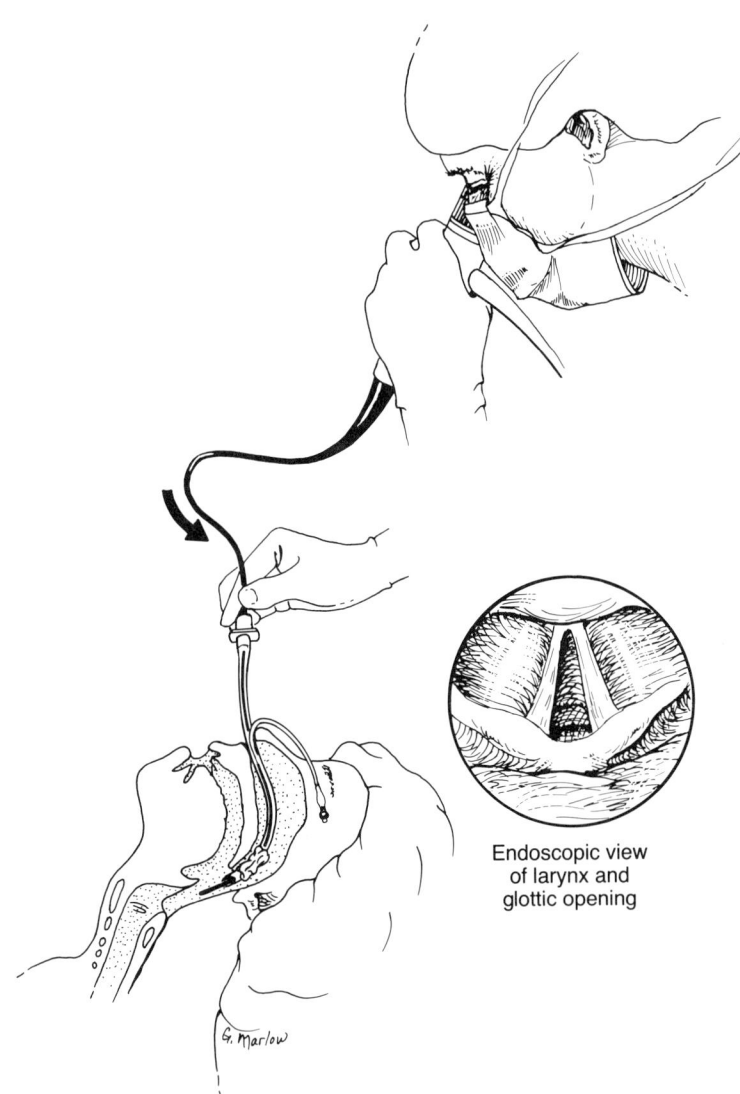

Endoscopic view of larynx and glottic opening

FIGURE 6–2

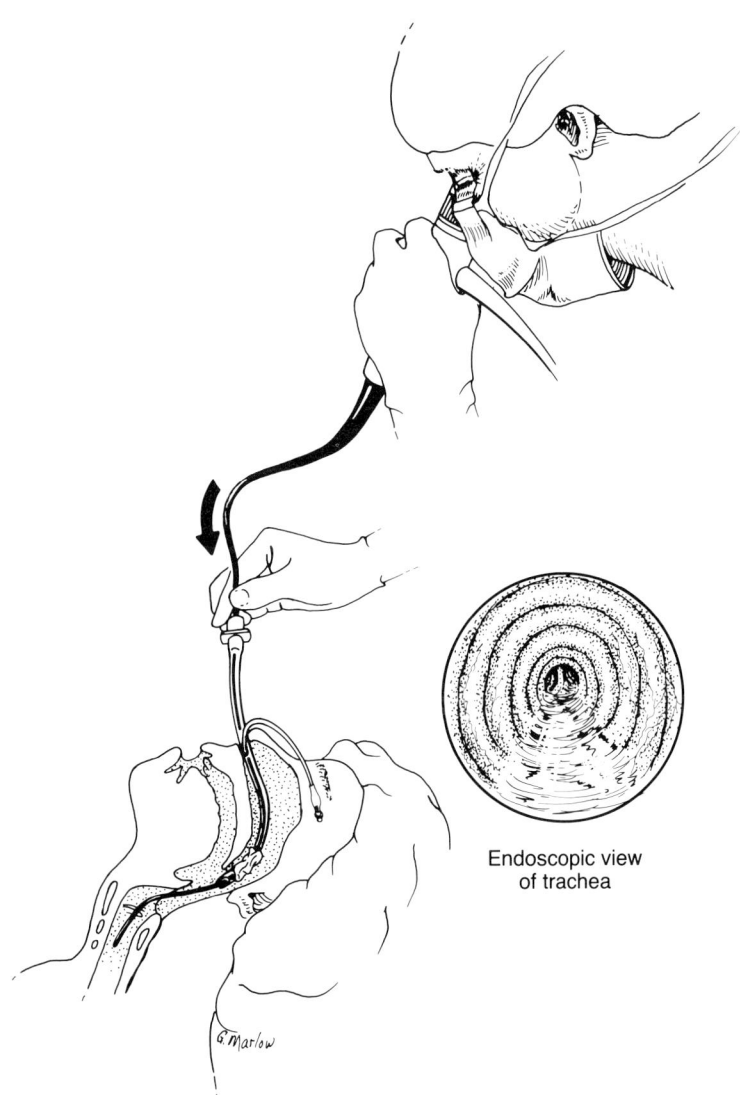

FIGURE 6–3

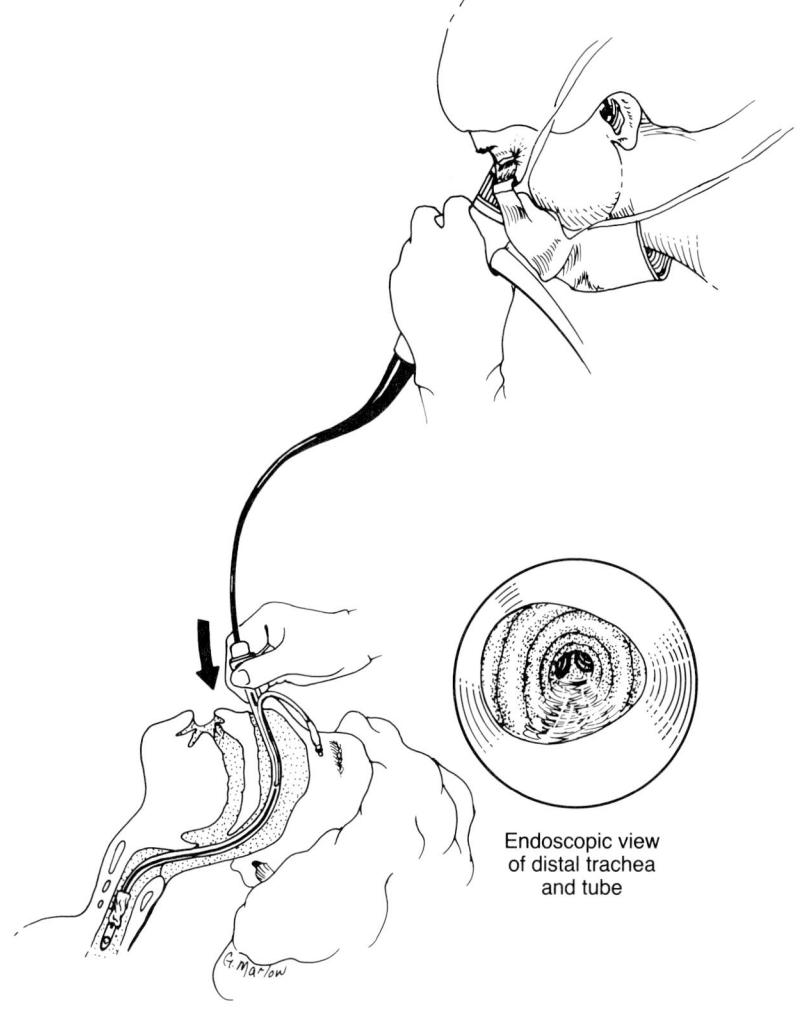

FIGURE 6-4

References

Ikeda S: Atlas of Flexible Bronchofiberoscopy, pp 31–51. Baltimore, University Park Press, 1974

Messeler KH, Petterson KI: Endotracheal intubation with the fiberoptic bronchoscope. Anaesthesia 35:294–298, 1980

Ovassapian A, Yelich SJ, Dykes MHM, Brunner EE: Fiberoptic nasotracheal intubation: Incidence and causes of failure. Anesth Analg 62:692–695, 1983

Patil VU, Stehling LC, Zander HL: Fiberoptic Endoscopy in Anesthesia, p 146. Chicago, Year Book Medical Publishers, 1983

Tucker HM: The Larynx, pp 163–179. New York, Thieme Medical Publishers, 1987

7

Transtracheal Jet Ventilation

Preparation of Equipment

Perhaps the most important consideration with the technique of transtracheal jet ventilation is to have the equipment prepared and readily available. It would be difficult to assemble the appropriate equipment quickly and correctly during an emergency. Thus, an inexpensive cricothyroid jet ventilation system should be available at all anesthetizing locations. The ventilation system used at my institution consists of a 15-mm endotracheal tube adapter (which fits into the fresh gas outflow of the anesthesia machine), a 3-foot length of high-pressure oxygen tubing, a 14 F suction catheter (cut to 6 to 9 inches), and a Luer-Lok male connector (connected to the suction cannula) (Fig. 7–1). This ventilation system connects the high-pressure oxygen source at the anesthesia machine to the 12-gauge or 14-gauge intravenous cannula, which will be placed into the airway through the cricothyroid membrane. By simultaneously depressing the oxygen flush button of the anesthesia machine and occluding the thumb hole on the suction cannula, a high-pressure flow of

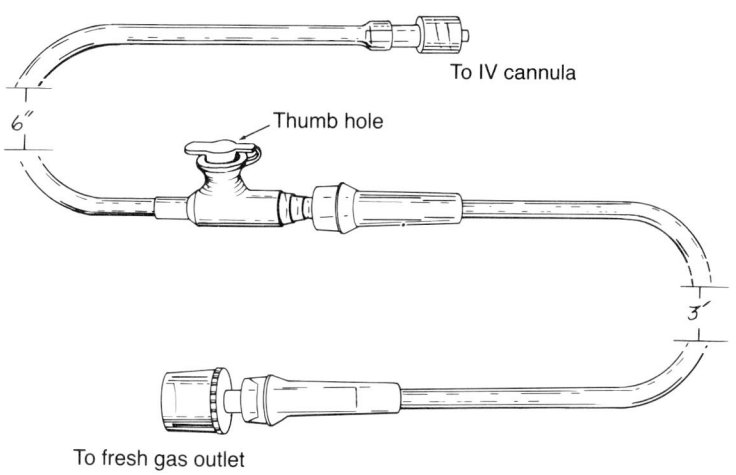

FIGURE 7–1

oxygen may be delivered to the patient's trachea. A system such as this is inexpensive and has been shown in laboratory studies to provide adequate ventilatory support. (If the anesthesia machine has an outlet that will not accept a 15-mm connector, the ventilation assembly may be connected to the Y-piece of the breathing circuit and the reservoir bag may be replaced with an occlusive strip of plastic tape.)

Technique

EQUIPMENT NEEDED

Sterile gloves
Antiseptic solution
12-gauge or 14-gauge intravenous cannula
Adapter for fresh gas outlet
Usual monitoring devices
Resuscitation drugs and equipment

PROCEDURE

Cleanse the skin overlying the cricothyroid membrane with antiseptic solution. Insert a 12-gauge or 14-gauge intravenous cannula through the cricothyroid membrane (Fig. 7–2). Confirm the proper location of the cannula (after removing the needle) by free aspiration of gas through the cannula. Connect the cannula to the Luer-Lok connector on the transtracheal ventilation system (Fig. 7–3). Connect the other end of the transtracheal ventilation system to the fresh gas outlet on the anesthesia machine. Intermittent or continuous depression of the oxygen flush valve on the anesthesia machine and intermittent occlusion of the thumb hole on the suction catheter flow will provide sufficient oxygen to maintain an adequate arterial oxygen saturation while the patient is awakened or is being prepared for tracheostomy or during additional attempts at intubation.

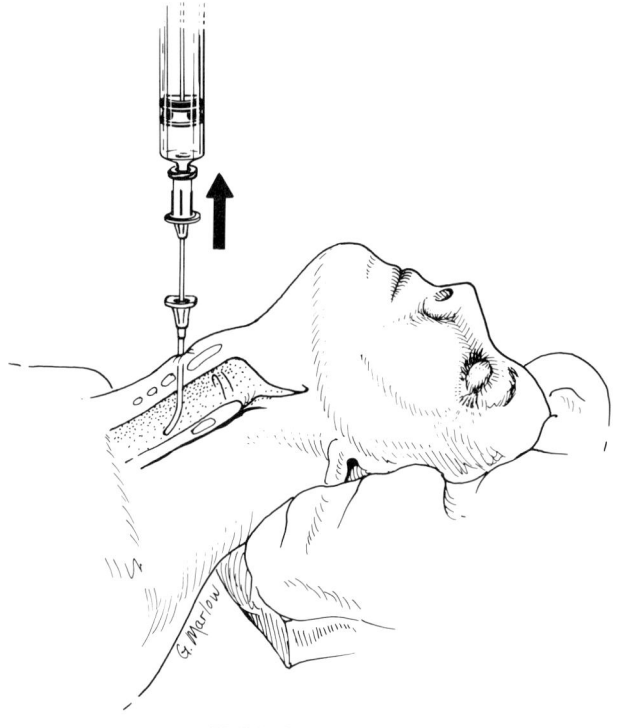

FIGURE 7–2

If transtracheal jet ventilation must be accomplished at a site where an anesthesia machine is not available, the transtracheal ventilation system may be connected directly to a wall oxygen flowmeter adapter adjusted to its highest flow setting.

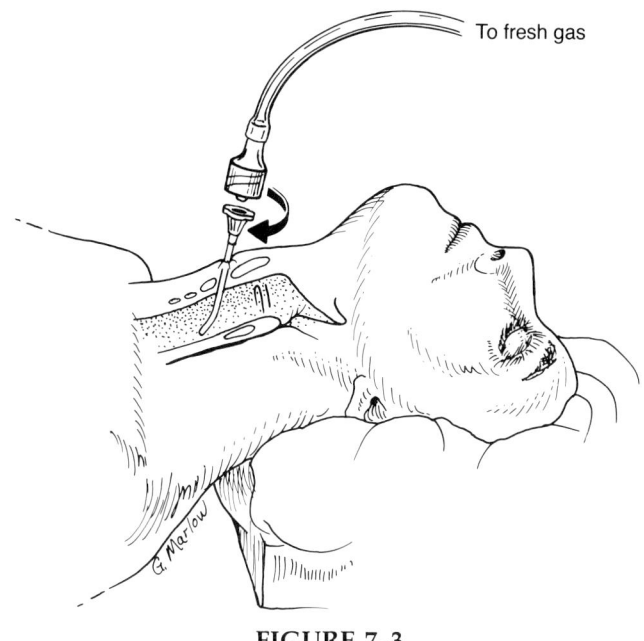

FIGURE 7–3

References

Benumof JL, Scheller MS: The importance of transtracheal jet ventilation in the management of the difficult airway. Anesthesiology 71:769–778, 1989

Scuderi PE, McLeskey CH, Comer PB: Emergency percutaneous transtracheal ventilation during anesthesia using readily available equipment. Anesth Analg 61:867–870, 1982

Smith RB, Schaer WB, Pfaeffle H: Percutaneous transtracheal ventilation for anaesthesia and resuscitation: A review and report of complications. Can Anaesth Soc J 22:607–612, 1975

8

Cricothyroidotomy

Although cricothyroidotomy has been used in the past when attempts at intubation and mask ventilation have failed, its use should be reserved for those instances when transtracheal jet ventilation cannot be accomplished. Given the high degree of familiarity that anesthesia personnel have for the Seldinger guide wire technique, my approach to cricothyroidotomy more closely resembles vascular cannulation than a traditional surgical tracheostomy.

Cricothyroidotomy is not a replacement for tracheostomy. If a surgeon will be available for tracheostomy, I recommend maintaining the patient with transtracheal jet ventilation, if possible, while tracheostomy is performed (if a permanent airway is needed), rather than proceeding directly to cricothyroidotomy. Tracheostomy probably never needs to be performed by an anesthetist; therefore, I will not describe the technique.

Technique

EQUIPMENT NEEDED

Sterile gloves
Antiseptic solution
Melker cricothyroidotomy set
5-ml syringe
25-gauge needle
5 ml lidocaine 1%
Usual monitoring devices
Resuscitation drugs and equipment

PREPARATION OF EQUIPMENT AND PATIENT

Position the patient supine on the operating room table with a blanket behind the shoulders (so that the head will be hyperextended). Attach the electrocardiographic leads, blood pressure cuff, and pulse oximeter probe for monitoring during the procedure (usually these will already be in place). Make sure that the necessary surgical instruments are available. Cleanse the skin of the patient's neck with antiseptic solution. Palpate the cricoid and thyroid cartilages to identify the cricothyroid membrane. Infiltrate local anesthetic in the skin overlying the cricothyroid membrane.

INCISION

Incise the skin horizontally with a No. 15 scalpel blade about 1 cm from the midline on either side, exposing the cricothyroid membrane (Fig. 8–1). Inject local anesthetic in the cricothyroid membrane and in the airway (transtracheal injection, see Chapter 2). Incise the cricothyroid membrane vertically about 1 cm. Insert the 18-gauge intravenous cannula through the cricothyroid membrane incision inferiorly into the airway. Confirm its position by free aspiration of gas (Fig. 8–2). Remove the needle, pass the rigid guide wire through the cannula inferiorly into the airway, and remove the cannula (Fig. 8–3).

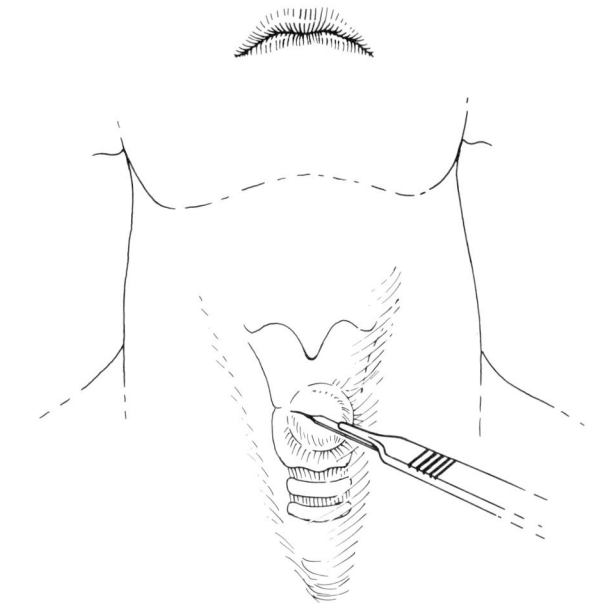

FIGURE 8–1

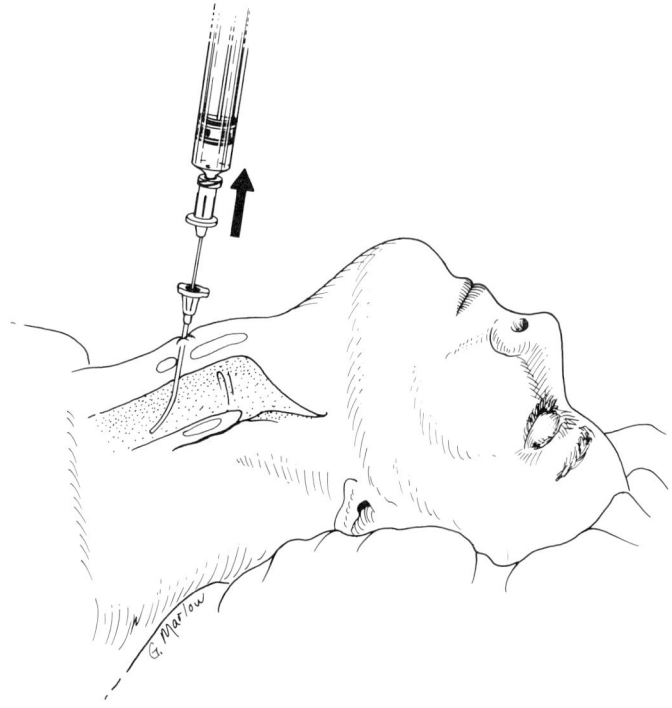

FIGURE 8–2

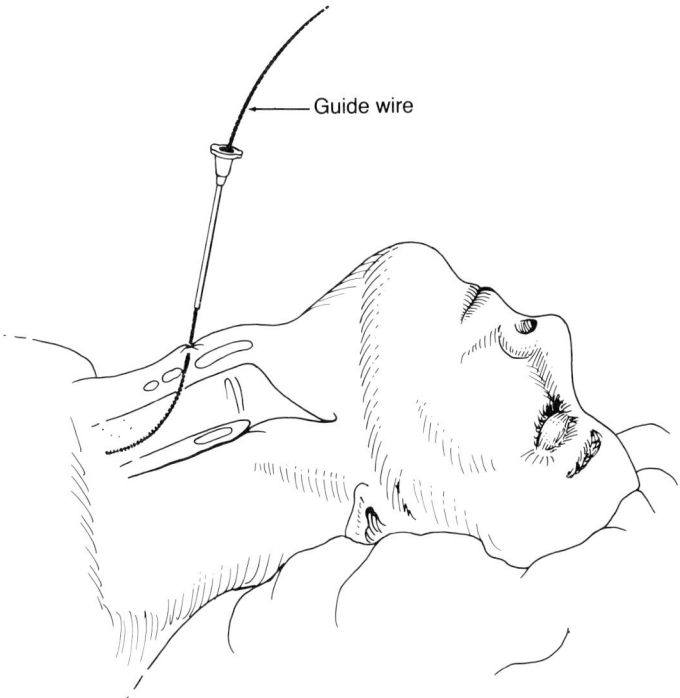

FIGURE 8–3

TUBE INSERTION

Pass the tracheal airway and smaller dilator over the guide wire inferiorly into the airway (Fig. 8–4). Remove the wire and the dilator (Fig. 8–5). Check the proper position of the tube with auscultation, capnometry, and pulse oximetry, or with

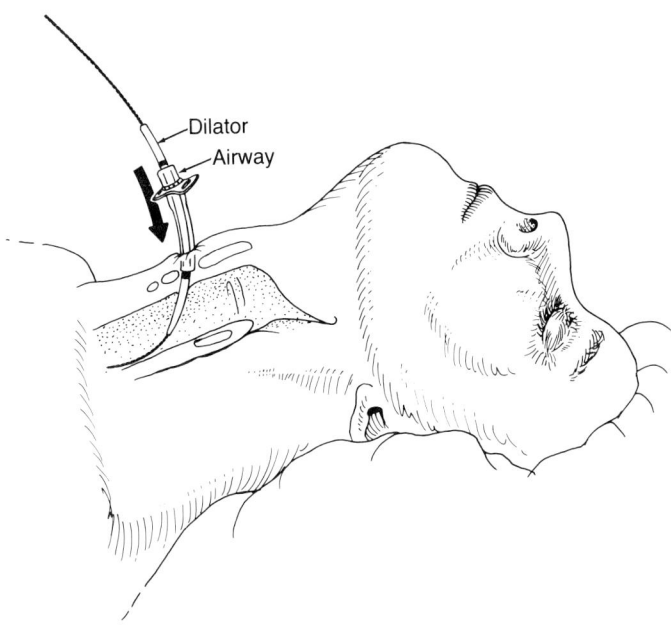

FIGURE 8–4

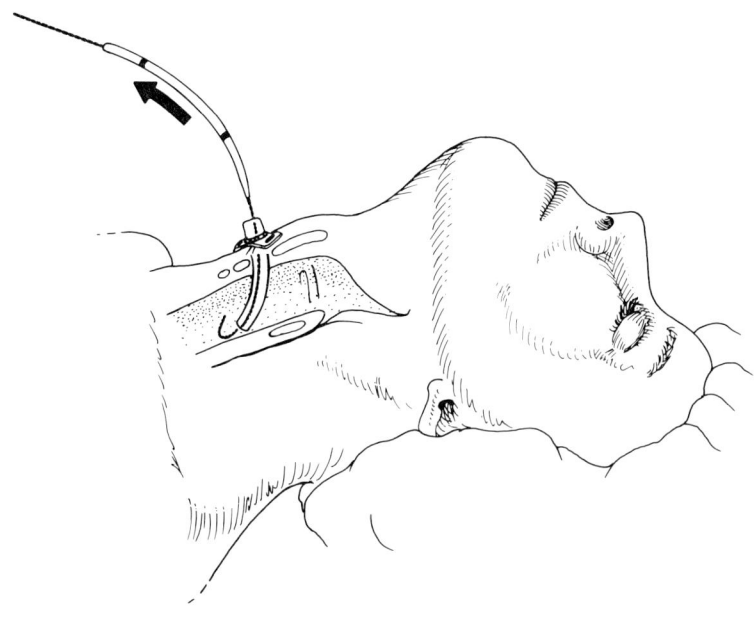

FIGURE 8–5

blood gas analysis and a chest radiograph. Finally, secure the tube to the patient either with two 3-0 black silk sutures or with an umbilical tape passed behind the patient's neck and tied to the sides of the tracheal tube.

References

Brantigan CO, Grow JB Sr: Cricothyroidotomy: Elective use in respiratory problems requiring tracheotomy. J Thorac Cardiovasc Surg 71:72–81, 1976

Cutler BS: Cricothyroidotomy for emergency airway. In Vander Salm TJ, Cutler BS, Wheeler HB (eds): Atlas of Bedside Procedures, pp 169–176. Boston, Little, Brown & Co, 1979

McGill J, Clinton JE, Ruiz E: Cricothyrotomy in the emergency department. Ann Emerg Med 11:361–364, 1982

Safar P, Penninckx J: Cricothyroid membrane puncture with special cannula. Anesthesiology 28:943–948, 1967

9

Retrograde Intubation

Occasionally, when direct laryngoscopy has proved unsuccessful, I have used a retrograde Seldinger technique with an intravenous cannula and a long, rigid guide wire. I have also substituted an epidural catheter (passed through the cricothyroid membrane through an epidural needle) for the guide wire.

Technique

EQUIPMENT NEEDED

Sterile gloves
Antiseptic solution
3-ml syringe
25-gauge needle
Lidocaine 1%
16-gauge intravenous cannula
Endotracheal tube changing stylet (or frozen gastric sump tube)
125-cm (length) 0.89-mm (0.035 in) guide wire
Endotracheal tube (anode or armored tube preferred)
Usual monitoring devices
Resuscitation drugs and equipment

PROCEDURE

Insert an intravenous cannula if one is not already present. Attach the pulse oximeter probe, electrocardiographic leads, and blood pressure cuff for monitoring during the procedure. Cleanse the skin of the neck with antiseptic solution. In awake patients, if there are no contraindications, perform superior laryngeal nerve blocks and transtracheal local anesthetic injections (see Chapter 2). Inject lidocaine 1% in the skin overlying the cricothyroid membrane. Local anesthesia may be omitted in anesthetized patients. Pass a 16-gauge or larger intravenous cannula through the cricothyroid membrane in an inferior to superior direction (Fig. 9–1). Remove the needle and confirm that the cannula is within the airway by free aspiration of gas. Pass the 0.035-inch 125-cm J-wire through the cannula, past the glottis, and into the mouth. Grasp the end of the guide wire as it passes out of the mouth (or occasionally, out through the naris) (Fig. 9–2). Pass the tube changing stylet over the wire into glottis (Fig. 9–3). Withdraw the J-wire through the stylet. Pass the armored (or

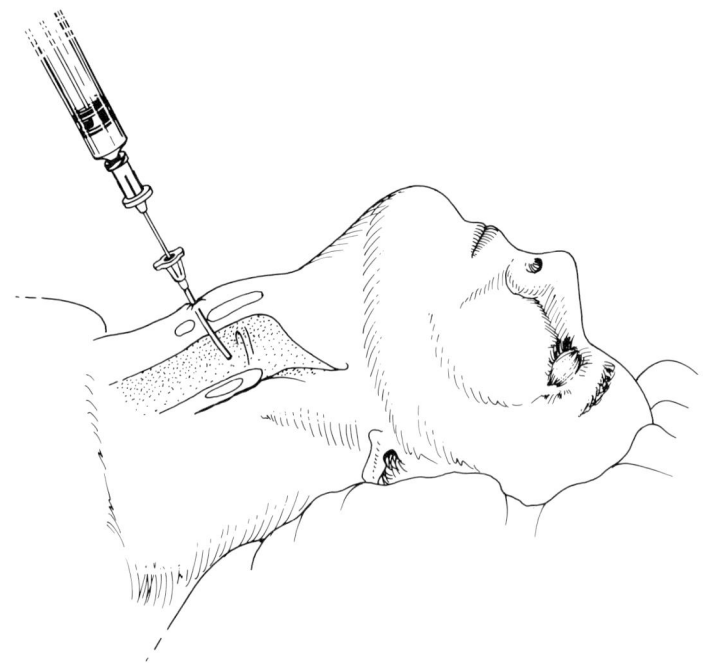

FIGURE 9–1

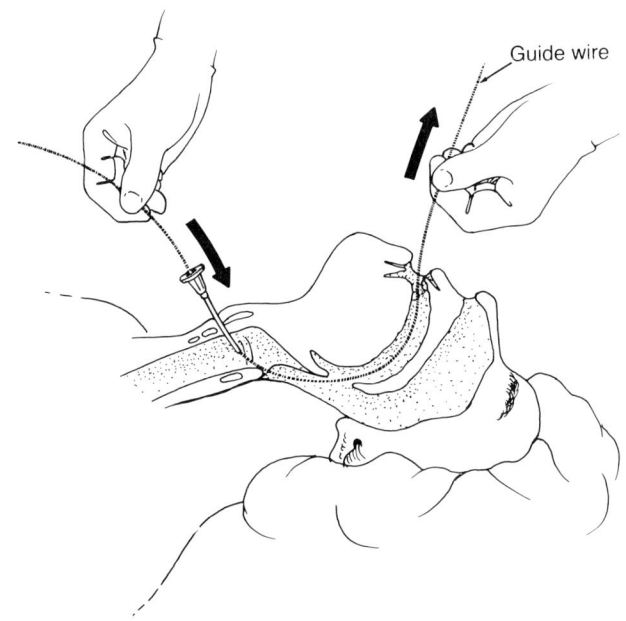

FIGURE 9–2

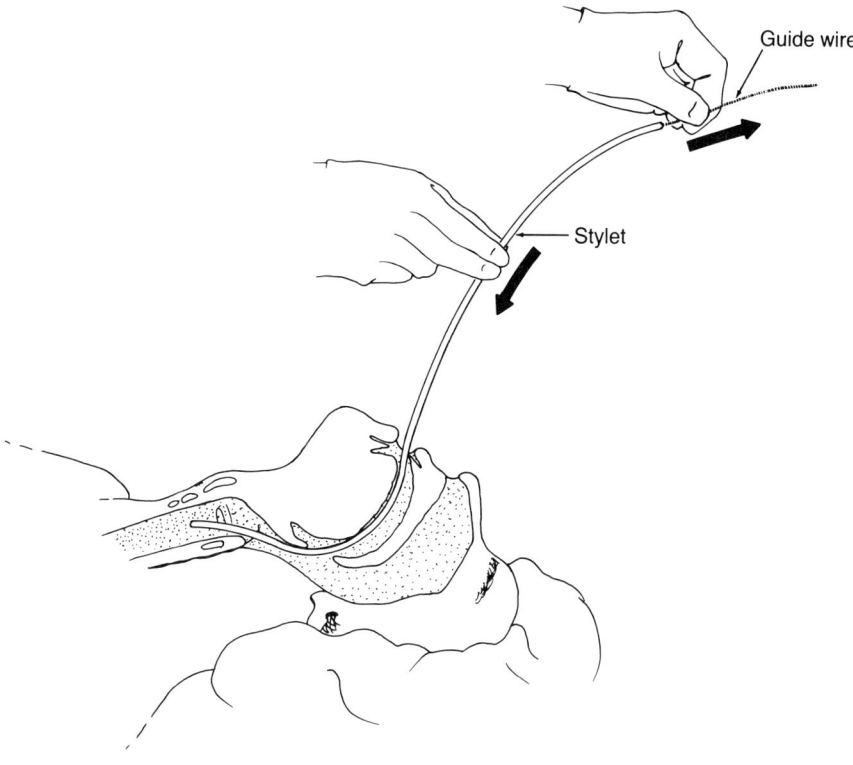

FIGURE 9–3

anode) endotracheal tube over the stylet into the trachea (Fig. 9–4). The anode (or armored) flexible tube is preferred because it conforms to the abnormal airway more readily than the semi-rigid polyvinyl endotracheal tube. Withdraw the stylet and

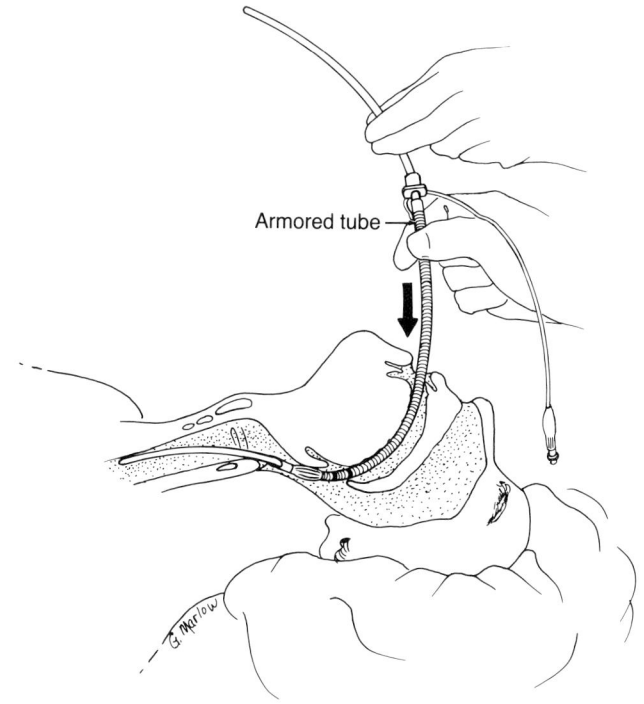

FIGURE 9–4

inflate the endotracheal tube cuff. Confirm the position of the tube by auscultation, capnometry, and finger pulse oximetry, or by blood gas analysis and a chest radiograph.

If the tube changing stylet is omitted, I recommend passing the guide wire through the Murphy eye of the endotracheal tube to facilitate the tube's passage into the glottis.

References

Abou-Madi MN, Trop D: Pulling vs. guiding: A modification of retrograde guided intubation. Can J Anaesth 36:336–339, 1989

Borland LM, Swan DM, Leff S: Difficult pediatric intubation: A new approach to the retrograde technique. Anesthesiology 55:577–578, 1981

Harmer M, Vaughan RS: Guided blind oral intubations. Anaesthesia 35:921, 1980

Hines MH, Meredith JW: Modified retrograde intubation technique for rapid airway access. Am J Surg 159:597–599, 1990

Powell WF, Ozdil T: A translaryngeal guide for tracheal intubation. Anesth Analg 46:231–234, 1967

Waters DJ: Guided blind endotracheal intubation for patients with deformities of the upper airway. Anaesthesia 18:158–162, 1963

10

Intubation with Lighted Stylet

The light wand can be used as a guide for intubation of patients with both normal and abnormal airways. The light wand is a stylet with a light on its distal tip. To use it effectively, the incident light in the operating room must be kept to a minimum.

Technique

EQUIPMENT NEEDED

Gloves
Lighted stylet
Endotracheal tube
Usual monitoring devices
Resuscitation drugs and equipment

PROCEDURE

Insert an intravenous cannula if one is not already present. Attach the pulse oximeter probe, electrocardiographic leads, and blood pressure cuff for monitoring during the procedure. In awake patients, superior laryngeal nerve blocks and transtracheal injection of local anesthetic should be performed, if there is no contraindication (see Chapter 2).

Insert the light wand through the endotracheal tube, and confirm that the light on the light wand functions. Insert the endotracheal tube and light wand into the patient's mouth. Extinguish all the operating room lights. Confirm that the light from the light wand is visible through the skin of the patient's neck. Advance the light wand and tube blindly down through the oropharynx and into the trachea (Fig. 10–1). When the light wand and tube pass into the trachea, the light from the light wand tip will be visible through the skin of the neck as a distinct, circumscribed glow in the midline. Should the light wand and tube be passed into the esophagus, the light will appear diffused through the skin of the neck (Fig. 10–2).

After passing the tube into the trachea, confirm that it is properly positioned by auscultation in the axillae, capnometry, and finger pulse oximetry, or with blood gas analysis and a chest radiograph.

50

Airway
Management

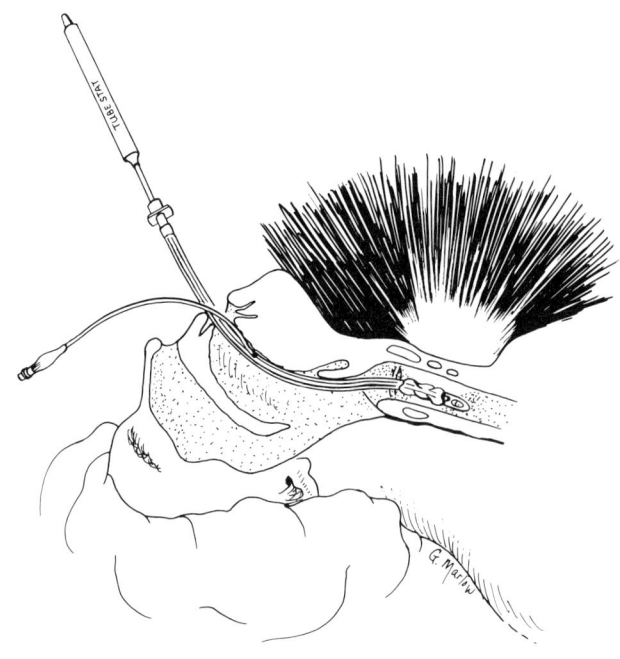

FIGURE 10–1

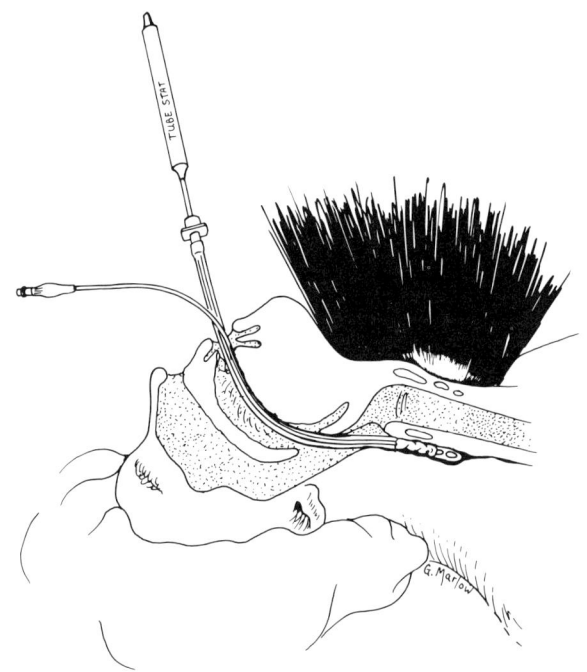

FIGURE 10–2

References

Ducrow M: Throwing light on blind intubation. Anaesthesia 33:827–829, 1978

Ellis DG, Jakymec A, Kaplan RM, Stewart RD, Freeman JA, Bleyaert A, Berkebile PE: Guided orotracheal intubation in the operating room using a lighted stylet: A comparison with direct laryngoscopic technique. Anesthesiology 64:823–826, 1986

MacIntosh R, Richards H: Illuminated introducer for endotracheal tubes. Anaesthesia 12:223–225, 1957

Stewart RD, Larose A, Stoy WA, Heller MB: Use of a lighted stylet to confirm correct endotracheal tube placement. Chest 92:900–903, 1987

Vollner TP, Stewart RD, Paris RD, Ellis DG, Berkebile PE: Use of the lighted stylet for guided orotracheal intubation in the prehospital setting. Ann Emerg Med 14:324–328, 1985

11

Intubation with Double-Lumen Endobronchial Tubes

Although the double-lumen endobronchial tube was devised for selective right and left lung bronchospirometry in awake patients, at present, double-lumen tubes are used most often to improve patient safety or operating conditions during general anesthesia, rather than as part of the diagnostic evaluation. Double-lumen tubes are used on rare occasions for positive-pressure ventilation of patients with bronchopleural fistulae or unilateral bullae (Table 11–1).

TABLE 11–1

INDICATIONS FOR DOUBLE-LUMEN TUBE PLACEMENT

Strong Indications
Unilateral pulmonary infection
Unilateral pulmonary hemorrhage
Bronchopleural fistula

Moderate Indications
Descending thoracic aortic surgery
Esophageal surgery
Pulmonary lobectomy
Transthoracic spine surgery

Weak Indication
Pneumonectomy

Types and Characteristics of Double-Lumen Tubes

The several available double-lumen tubes may be identified by the following characteristics: (1) presence or absence of a carinal hook, (2) shape of the bronchial lumen, and (3) side of intended endobronchial intubation. Double-lumen tubes are available in four sizes, ranging from 35 F to 41 F. A 35 F tube has roughly the same external diameter as an 8.0-mm conventional endotracheal tube; a 41 F tube has roughly the same external diameter as an 11.0-mm conventional endotracheal tube.

I prefer not to use the 35 F tube because of its greater tendency to become clogged by secretions. I usually put 37 F tubes in women and 39 F or 41 F tubes in men. When lung isolation is required during pediatric thoracic surgery, I place a Fogarty embolectomy cannula in the operative lung (using the fiberoptic endoscope) and provide ventilation through a conventional endotracheal tube.

The Carlens tube is designed to have its bronchial limb inserted into the left mainstem bronchus. For optimal positioning, it should be advanced until its carinal hook "catches" on the carina. The tracheal and bronchial lumina of the Carlens tube are cylindrical and relatively small for the external diameter of the tube. The White tube resembles the Carlens tube but is intended for insertion into the right mainstem bronchus. The right upper lobe bronchus branches from the right mainstem bronchus within 2 to 3 cm of the carina, necessitating that the White tube (and other right-sided designs) have a slit in the bronchial cuff to permit right upper lobe ventilation when the cuff is inflated. Because of the relatively small, cylindrical air passages of both the White and the Carlens tubes, obstruction by secretions is a common problem (Fig. 11–1).

Robertshaw tubes incorporate a number of design features that may make them superior to the Carlens or White designs. First of all, Robertshaw tubes have no carinal hook. Many anesthetists believe that carinal hooks often impede tube insertion through the vocal cords. The tracheal and bronchial lumina of Robertshaw tubes are oval and larger for a given external tube diameter than the lumina of either Carlens or White tubes. Reusable and disposable Robertshaw tubes are available for both right-sided and left-sided endobronchial insertion. The right-sided disposable tube's bronchial cuff is eccentrically located, which more effectively provides unobstructed ventilation of the right upper lobe bronchus than any other right-sided design.

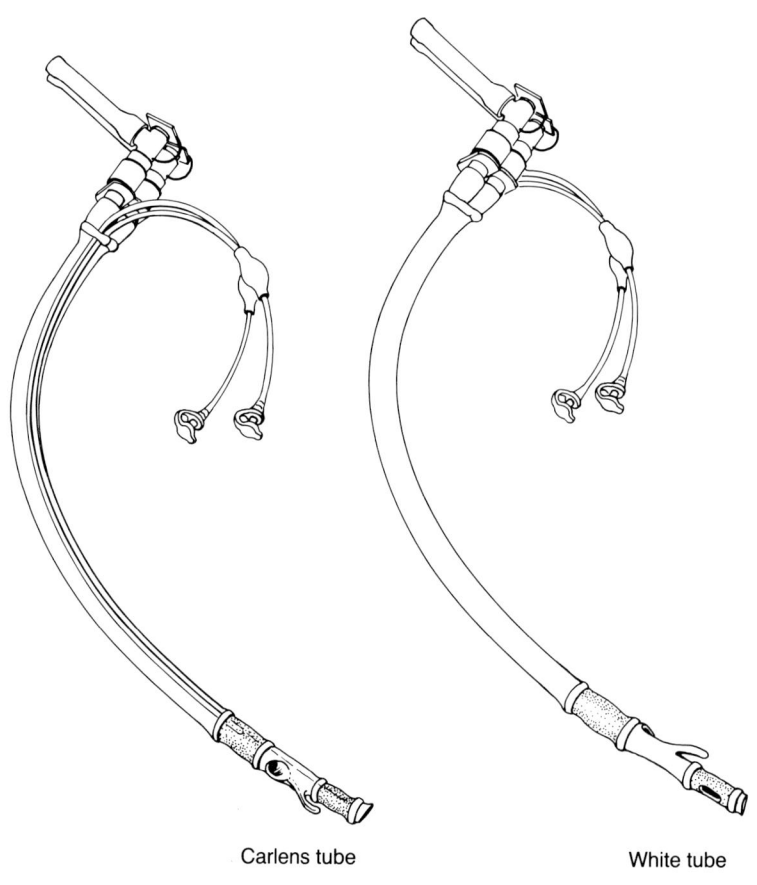

Carlens tube   White tube

FIGURE 11–1

Owing to problems ventilating the right upper lobe with right-sided endobronchial tubes, some anesthetists routinely use left-sided endobronchial tubes for one-lung anesthesia, regardless of the lung they will selectively ventilate during surgery. I disagree with this approach. I prefer to place the bronchial limb of the double-lumen tubes into the bronchus of the lung that I intend to ventilate during surgery, believing that the bronchial limb more effectively and reliably provides selective ventilation of the lung on the nonoperative side.

Technique

EQUIPMENT NEEDED

Gloves
Suction device and Yankauer suction tip
Laryngoscope and laryngoscope blades
Pediatric flexible fiberoptic bronchoscope (primarily for right-sided tube placement)
Double-lumen tubes of various sizes
Single-lumen tubes of appropriate sizes
Stylet
Oral and nasal airways
Magill forceps
Continuous positive airway pressure valve (for CPAP of nonventilated lung)
Oxygen tank and Mapleson circuit (for CPAP of nonventilated lung)
Stethoscope
Kelly clamp
Tincture of benzoin
Adhesive tape
Drugs and equipment for induction of general anesthesia
Usual monitoring devices
Resuscitation drugs and equipment

PREPARATION

Position the patient supine on the operating table in the "sniffing" position for laryngoscopy. Attach the standard monitoring devices to the patient. After inducing general anesthesia, paralyze the patient with a nondepolarizing neuromuscular blocking agent or with a succinylcholine bolus and infusion. Laryngoscopy for double-lumen tube placement will often be more time consuming than with a conventional single-lumen endotracheal tube and may exceed the duration of paralysis provided by a bolus dose of succinylcholine. I recommend exposing the glottis with the MacIntosh laryngoscope blade rather than the Miller laryngoscope blade because the curved design seems to provide more room between the laryngoscope blade and the lower teeth for passing the large double-lumen tube.

LARYNGOSCOPY AND TUBE INSERTION

Insert the double-lumen tube (with stylet in place) through the vocal cords under direct vision (Fig. 11–2). The bronchial lumen should be uppermost as the tube goes through the vocal cords; then the entire double-lumen tube should be turned so that the bronchial lumen is pointed toward the desired side of bronchial intubation (Fig. 11–3). Withdraw the stylet slightly and advance the tube as far as possible.

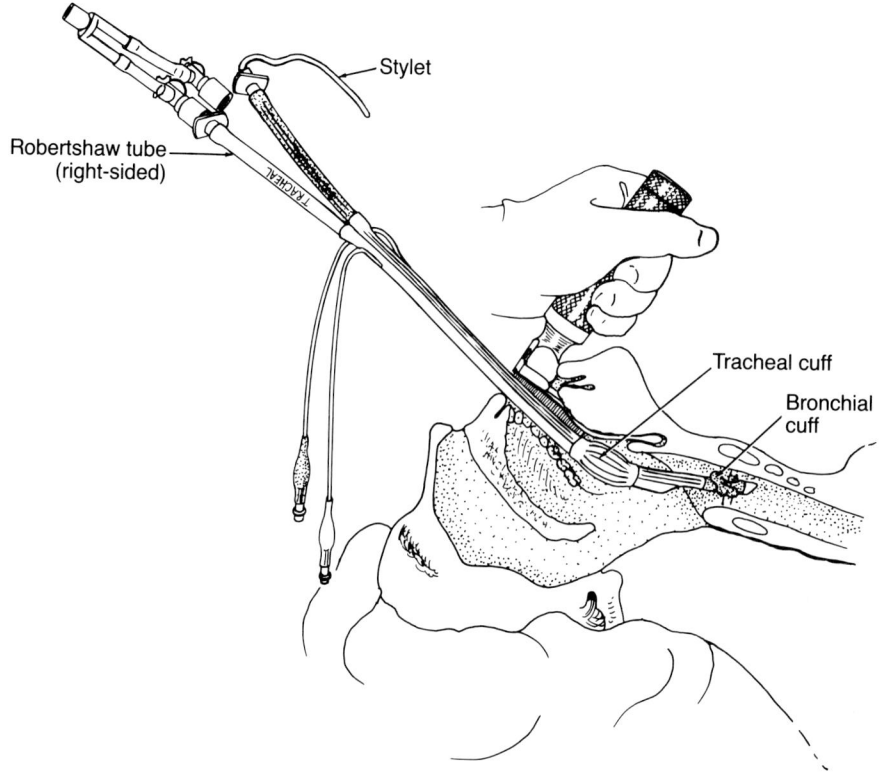

FIGURE 11–2

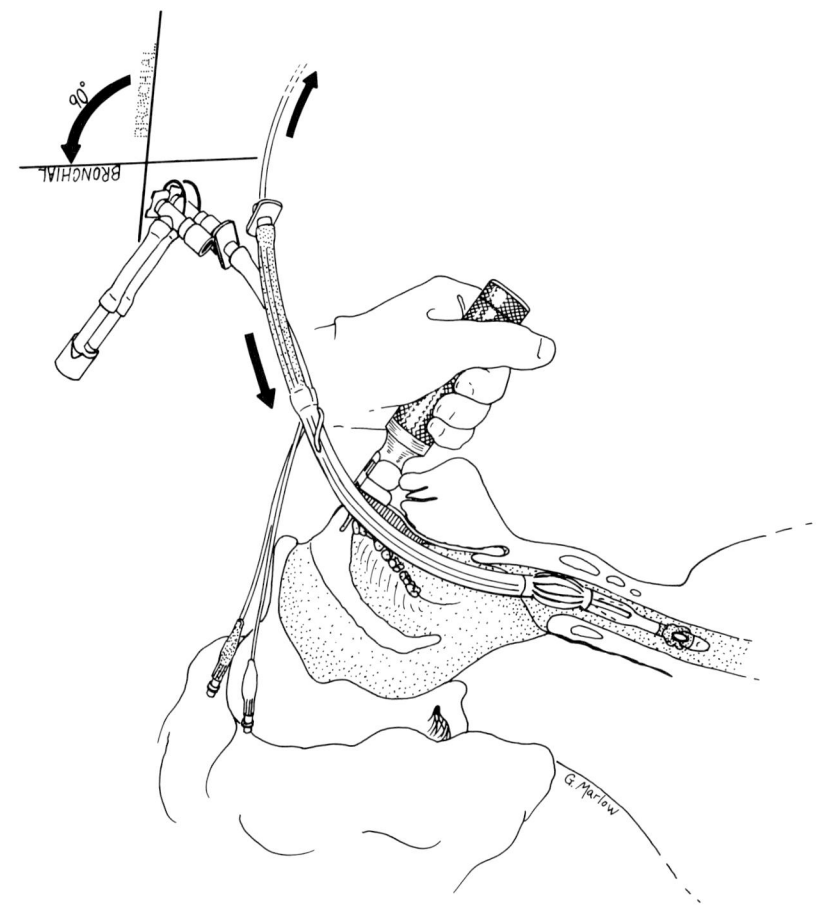

FIGURE 11–3

CHECKING THE TUBE POSITION

Inflate the tracheal cuff (this usually requires less than 5 ml of air) and connect the tube to the breathing circuit for capnographic confirmation that the tube is within the trachea. Next, inflate the bronchial cuff with 3 ml (or less) of air. Clamp the proximal tracheal channel (coming from the breathing circuit) and disconnect the distal tracheal channel (coming from the patient) (Fig. 11–4). Auscultation should

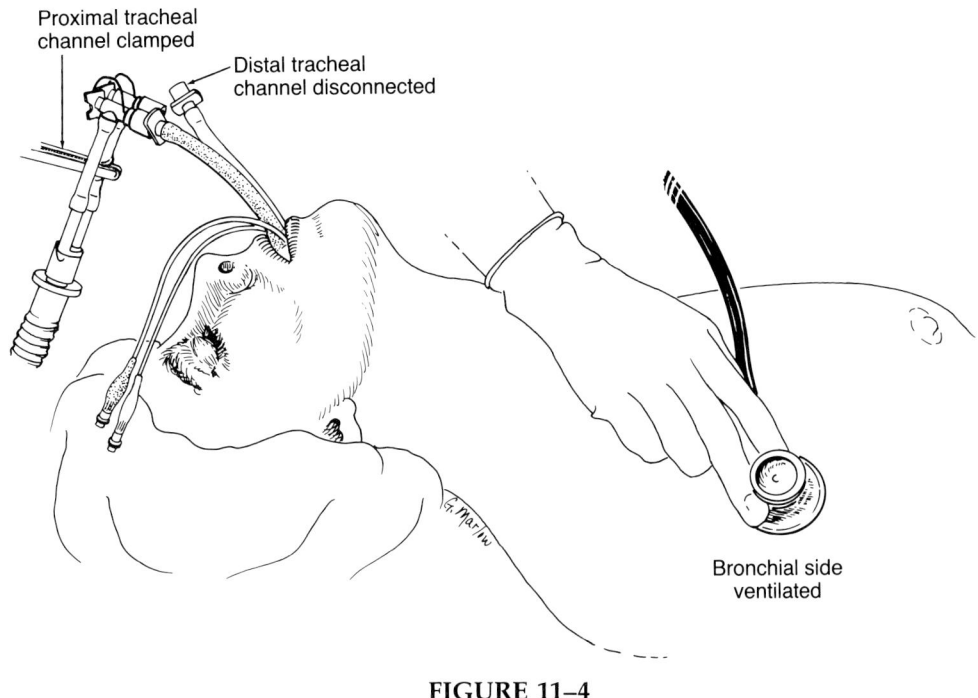

FIGURE 11–4

reveal breath sounds in the axilla on the side of endobronchial intubation and minimal breath sounds (only those transmitted from the ventilated lung should be heard) in the contralateral axilla. Next, occlude the proximal bronchial lumen of the tube (coming from the breathing circuit) and disconnect the distal bronchial channel (coming from the patient) (Fig. 11–5). Ventilate the patient through the unclamped tracheal channel. Breath sounds should be heard in the axilla contralateral to the side of endobronchial intubation; minimal transmitted sounds should be heard in the axilla ipsilateral to endobronchial intubation.

SECURING THE TUBE

Secure the tube to the patient's face with adhesive tape and tincture of benzoin. If the patient must be moved prior to surgical incision (usually to a lateral decubitus position), check the ability of the tube to selectively ventilate the nonoperative lung one last time before surgery begins.

PREVENTION OF RIGHT UPPER LOBE ATELECTASIS

When I insert a right-sided endobronchial tube, I routinely confirm with fiberoptic endoscopy (see Chapter 6) that the right upper lobe bronchus is not obstructed by the right bronchial cuff. I do not view the auscultatory finding of right upper lobe hypoventilation (decreased breath sounds above the clavicle) as a definitive test. I insert a pediatric bronchoscope through the bronchial lumen and advance it slowly

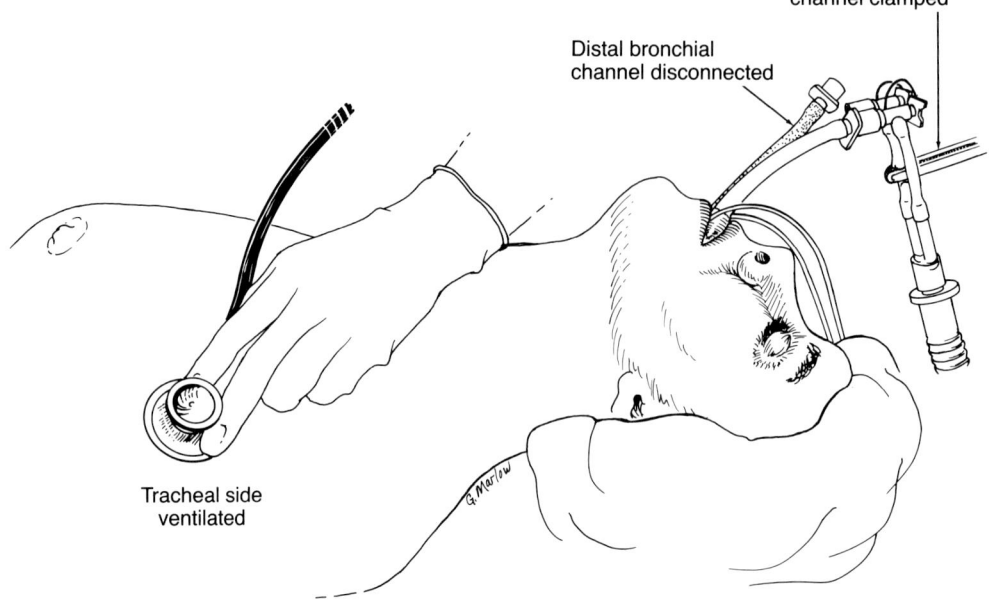

FIGURE 11–5

past the carina (Fig. 11–6). The right upper lobe bronchus should be visible through the slit in the right bronchial cuff, if the tube is properly positioned for right upper lobe ventilation. If, on the other hand, no lumen is visible, deflate the bronchial and tracheal cuffs so that the tube can be slowly advanced (or withdrawn, if necessary) under direct vision with the bronchoscope until the right upper lobe bronchial opening can be seen clearly through the hole in the cuff. Since the tube position often shifts when the patient is turned, I commonly do not check the location of the right upper lobe orifice until after turning the patient into the lateral decubitus position, so as to increase time efficiency in the operative suite.

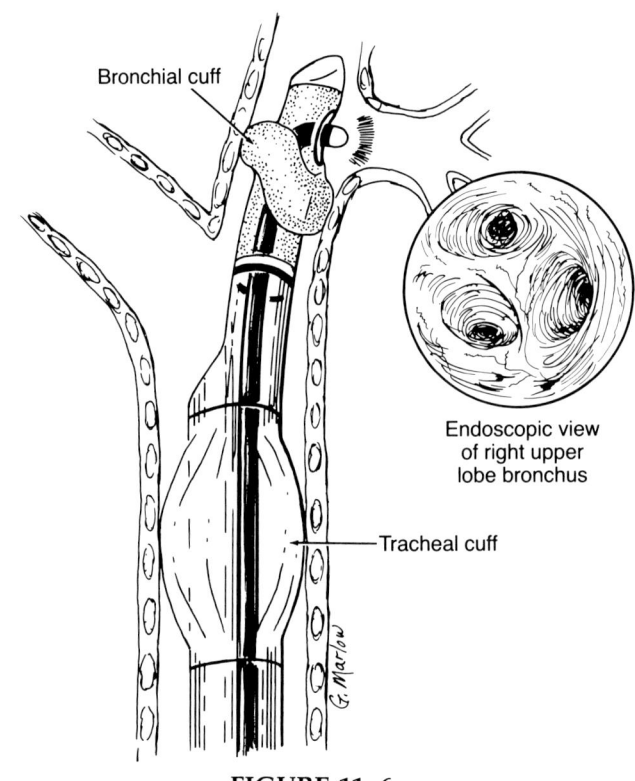

FIGURE 11–6

Malpositioned Double-Lumen Tubes

I do not routinely use the fiberoptic bronchoscope to position left-sided double-lumen tubes; however, I do not hesitate to use endoscopy when I have difficulty selectively ventilating a lung, if simpler maneuvers have failed.

If both lungs can be ventilated with the bronchial cuff deflated and the tracheal cuff inflated, but selective ventilation of neither lung can be accomplished, the tube may not have been inserted far enough. Alternatively, the bronchial cuff may have failed. In this situation, I first determine whether either cuff leaks. If both cuffs appear functional, I deflate both cuffs, advance the tube, and then attempt selective ventilation. If neither maneuver is successful, I perform fiberoptic endoscopy to check the position of the bronchial and tracheal cuffs.

When the tube passes into the "wrong" bronchus, attempts at selective ventilation may be successful in ventilating the "wrong" lung. If the bronchial limb repeatedly passes into the "wrong" bronchus, I withdraw the bronchial limb proximal to the carina and pass the endoscope through the bronchial lumen past the carina and into the bronchus of the lung I wish to ventilate (Fig. 11–7). I then slide the bronchial limb of the tube over the endoscope into the bronchus. The right and left mainstem bronchi can be distinguished during endoscopy by the angle of takeoff from the carina (shallower for the right side than the left) and by the very proximal origin of the right upper lobe bronchus compared with the more distal tube off of the left upper lobe bronchus from the left mainstem bronchus.

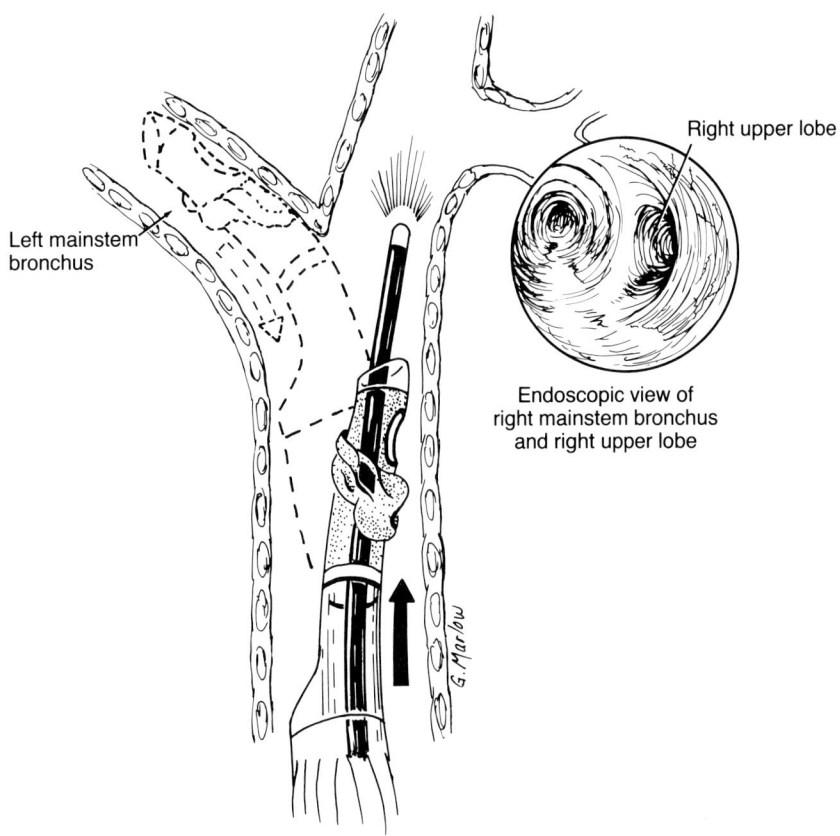

FIGURE 11–7

Sometimes the appropriate lung can be selectively inflated, but deflation is impeded. Excessive inflation of the bronchial cuff may be the cause, leading to a "ball-valve" type of obstruction. Endoscopy may reveal cuff herniation over the tip of the bronchial limb. Slight deflation of the cuff (withdrawing 1 to 2 ml of air) may be curative. Alternatively, partial occlusion of the lumen by secretions or blood may be the cause.

I have had difficulty selectively ventilating the *right* lung with a *left*-sided tube (and vice versa) when the tube has been inserted too far. When the tracheal cuff abuts the carina, inspired gas may be forced past an inflated bronchial cuff, if inspiratory pressures are high enough. Conversely, one can often selectively ventilate the lung into which the bronchial limb has been inserted. Endoscopy through the tracheal lumen will reveal the exceedingly distal location of the tracheal cuff. The solution is to deflate the cuffs and withdraw the tube by 1 to 2 cm, reinflate the cuffs, and retest.

One-Lung Ventilation

When I switch from two-lung to one-lung ventilation, I normally do *not* alter the ventilator settings. I pay careful attention to peak inspiratory pressure and arterial oxygen saturation. If peak inspiratory pressures exceed 35 cm H_2O, I consider reducing the tidal volume and increasing the respiratory rate, maintaining a constant minute ventilation.

Oxygen Saturation during One-Lung Anesthesia

In most cases, when the switch is made from two-lung to one-lung ventilation, the PaO_2 will fall as a consequence of blood flow through the unventilated lung. I routinely use an anesthetic technique in which I can employ nearly 100% inspired oxygen. Patients having parenchymal disease in the collapsed lung seem to have a lesser decrease in PaO_2 during one-lung anesthesia than those with normal lungs. Pulmonary blood flow is partially regulated by the alveolar oxygen tension. So-called hypoxic pulmonary vasoconstriction serves to help the anesthetist during one-lung anesthesia by reducing blood flow to the nonventilated lung. Unfortunately, all vapor general anesthetic agents inhibit hypoxic pulmonary vasoconstriction.

If hypoxemia develops during one-lung anesthesia with a properly positioned double-lumen tube, I find it helpful to determine by auscultation and capnography whether the dependent lung is being properly ventilated. Suctioning may remove blood or mucus impeding lobar ventilation. Manual ventilation and the neuromuscular stimulator can determine whether additional neuromuscular relaxant is required. If these maneuvers are unsuccessful, the nonventilated lung can be subjected to continuous positive airway pressure (Fig. 11–8). If hypoxemia persists, the patient must be returned to two-lung ventilation. Often, the oxygen saturation can be well maintained merely by ventilating the lung on the operative side for 1 to 2 minutes, on a 15-minute schedule interspersed with one-lung ventilation.

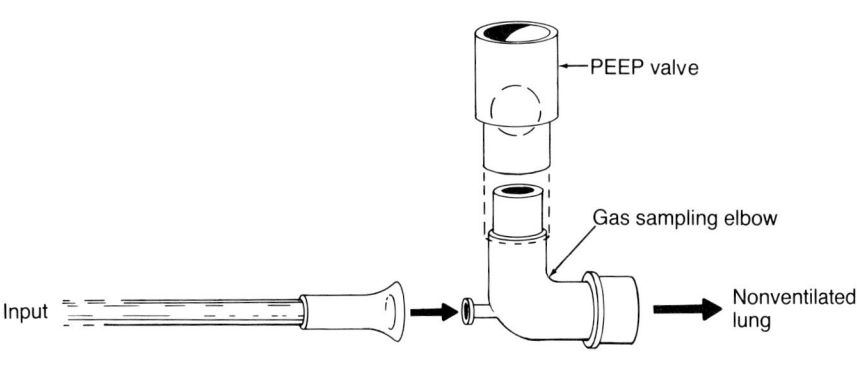

FIGURE 11–8

References

Benumof JL: Anesthesia for Thoracic Surgery, pp 223–259. Philadelphia, WB Saunders, 1987

Benumof JL: One-lung ventilation and hypoxic pulmonary vasoconstriction: Implications for anesthetic management. Anesth Analg 64:821–833, 1985

Black AMS, Harrison GA: Difficulties with positioning Robertshaw double lumen tubes. Anaesth Intens Care 3:299–311, 1975

Brodsky JB: Isolation of the lungs. In Brodsky JB (ed): Thoracic Anesthesia, pp 264–281. Philadelphia, JB Lippincott, 1990

Capan LM, Turndoff HM, Miller S: Maximizing oxygenation during one-lung anesthesia. In Brodsky JB (ed): Thoracic Anesthesia, pp 282–305. Philadelphia, JB Lippincott, 1990

Cutaia M, Rounds S: Hypoxic pulmonary vasoconstriction: Physiologic significance, mechanism and clinical relevance. Chest 97:706–718, 1990

Ikeda S: Atlas of Flexible Bronchofiberoscopy, pp 31–52. Baltimore, University Park Press, 1974

Kerr JH: Physiologic aspects of one-lung (endobronchial) anaesthesia. In Norlander O (ed): Anaesthesia in Thoracic Surgery. Int Anesthesiol Clin 10:61–78, 1972

Kerr JH, Smith AC, Prys-Roberts C, Meloche R: Observations during endobronchial anaesthesia: I. Ventilation and carbon dioxide clearance. Br J Anaesth 45:159–167, 1973

Kerr JH, Smith AC, Prys-Roberts C, Meloche R, Foëx P: Observations during endobronchial anaesthesia: II. Oxygenation. Br J Anaesth 46:84–92, 1974

Vaughan RS: Endobronchial intubation. In Latto IP, Rosen M (eds): Difficulties in Tracheal Intubation, pp 156–172. Philadelphia, Baillière Tindall, 1984

Wilson RS: Endobronchial intubation. In Kaplan JA (ed): Thoracic Anesthesia, pp 389–402. New York, Churchill Livingstone, 1982

12

Replacement of an Endotracheal Tube

Patients undergoing mechanical ventilation in the intensive care unit may require replacement of their endotracheal tubes, usually for cuff leaks. This often occurs in patients requiring prolonged intubation, who are usually dependent on high inspired concentrations of oxygen. These patients may not tolerate even brief periods of hypoventilation during tube changes. Other patients requiring tube replacement may have been intubated with great difficulty owing to anatomic abnormalities, airway edema, or airway trauma. In short, endotracheal tube replacement cannot be approached in a cavalier fashion. Assume that the worst may happen and have a contingency plan in case the first attempt at reintubation is unsuccessful. I recommend replacing endotracheal tubes over a rigid plastic "tube changer" or under direct vision with either a fiberoptic endoscope or a conventional laryngoscope. The semi-rigid plastic stylets for endotracheal tube changes are vastly superior to the gastric and suction tubes that have been used for this purpose in the past. If the patient has been sedated and paralyzed for mechanical ventilation, ensure that the patient is *fully* paralyzed before attempting to change the endotracheal tube.

Technique

EQUIPMENT NEEDED

Gloves
Endotracheal tubes of appropriate sizes
Laryngoscope handle and blades
Tube changer or Eschmann stylet
Equipment for ventilation with bag and mask
Fiberoptic bronchoscope (optional)
Usual monitoring devices
Resuscitation drugs and equipment

USE OF TUBE CHANGER

Ensure that all necessary equipment for ventilation with bag and mask and for orotracheal intubation is present and in working condition. Hyperventilate the patient with 100% oxygen through the existing tube. Untape the existing tube, and then deflate the tracheal cuff. Insert the tube changer to approximately half its length into the existing tube (Fig. 12–1). Remove the existing tube and replace it with a new one over the tube changer (Fig. 12–2). Remove the tube changer and inflate the cuff on the new tube. Confirm that the new endotracheal tube is correctly placed within the trachea by auscultation in both axillae, capnometry, and pulse oximetry, or with blood gas analysis and a chest radiograph. Tape the new endotracheal tube in place.

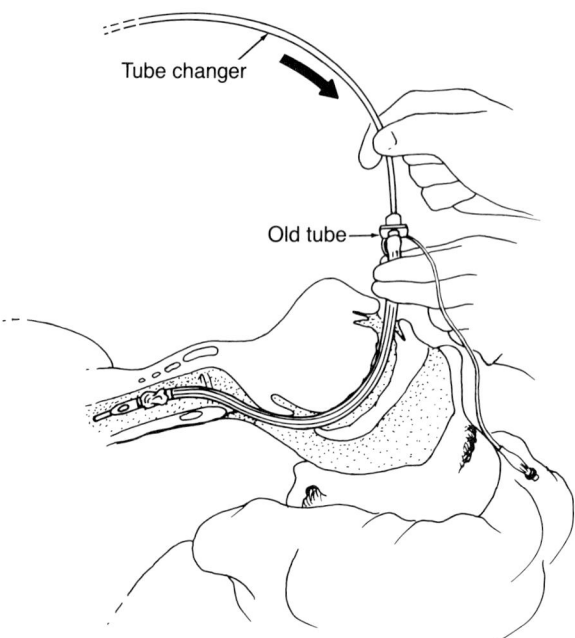

FIGURE 12–1

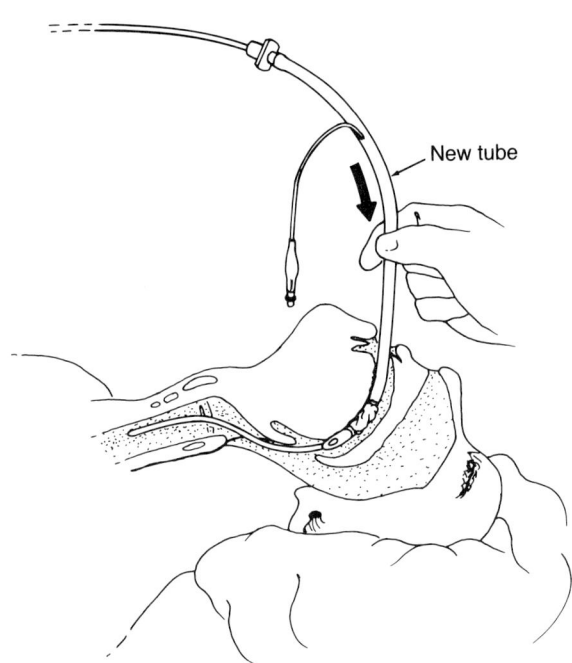

FIGURE 12–2

REPLACEMENT OF ENDOTRACHEAL TUBE UNDER DIRECT VISION

Confirm that the laryngoscope handle, blades, light bulbs, and all necessary equipment for ventilation with bag and mask are present and function properly. Hyperventilate the patient with 100% oxygen. Insert the laryngoscope blade and visualize the glottis. When the endotracheal tube can be seen passing between the cords into the glottis, the tube should be untaped, the cuff deflated, and the tube removed. In critical situations an assistant should untape and remove the old tube so that the laryngoscopist can concentrate on placing the new tube expeditiously (Fig. 12–3). After inserting the new tube, remove the laryngoscope from the mouth, inflate the tube cuff, and ventilate the patient with oxygen. Confirm that the tube is correctly placed within the trachea using capnometry, pulse oximetry, and auscultation in both axillae, or with blood gas analysis and a chest radiograph.

Alternatively, visualize the glottis with a fiberoptic endoscope (passed either orally or nasally) over which a fresh endotracheal tube has previously been passed. Remove the malfunctioning endotracheal tube, advance the endoscope into the glottic opening, and pass the fresh tube over the endoscope into the glottis (Fig. 12–4). Remove the endoscope, inflate the cuff, and connect the tube to a source of oxygen. Confirm the correct placement of the tube as described earlier.

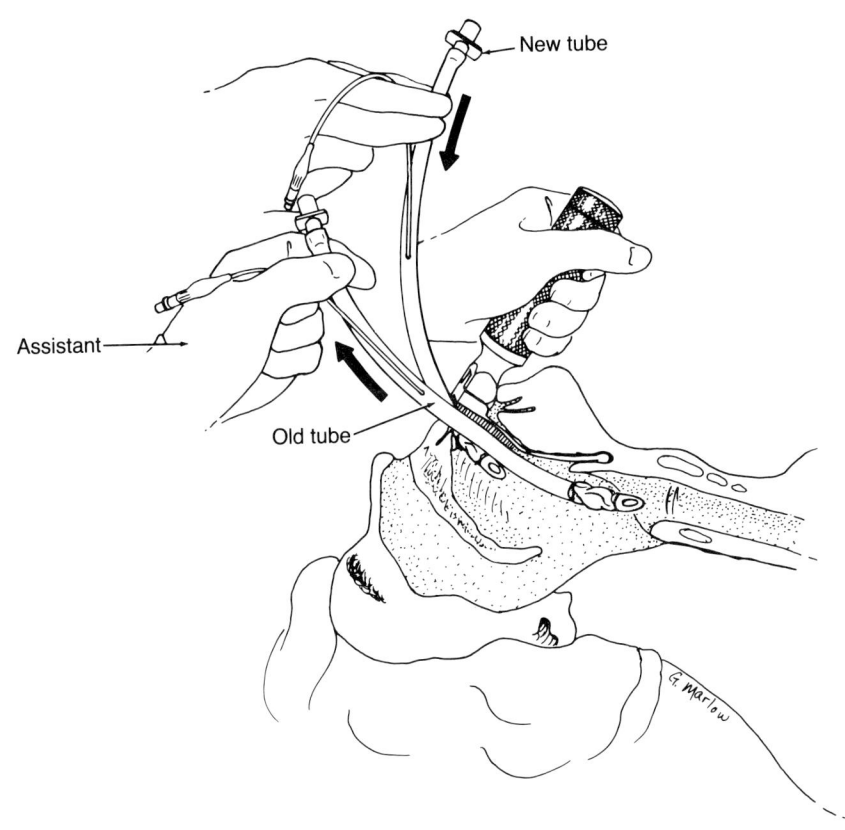

FIGURE 12–3

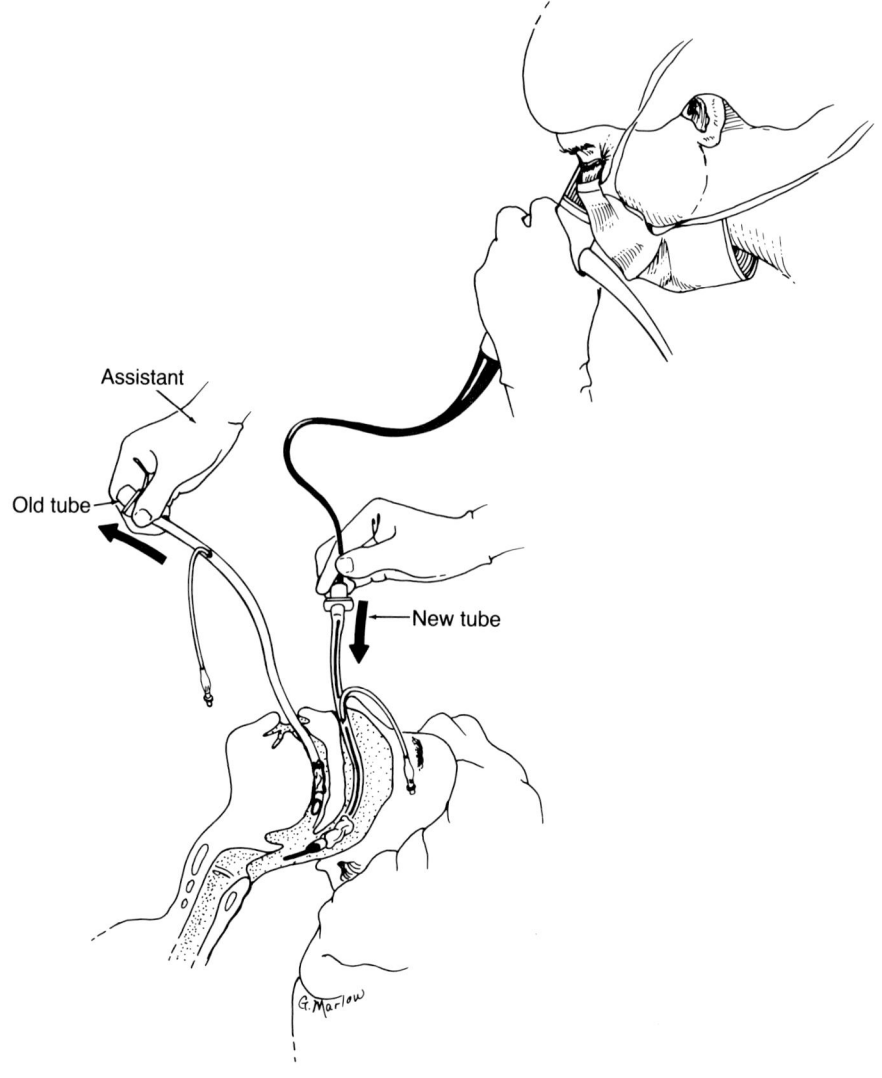

FIGURE 12–4

13

Emergency Needle Thoracentesis

Although elective thoracostomy tube placement will nearly always be performed by a surgeon, every practitioner of anesthesia and intensive care needs to know how to perform emergency needle thoracentesis. Such standard anesthetic and intensive care practices as positive-pressure ventilation (particularly in patients with pulmonary bullae), supraclavicular block, subclavian vein cannulation, or internal jugular vein cannulation all carry a significant risk of pneumothorax. It is unreasonable to expect that a surgeon will be immediately available whenever an undetected pneumothorax may progress to a tension pneumothorax. Emergency needle thoracentesis will convert a tension pneumothorax into a simple pneumothorax, reducing the likelihood of cardiopulmonary arrest. If no pneumothorax is present, needle thoracentesis carries a 10% to 20% risk of inducing a new pneumothorax.

Technique

EQUIPMENT NEEDED

Sterile gloves
Antiseptic solution
14-gauge or 16-gauge intravenous cannula
20-ml syringe

PREPARATION

Cleanse the skin of the anterior chest with antiseptic solution on the side of the suspected pneumothorax. Identify the second intercostal space as the intercostal space beneath the first and second palpable ribs caudad to the clavicle.

NEEDLE INSERTION

Insert a large-bore intravenous cannula with a syringe attached through the intercostal space in the midclavicular line, keeping the intravenous needle closer to the lower rib to avoid lacerating the intercostal artery or vein (Fig. 13–1). As the needle and cannula pass into the pleural space, a characteristic "pop" is usually felt. If a pneumothorax is present, the operator will instantly be able to aspirate air. If a

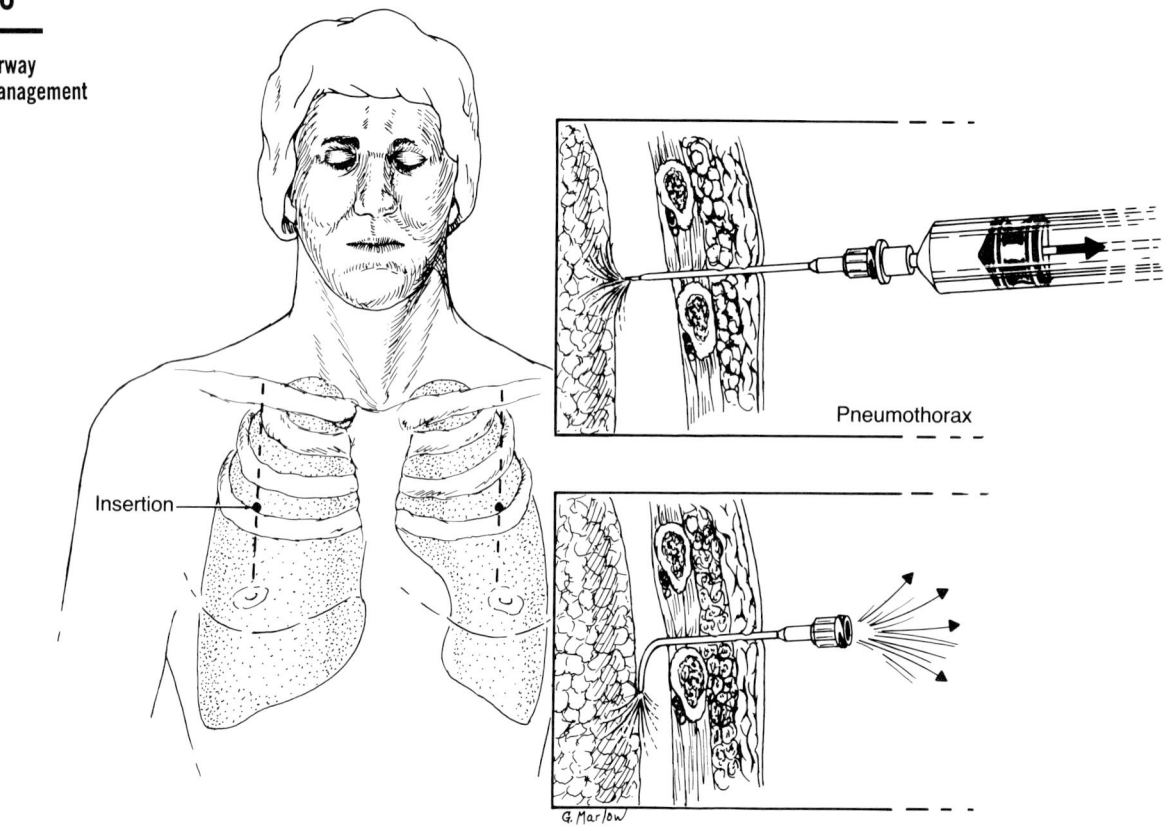

FIGURE 13–1

tension pneumothorax is present, pass the cannula over the needle, remove the needle, and allow the pressurized gas to escape. If no air can be aspirated, indicating that tension pneumothorax is not present, remove the needle and cannula.

DISPOSITION

Since placement of an intravenous cannula into the pleural space is (at best) a temporizing technique, a surgeon should be notified to perform follow-up examinations and to determine whether chest tube thoracostomy is required.

Reference

Kovarik JL, Brown RK: Tube and trocar thoracostomy. Surg Clin North Am 49:1455–1460, 1969

II

INTRAVASCULAR CANNULATION

14

Intravenous Cannulation

Intravenous cannulation may be considered the most basic anesthesia procedure, since, in general, no other procedure (other than those related to airway management) can be performed until an intravenous infusion line is obtained. The site of choice for intravenous cannulation of nearly every adult patient will be found on the back of the hand or on the forearm. In small children, in addition to these sites, I also include veins in the foot and the scalp (in infants). I have sometimes been forced to use central venous cannulation (see Chapter 15) as my primary intravenous technique, particularly in intravenous drug abusers and chemotherapy patients.

Technique

EQUIPMENT NEEDED

Gloves
Antiseptic solution
Intravenous cannulae
Intravenous infusion and tubing
Venous tourniquet
3-ml syringe
25-gauge needle
Lidocaine 1%

PROCEDURE

Apply a venous tourniquet to the upper arm (Fig. 14–1). Cleanse the skin overlying a visible vein with antiseptic solution. Inject lidocaine 1% in the skin overlying this vessel. Be careful not to insert the needle into the vessel itself (Fig. 14–2). Next, insert the intravenous cannula and needle through the skin and carefully advance the point of the needle into (but not through) the vein (Fig. 14–3). When blood returns into the needle hub, carefully advance the cannula over the needle into the vessel itself and remove the needle from the cannula (Fig. 14–4). Attach the intravenous infusion tubing to the cannula and tape both to the skin. If the cannula cannot be advanced over the needle, sometimes the resistance can be overcome by advancing the needle a fraction of a millimeter farther. Be careful not to advance the needle through the back wall of the vein.

Intravascular Cannulation

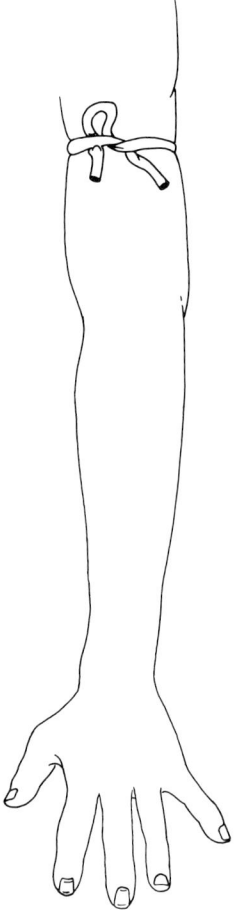

FIGURE 14–1

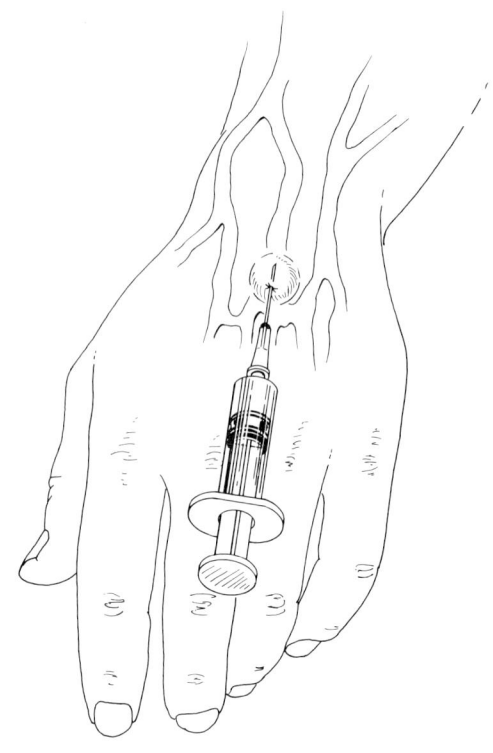

FIGURE 14–2

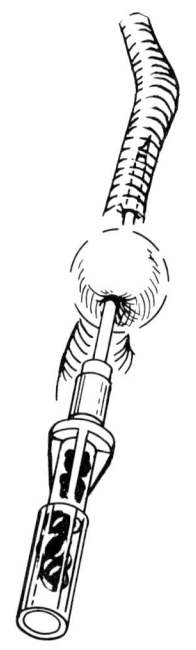

FIGURE 14–3

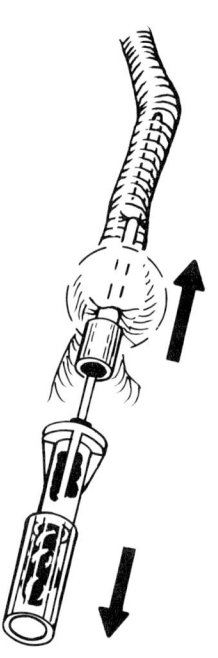

FIGURE 14–4

If the initial cannulation attempt is unsuccessful and an additional attempt is to be made in the same extremity, do not remove the cannula before replacing the venous tourniquet on the upper arm. If the venous cannula from the first unsuccessful attempt is removed, a hematoma may appear while the second cannulation attempt is in progress.

Reliable locations where veins can usually be found (in addition to the back of the hand) also include the so-called intern's vein at the base of the thumb along the lateral surface of the radius and the basilic and cephalic veins in the antecubital fossa. I usually do not cannulate veins in the antecubital fossa unless I cannot insert a venous cannula at a more distal site on the upper extremity, particularly in those patients who may remain in hospital for long periods of time after their surgery. I anticipate that the venous cannula will have to be replaced and that ever more proximal sites will have to be used.

15

Central Venous Cannulation

Central venous cannulation became popular during the 1960s and 1970s when widespread application of total parenteral nutrition popularized subclavian cannula placement, the Seldinger technique and J-wires made central venous cannulation through the external jugular veins practical, and the balloon-tipped pulmonary artery catheter was introduced and accepted.

Indications

Central venous cannulae may be used for *monitoring* right atrial pressure to provide a guide for right ventricular filling and function, for *treatment* of venous air emboli by aspiration, and for *infusion* of blood products, medicinals, or intravenous fluids. Central venous cannulation is the preliminary step to percutaneous placement of a pulmonary artery catheter.

Sites

The most popular sites for placement of central venous cannulae during anesthesia are the internal and external jugular veins (Fig. 15-1). Less popular options include the subclavian veins, the basilic veins, and the femoral veins. During cardiac surgery, cannulae may be placed surgically in the right atrium under direct vision.

Location of the Cannula Tip

When central venous cannulae are placed for aspiration of venous air emboli (most commonly during neurosurgical operations conducted in the sitting position), the orifice of the cannula is best placed at the junction of the superior vena cava and the right atrium. This may be accomplished using intravascular electrocardiography (see Chapter 16). In most other settings, the ideal location for the cannula tip is within the superior vena cava.

Following placement of any central venous cannula, it is essential that the final location of the cannula tip be confirmed to be within the intrathoracic venous system and *not* within the heart. Thus, a chest radiograph is usually obtained as soon as is practical to ensure that the cannula is in a safe position.

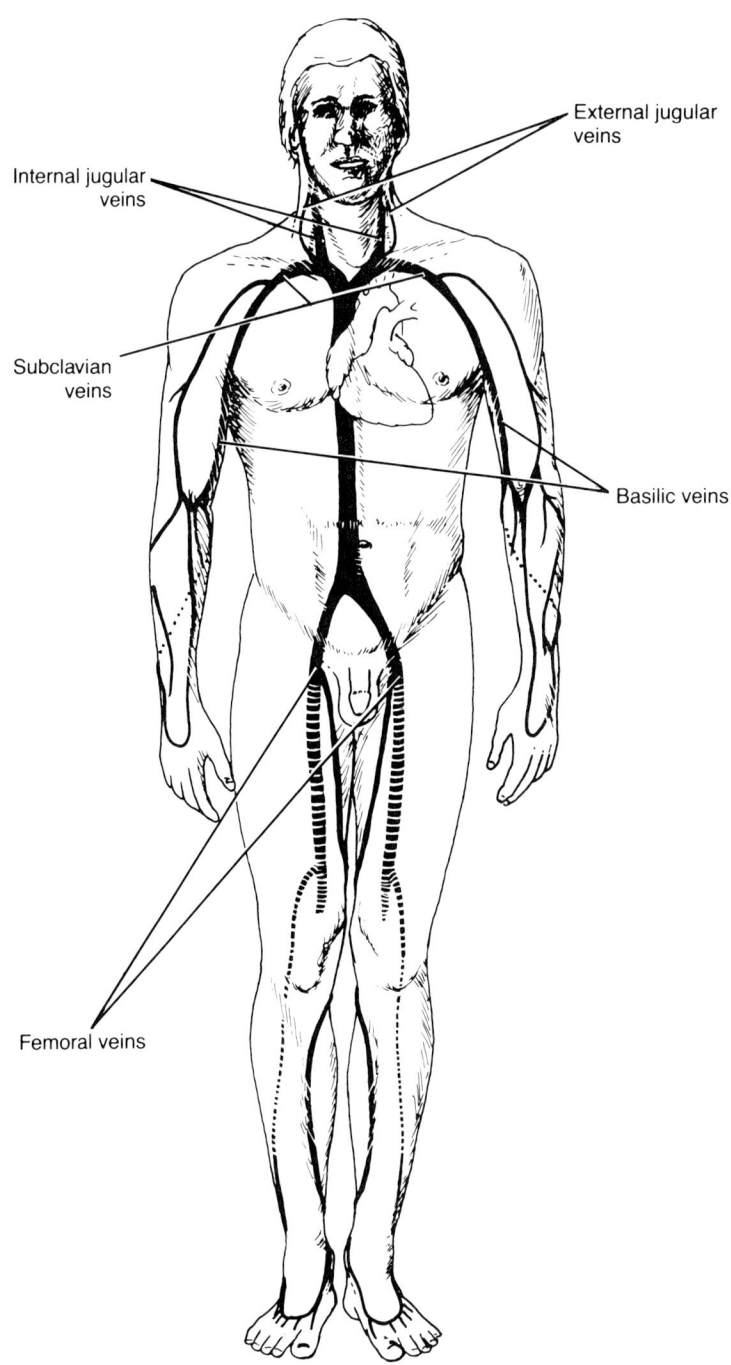

FIGURE 15–1

Central Venous Pressure Monitoring

Transduced central venous cannulae demonstrate three characteristic rises in pressure during a cardiac contraction cycle, termed the a, c, and v waves. The a wave corresponds to atrial contraction; the c wave corresponds to closure of the tricuspid valve during right ventricular contraction; the v wave corresponds to diastolic filling of the atrium during right ventricular diastole (Fig. 15–2).

The transduced central venous pressure may be used as a guide to fluid transfusion therapy (i.e., a decrease in the central venous pressure indicates a decrease in circulatory blood volume); however, numerous authors have pointed out the frequent lack of correlation between changes in left ventricular filling and central venous pressure. For this reason, I find central venous pressure to be useful only in combination with clinical assessment in determining the fluid volume needs of critically ill patients.

The central venous pressure waveform can be used as a guide to the diagnosis of arrhythmias. Junctional arrhythmias characteristically produce "cannon" a waves owing to the concurrent contraction of the right atrium and right ventricle.

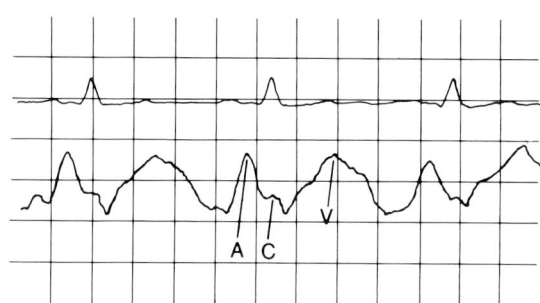

FIGURE 15–2

Internal Jugular Vein Cannulation

The internal jugular vein is ideally suited for central venous cannulation during anesthesia. The head and neck are usually conveniently accessible to the anesthetist throughout surgery, allowing the internal jugular vein to be cannulated at almost any time. Finally (and perhaps most importantly) the pathway from the right internal jugular vein to the superior vena cava is nearly a straight line, limiting the ability of the cannula to wander off its intended course and making it feasible to defer chest radiographic confirmation of cannula location until the end of surgery (provided blood can be aspirated from the cannula and appropriate pressures are measured).

EQUIPMENT NEEDED

Sterile gloves
Antiseptic solution
Intravenous infusion set
Central venous cannula tray (2-ml syringe, 1% lidocaine, 22-gauge needle, 5-ml syringe, J-wire, central venous cannula of appropriate length, 3-0 nonabsorbable suture on a cutting needle)
Means for placing patient in Trendelenburg position (e.g., "shock blocks")
Usual monitoring devices
Resuscitation drugs and equipment

PREPARATION AND POSITIONING

Attach the electrocardiographic leads, blood pressure cuff, and pulse oximeter probe for monitoring during the procedure. Position the patient supine on the operating table in the Trendelenburg position (with the head below the level of the heart) to increase the central venous pressure and distend the internal jugular vein. This increases the likelihood of successful cannulation and reduces the risk of an air embolus. Patients with dyspnea from chronic lung disease or congestive heart failure may not tolerate the Trendelenburg position. The patient's head should be turned to the side opposite the site of intended cannulation (Fig. 15–3).

Cleanse the skin overlying the puncture site with antiseptic solution and place a sterile fenestrated drape (or three folded surgical towels) so that the puncture site and pertinent landmarks are clearly visible.

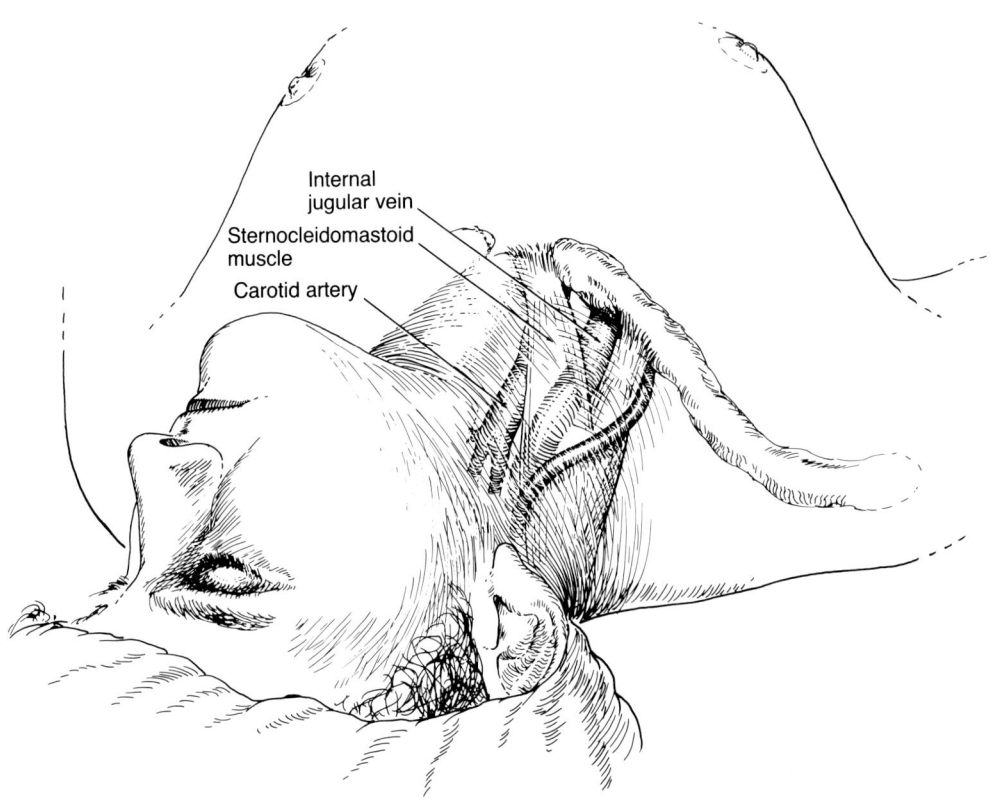

FIGURE 15–3

LOCATION OF INTERNAL JUGULAR VEIN

The internal jugular vein is located by reference to visible and palpable landmarks. I use either of two techniques for internal jugular vein cannulation, which I will refer to as the *medial* and *triangle* approaches. In the medial approach, the exploring needle enters the skin medial to the sternocleidomastoid muscle at about the level of the thyroid cartilage. Insert the needle lateral and dorsal to the carotid pulse, where the internal jugular vein lies within the carotid sheath (Fig. 15–4). When approaching the internal jugular vein from the top of the triangle formed by the junction of the sternal and clavicular heads of the sternocleidomastoid muscle and the clavicle, aim the exploring needle at the ipsilateral nipple (Fig. 15–5). I choose the approach that appears easiest in a given patient. For example, although I normally favor the medial approach, I use the triangle approach when the carotid

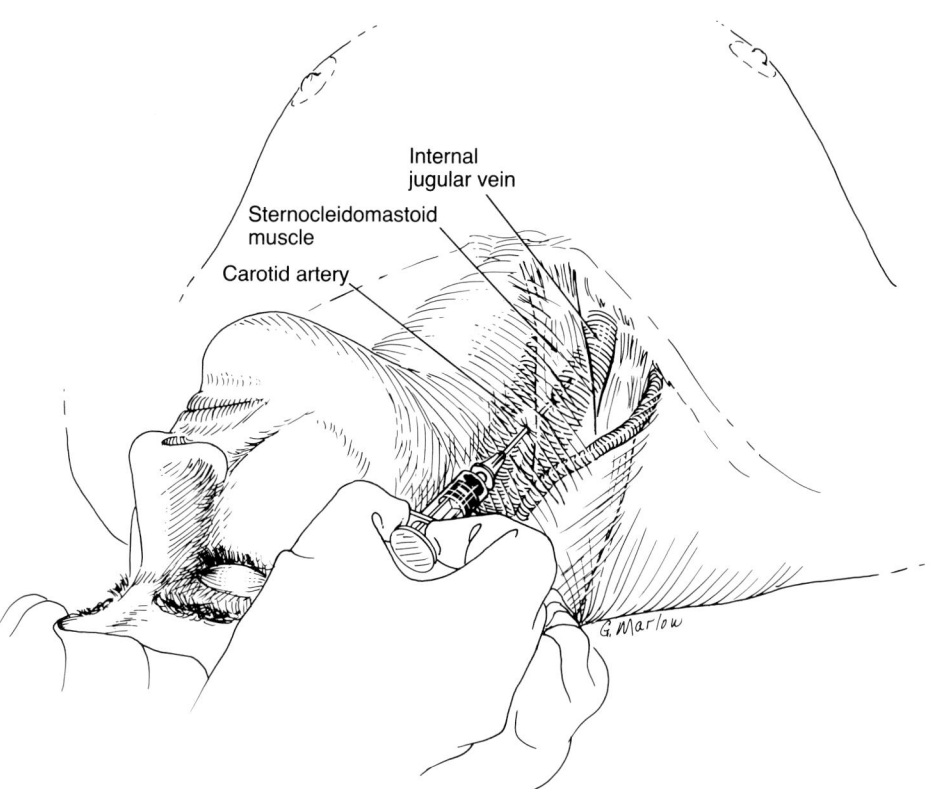

FIGURE 15–4

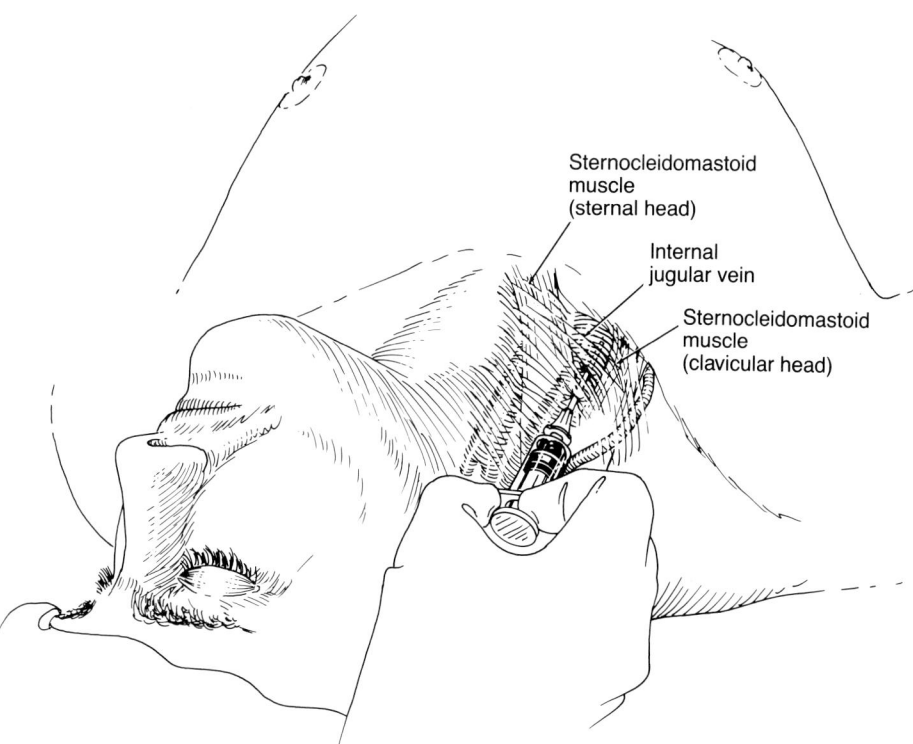

FIGURE 15–5

pulse is not palpable or the patient has a short neck. Then, if the technique chosen initially proves unsuccessful in two to three passes of the exploring needle, I try the other.

Inject 1% lidocaine in the skin and subcutaneous tissue before probing with the exploring needle. Check placement by aspiration before injecting any local anesthetic owing to the close proximity of so many arterial and venous structures. Identify the vein by aspirating venous blood through a 22-gauge exploring needle attached to a 3-ml syringe.

CANNULATION OF INTERNAL JUGULAR VEIN

After locating the internal jugular vein with the exploring needle, cannulate it with an intravenous cannula (or with a thin-walled needle large enough to permit passage of the J-wire), approaching the vein in the same way as proved successful with the exploring needle (Fig. 15–6). I do not recommend leaving the exploring needle and syringe in place while attempting cannulation with the larger needle; the extra needle and syringe usually get in the way.

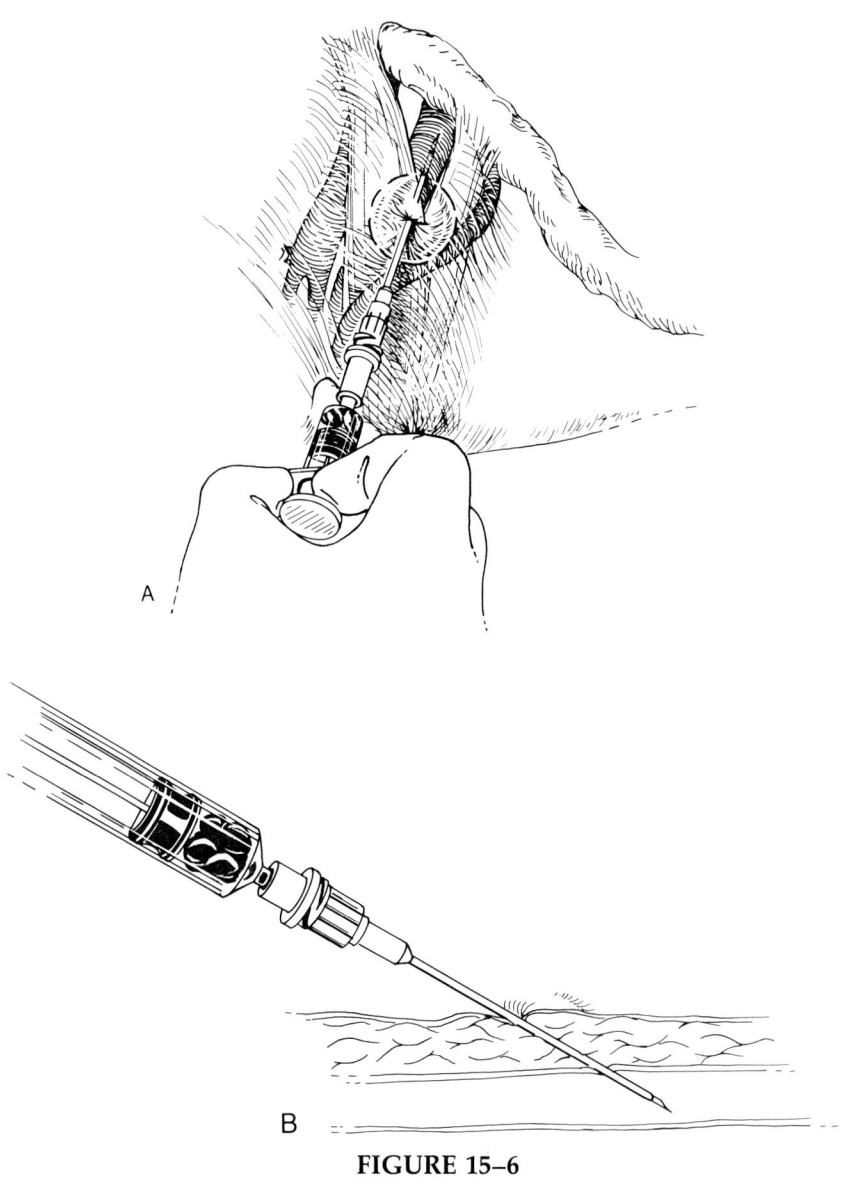

FIGURE 15–6

After the internal jugular vein has been entered with the intravenous needle, advance the 18-gauge (or 16-gauge) intravenous cannula over the needle into the vein and withdraw the needle so that the guide wire can be inserted (Fig. 15–7). *It is extremely important that there be no question as to whether the intravenous cannula is located within the jugular vein before it is replaced over the guide wire by a large introducer sheath (for pulmonary arterial catheterization).* Cannulae placed within the carotid artery usually emit pulsatile jets of bright red blood. Cannulae correctly placed within the internal jugular vein usually yield drops of dark blood, the rate of flow of which will depend on the phase of the respiratory cycle (flow is more rapid during expiration than inspiration) and the central venous pressure. When there is *any* doubt, compare the color of blood aspirated from the putative internal jugular cannula with that of a concurrently obtained arterial sample. Alternatively, transduce the pressure within the cannula either with an electrical transducer or a standard intravenous extension tubing (used as a "water" manometer). If the carotid has been entered with a small cannula or finder needle, remove the cannula or needle and apply manual pressure to the puncture site for several minutes to reduce the likelihood of hematoma formation (particularly if the patient is currently being given an anticoagulant or will be given heparin intraoperatively, as for vascular or cardiac surgery) before making another attempt to cannulate the internal jugular vein.

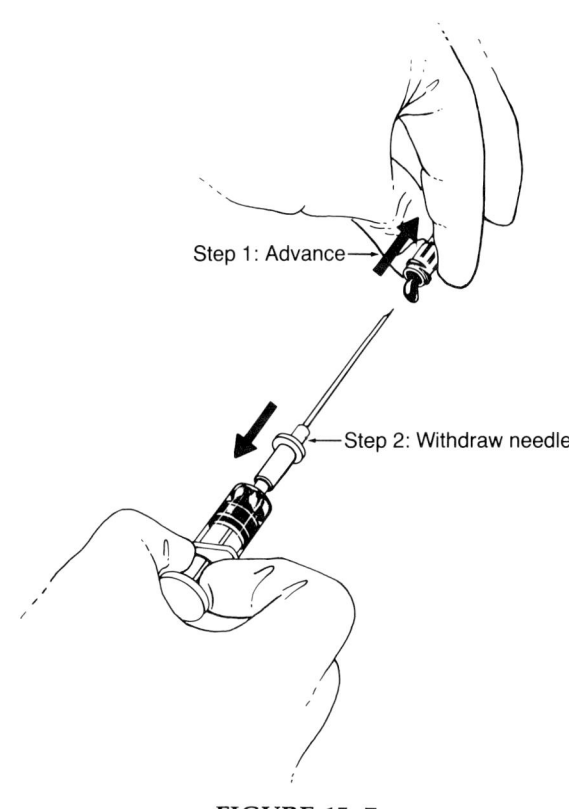

FIGURE 15–7

PASSAGE OF GUIDE WIRE

Insert the guide wire through the intravenous cannula into the central venous circulation (Fig. 15–8). Passage of the wire will often result in the appearance of premature beats on the electrocardiogram, particularly when the wire is passed (unnecessarily) more than half its length into the patient. Resistance to passing the wire is almost never encountered during right internal jugular cannulation and, if present, is usually a sign that the wire has passed outside the vein.

After the wire has been successfully placed and the initial intravenous cannula removed (Fig. 15–9), incise the skin (parallel to the Langer lines on the skin) at the site of skin puncture to ease the passage of the 6-inch (for right internal jugular approach) central venous cannula (Fig. 15–10). Some specialty trays include a rigid plastic dilator (to be passed over the guide wire at this point), which aids in inserting the jugular catheter through skin and fascia.

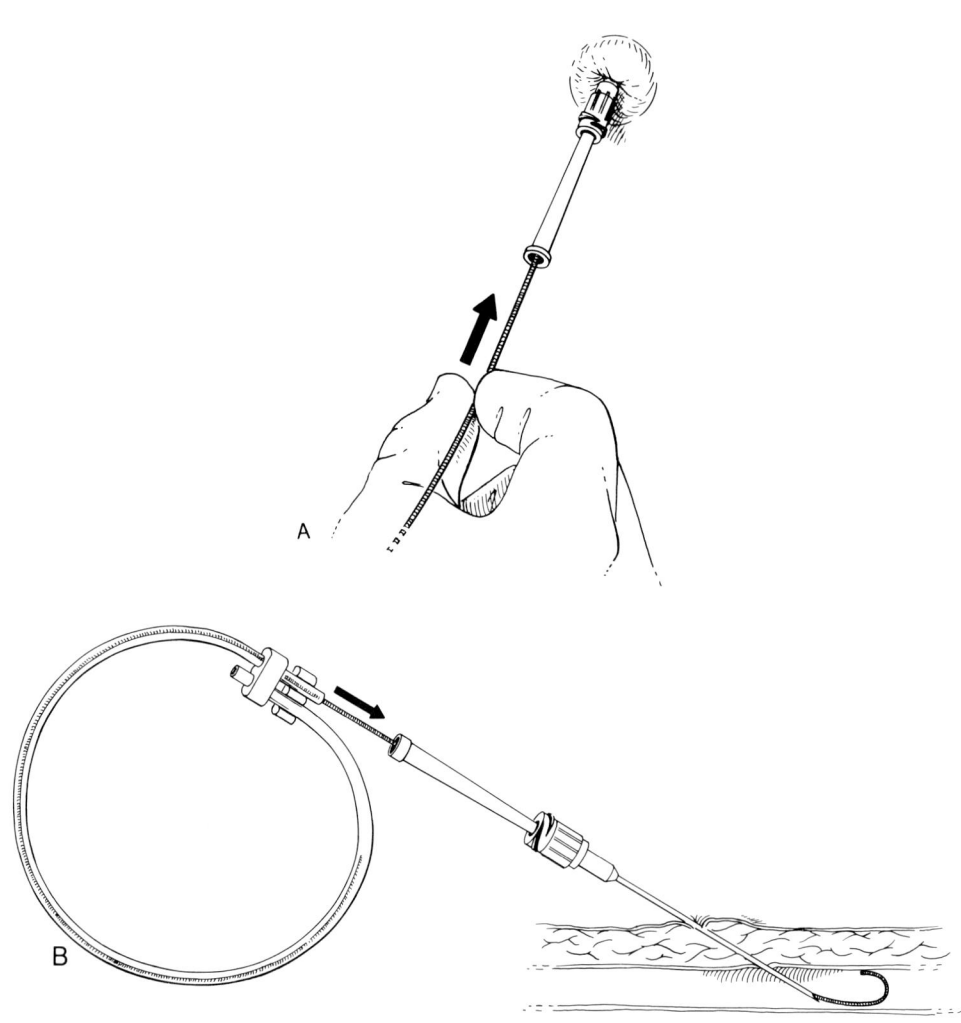

FIGURE 15–8

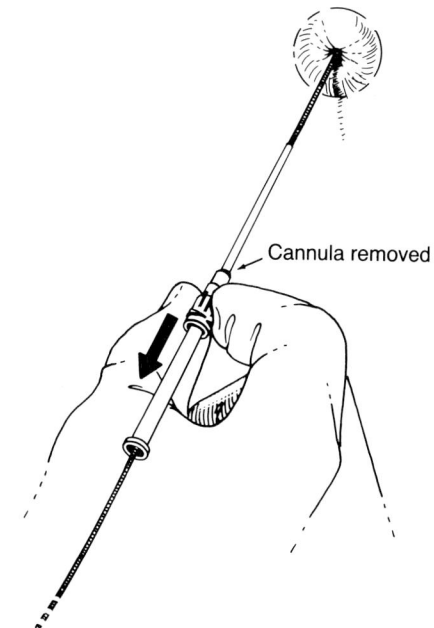

FIGURE 15–9

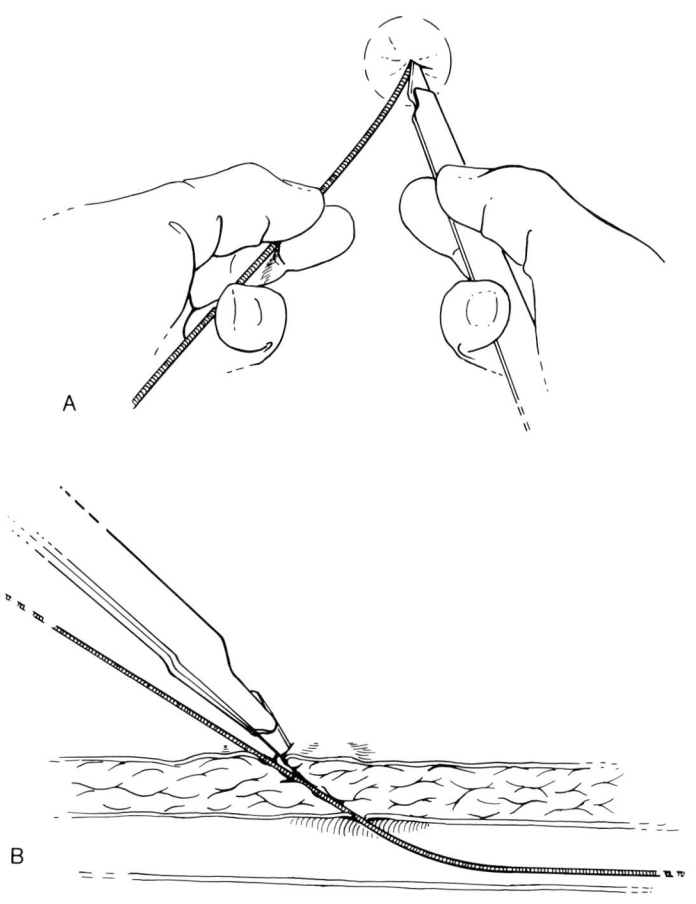

FIGURE 15–10

INSERTION OF CENTRAL VENOUS CANNULA

Advance the central venous cannula over the guide wire into the patient; then withdraw the guide wire and aspirate all air (Fig. 15–11). Connect the cannula to a transducer or to an intravenous infusion set. I favor sewing the cannula in place with a single 3-0 nylon stitch (Fig. 15–12).

Confirm with a chest radiograph that the cannula tip is located in the thoracic venous system and more than 1 cm from the cavoatrial junction. Examine the peripheral lung fields carefully for subtle signs of pneumothorax.

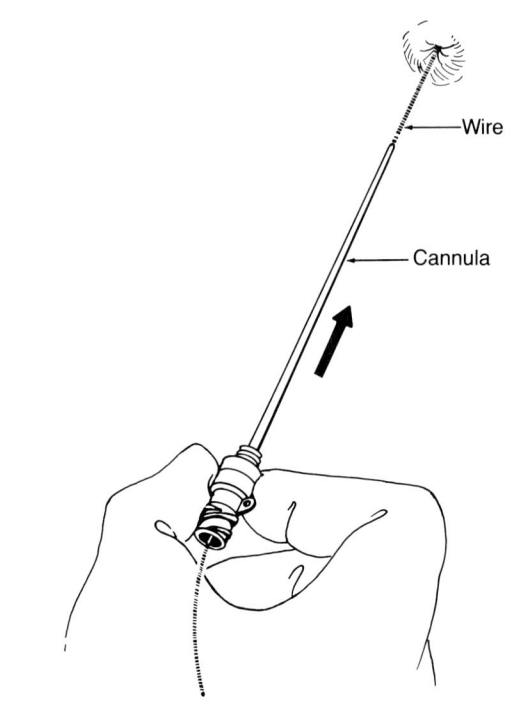

FIGURE 15–11

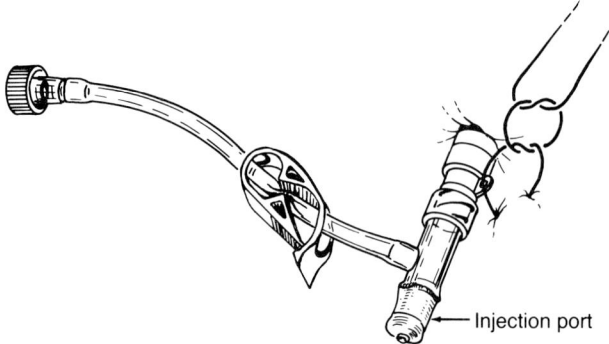

FIGURE 15–12

External Jugular Vein Cannulation

Central venous cannulation through the external jugular remained unpredictable and unpopular until J-wires were introduced. With the use of a J-wire, success rates of more than 90% have been reported for placement of central venous cannulae through the external jugular veins. The technique and equipment I use are very similar to those used for internal jugular vein cannulation; therefore, only the important differences between the two approaches will be highlighted in this section.

The external jugular veins are nearly always visible when a patient is placed in the head-down position. The veins run from medial to lateral, cross the lateral border of the sternocleidomastoid muscles, and then dive deep to reach the brachiocephalic veins on each side.

PREPARATION AND POSITIONING

Attach the electrocardiographic leads, blood pressure cuff, and pulse oximeter probe for monitoring during the procedure. Position the patient supine with the head turned to the side opposite the intended site of cannulation (Fig. 15–13).

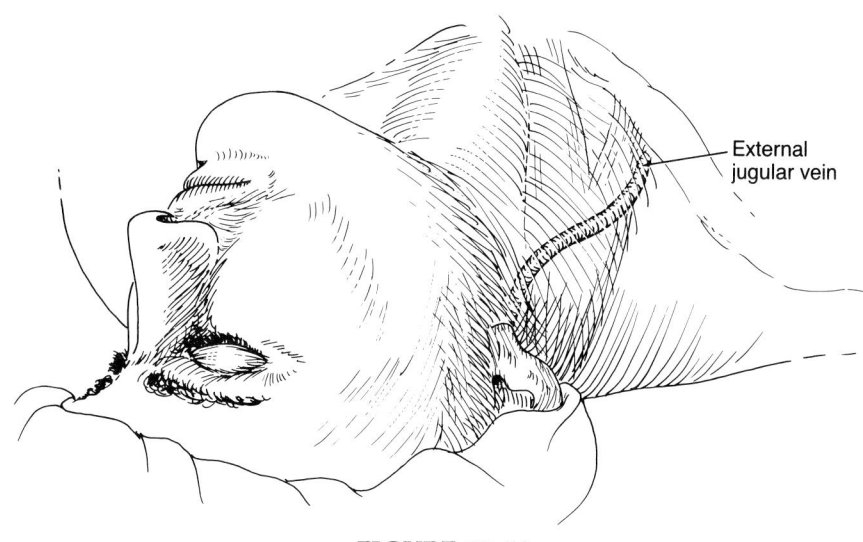

FIGURE 15–13

LOCATION OF EXTERNAL JUGULAR VEIN

After cleansing and anesthetizing the overlying skin, enter the vein with an 18-gauge (or 16-gauge) intravenous cannula (Fig. 15–14). A common mistake is to accidentally advance the needle and cannula straight through the front and back walls of the vein. I recommend advancing the cannula and needle carefully through the skin as an initial step, and only then carefully (and deliberately) cannulating the external jugular vein.

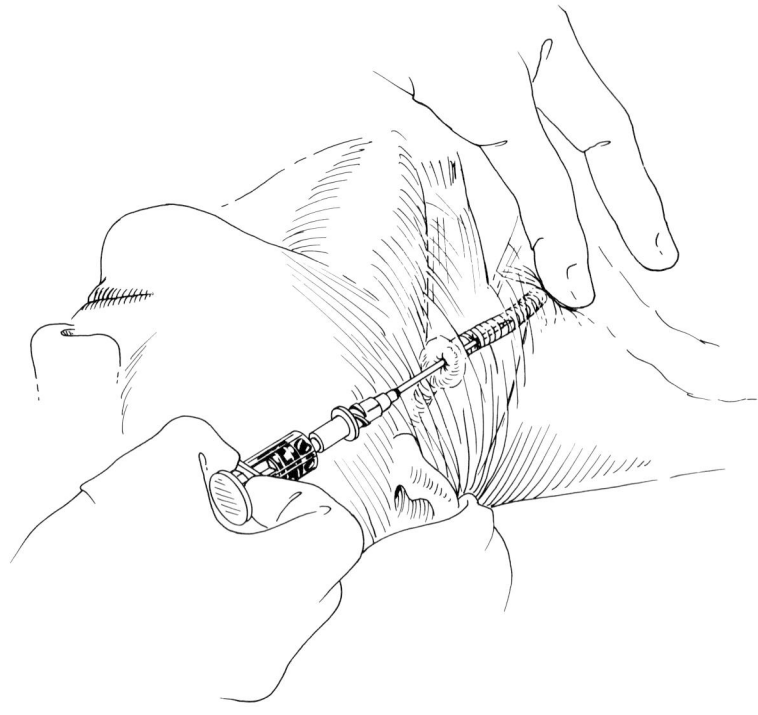

FIGURE 15-14

CANNULATION OF EXTERNAL JUGULAR VEIN

Slide the cannula off the needle into the vein (Fig. 15–15). Remove the needle, and pass the J-wire through the intravenous cannula down through the external jugular vein into the brachiocephalic vein (Fig. 15–16). Sometimes difficulty is encountered in passing the J-wire within the external jugular vein under the clavicle into the

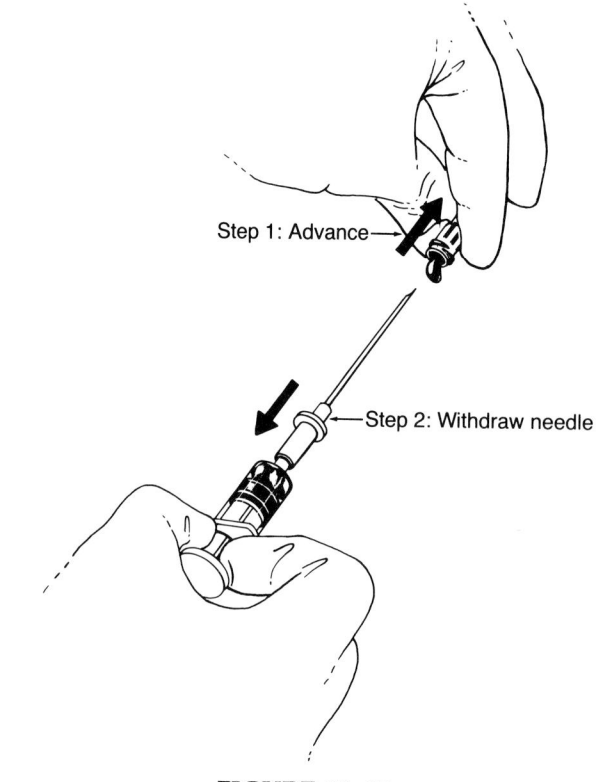

FIGURE 15-15

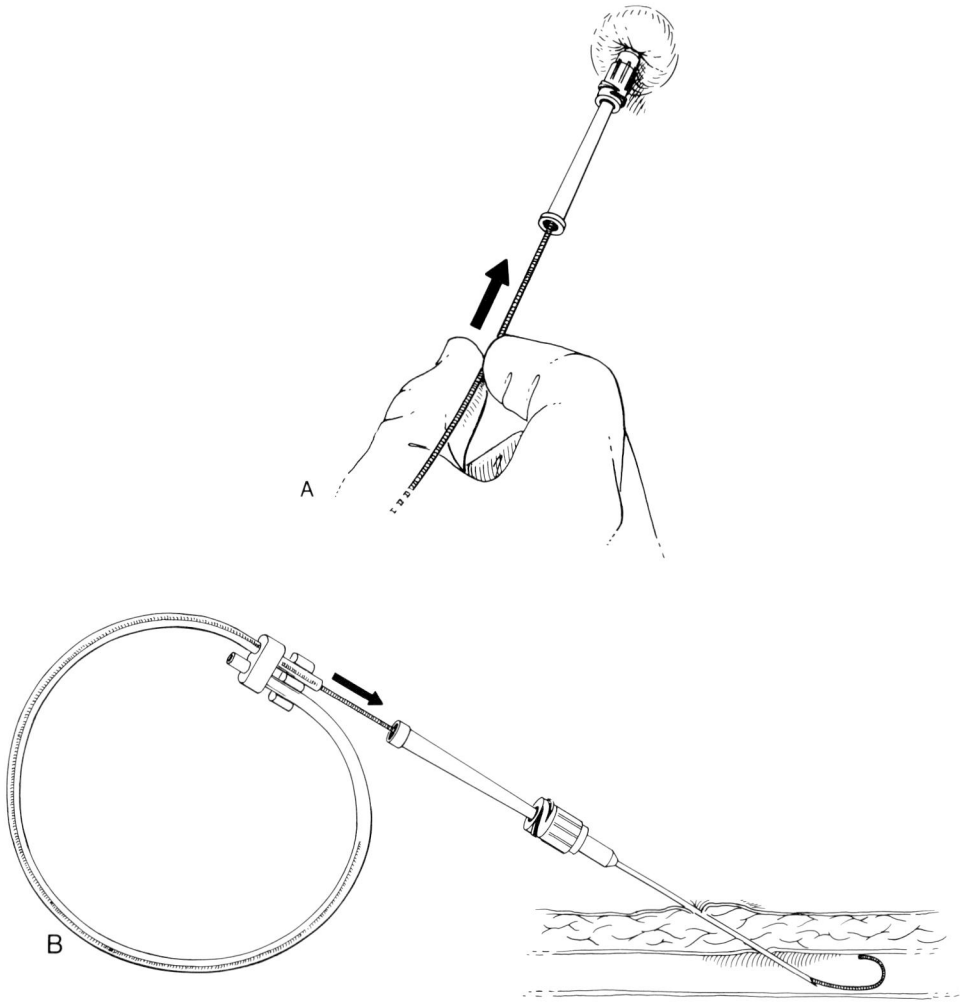

FIGURE 15–16

brachiocephalic vein. I have found that I can usually bypass this "obstruction" by slowly rotating the wire as I attempt to advance it. Sometimes it is necessary to have an assistant pull down on the patient's ipsilateral arm (or to have the patient reach for the ipsilateral knee), lowering the clavicle and thus permitting the wire to advance beyond the external jugular vein.

With the J-wire in place, remove the short venous cannula (Fig. 15–17). A skin nick is usually unnecessary. Most often, the central venous cannula will pass easily over the wire into the superior vena cava (Fig. 15–18).

After all air is aspirated from the cannula, connect it to an intravenous infusion or transducer tubing and suture it to the skin with 3-0 nylon (Fig. 15–19). Confirm the position of the cannula with a chest radiograph as soon as is practical.

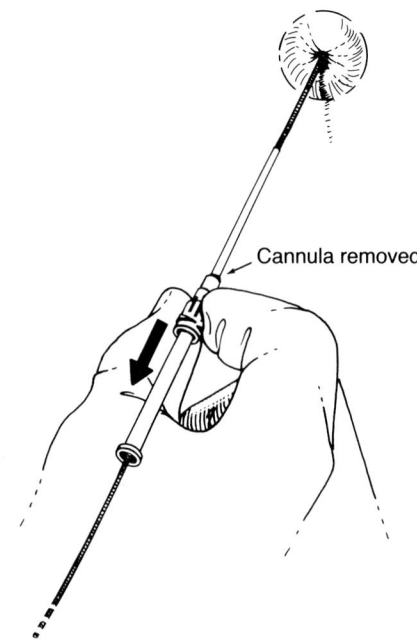

FIGURE 15–17

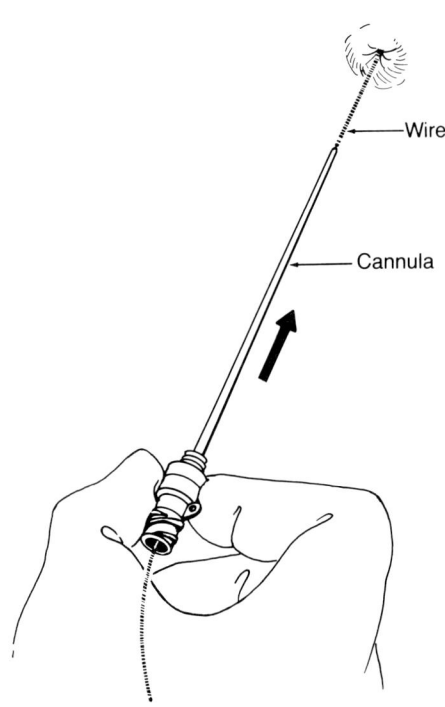

FIGURE 15–18

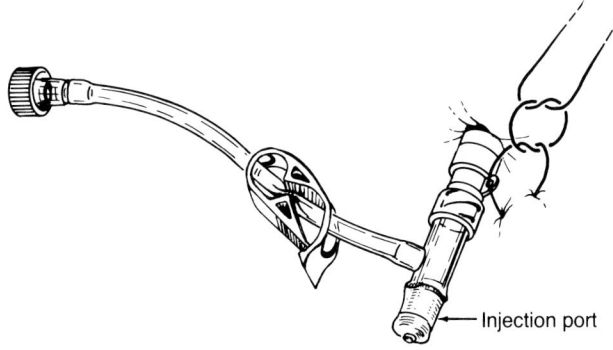

FIGURE 15-19

Subclavian Vein Cannulation

The subclavian vein should be cannulated in preference to other central venous sites whenever a central venous cannula will be required for more than 48 hours, for example, when total parenteral nutrition is administered. Subclavian cannula sites are easier to dress and the cannulae are easier to maintain in sterile condition and are more comfortable for awake patients than jugular venous cannulae. During cardiopulmonary resuscitation, one can more quickly place a cannula in the central circulation with a subclavian approach than with any other. Unfortunately, the risk of pneumothorax is also higher with the subclavian approach than with any other central venous cannulation approach.

EQUIPMENT NEEDED

Sterile gloves
Antiseptic solution
Intravenous infusion set
Central venous cannula tray (2-ml syringe, 25-gauge needle, 1% lidocaine, 22-gauge needle, 5-ml syringe, J-wire, central venous cannula of appropriate length, 3-0 nonabsorbable suture on a cutting needle) to which may be added a 14-gauge Intracath needle with its 16-gauge cannula, if the cannula-through-needle approach will be used
Means for placing patient in Trendelenburg position (e.g., "shock blocks")
Usual monitoring devices
Resuscitation drugs and equipment

PREPARATION AND POSITIONING

Attach the electrocardiographic leads, blood pressure cuff, and pulse oximeter probe for monitoring during the procedure. Position the patient supine on the operating room table in the head-down (Trendelenburg) position. Place a rolled towel under the patient between his scapulae. Cleanse the skin of the neck and upper chest with antiseptic solution. Place a sterile fenestrated drape (or three folded surgical towels) so that the puncture site and pertinent landmarks (clavicle and sternal notch) are clearly visible.

CANNULATION OF SUBCLAVIAN VEIN

Inject 1% lidocaine in the skin and underlying tissue immediately caudad to the clavicle, at the junction between the outer and middle thirds of the clavicle.

Opinion is divided as to whether a "cannula-through-needle" or a Seldinger technique using a guide wire works best for subclavian venipuncture. The former technique is particularly well suited for subclavian venipuncture owing to the difficulty sometimes encountered (when using a Seldinger technique) in persuading cannulae to negotiate their way underneath the clavicle and into the subclavian vein without kinking the guide wire.

Cannula-Through-Needle-Technique

Using the cannula-through-needle approach, advance the 14-gauge thin wall (Fig. 15–20) (e.g., Intracath) needle (with syringe attached) through the skin wheal and beneath the clavicle, aiming the needle medial, dorsal, and cranial toward the suprasternal notch. Maintain negative pressure on the syringe so that you will know when it enters the vein. A "pop" can usually be felt as the needle tip enters the subclavian vein.

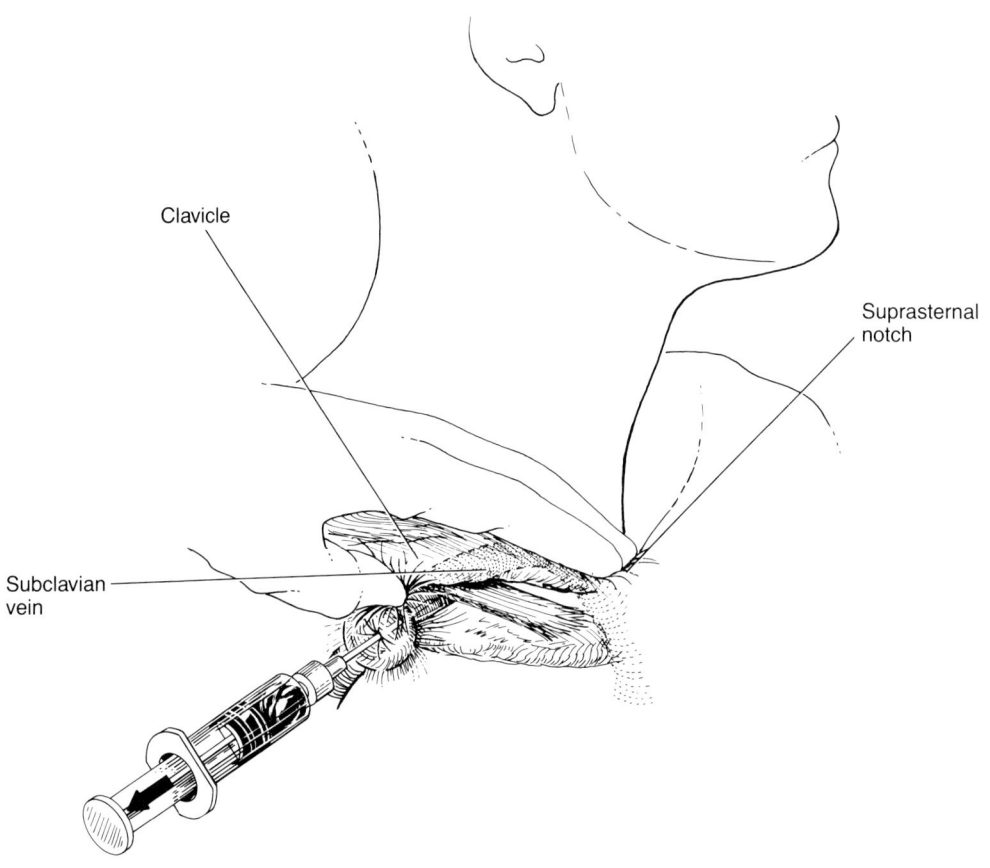

FIGURE 15–20

Remove the syringe from the needle and replace it with a gloved finger tip (to prevent both aspiration of air and excessive loss of blood). Pass the cannula through and at least 5 cm beyond the needle tip (Fig. 15–21). Withdraw the needle over the cannula while the cannula is held in place (Fig. 15–22). Some cannulae permit the complete removal of the 14-gauge needle; others allow the needle to be withdrawn back to the hub and require that a plastic adapter (level cover) be snapped over the needle to prevent it from shearing off the cannula (Fig. 15–23). Remove the guide wire (if one is present), aspirate all air from the cannula, and attach the cannula to an intravenous infusion.

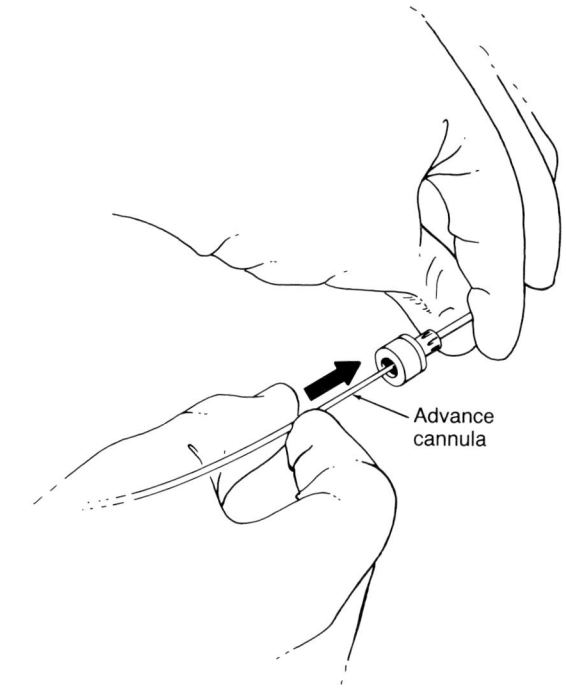

FIGURE 15–21

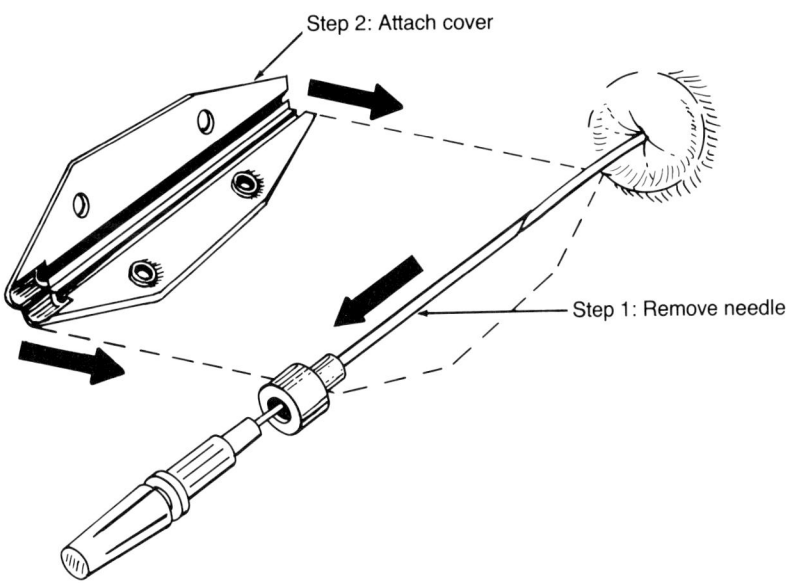

FIGURE 15–22

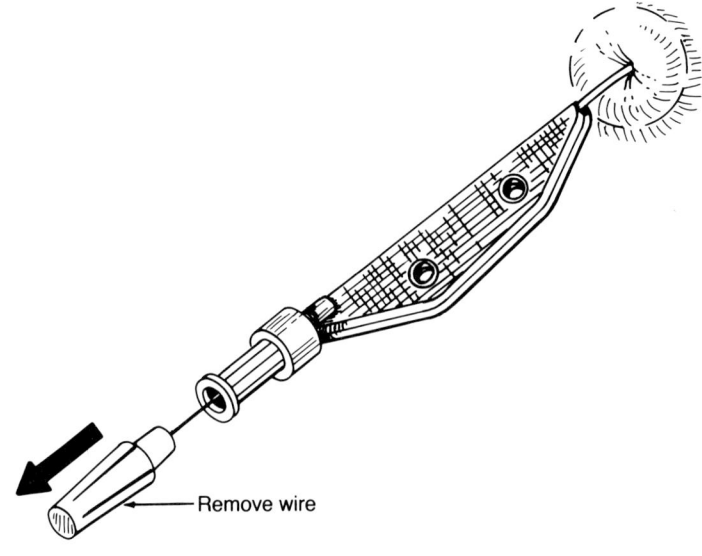

FIGURE 15–23

Seldinger Technique

Alternatively, one may use a Seldinger technique. Place an 18-gauge (or 16-gauge) intravenous cannula in the subclavian vein using an identical approach to that described earlier for the "cannula-through-needle" technique. Next, thread a J-wire through the cannula and remove the cannula over the J-wire. Incise the skin at the puncture site, and pass the central venous cannula over the wire and into the patient. Finally, remove the wire, leaving the central venous cannula in place.

Following either approach, suture the subclavian cannula to the skin with 3-0 nylon. Obtain a chest radiograph as soon as practical to confirm that the cannula is located in a central vein and not in the heart, axillary or jugular veins, or inferior vena cava, and to be sure that there is no pneumothorax.

Basilic Vein Cannulation

Central venous cannulation through the basilic vein has the advantage over the internal jugular and subclavian approaches of carrying a negligible risk of carotid artery puncture or pneumothorax. Unfortunately, cannulae inserted from the basilic vein do not as reliably enter the central venous circulation as those inserted from the external jugular, internal jugular vein, or subclavian veins. Moreover, the position of a successfully placed cannula tip within the thoracic cavity will change when the patient moves his arm. Nonetheless, in craniotomies (in which there may be a desire to avoid inserting cannulae where they might impede venous drainage of the brain) or in anticoagulated patients (in which the risk of accidental carotid or subclavian artery puncture may carry a greater risk than in the usual patient) basilic vein cannulation has a role.

Long cannulae are threaded far more easily into central circulation from the basilic than from the cephalic veins in the antecubital fossa. Thus, one must use the most medial vein in the antecubital fossa that appears large enough to permit cannulation.

EQUIPMENT NEEDED

Sterile gloves
Antiseptic solution
Intravenous infusion
3-ml syringe
25-gauge needle
Lidocaine 1%
24-inch central venous cannula with *external* introducing needle
Adhesive tape
Tincture of benzoin
Usual monitoring devices
Resuscitation drugs and equipment

PREPARATION AND POSITIONING

Attach electrocardiographic leads, blood pressure cuff (on the opposite arm), and pulse oximeter probe for monitoring during procedure. Position the patient supine on the operating room table. Place a venous tourniquet around the upper arm. Cleanse the antecubital fossa on the side of intended cannulation with antiseptic solution.

IDENTIFICATION OF BASILIC VEIN

Identify the basilic vein on the medial side of the antecubital fossa and distinguish it from the cephalic vein on the lateral side of the antecubital fossa. Anesthetize the skin overlying the basilic vein with 1% lidocaine. Enter the vein with the large (usually 14-gauge or 16-gauge) needle packaged with the central venous cannula (Fig. 15–24). Be careful not to advance the needle through the back wall of the vein.

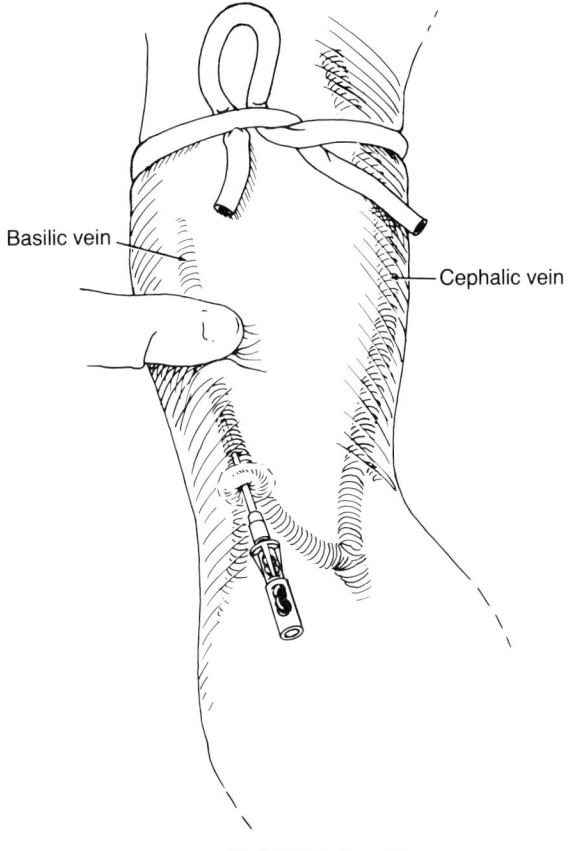

FIGURE 15–24

CANNULA-THROUGH-NEEDLE TECHNIQUE

Once the larger needle has entered the vein, release the tourniquet and thread the long (24-inch) cannula through the needle into the basilic vein, up the arm, and into the thoracic venous system (Fig. 15–25). Withdraw the larger needle over the cannula and remove the wire stylet (Figs. 15–26 and 15–27). By laying the stylet along the arm, along the course of the cannula within the patient, one can estimate the position of the cannula within the thoracic venous system.

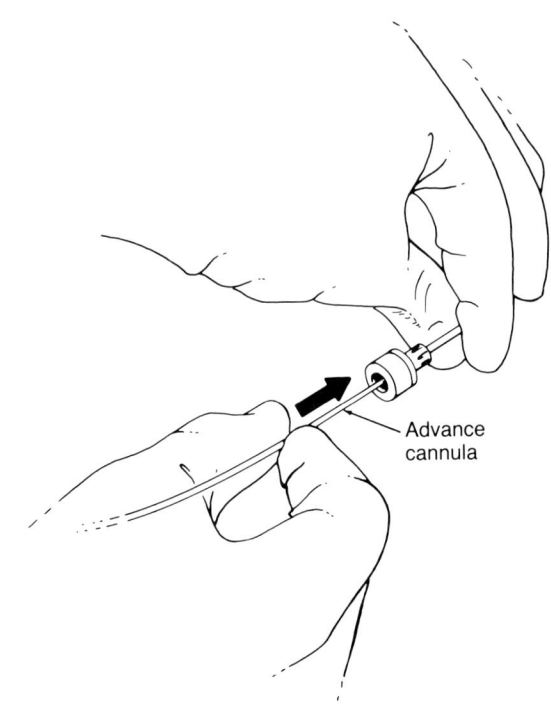

FIGURE 15–25

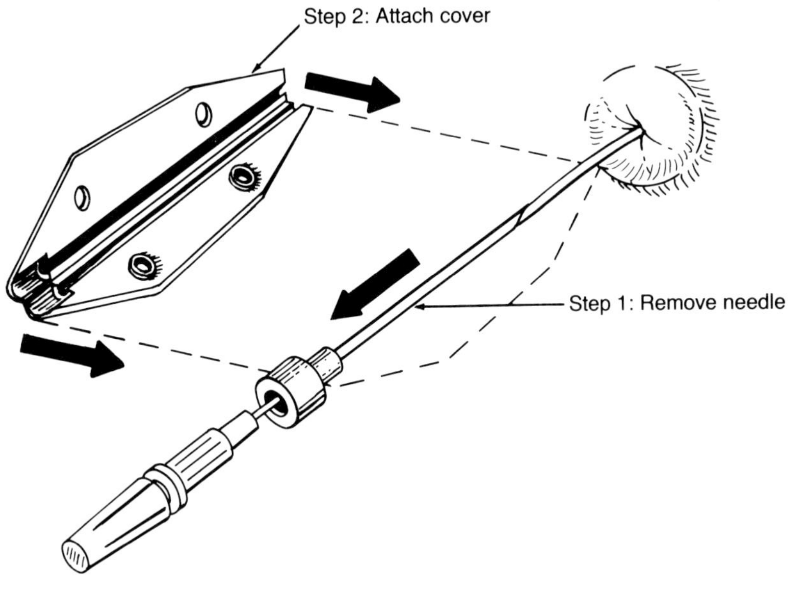

FIGURE 15–26

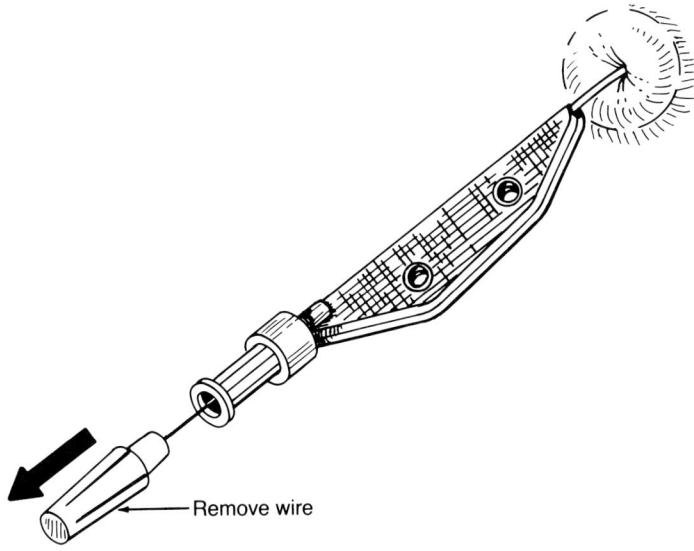

FIGURE 15–27

Remove all air from the cannula before connecting it to an intravenous infusion or to transducer tubing. Apply a sterile dressing to the puncture site and secure the cannula to the skin with tincture of benzoin and adhesive tape.

Obtain a chest radiograph to determine the location of the tip of the cannula. Long cannulae inserted from the arm do not always find their way into an appropriate part of the central circulation. I have seen them pass into ipsilateral and contralateral jugular veins, right ventricle, contralateral axillary vein, and even back out the ipsilateral basilic vein after coiling within the subclavian vein.

Femoral Vein Cannulation

Although femoral veins are commonly used during diagnostic right heart catheterization, particularly when the femoral artery is used for diagnostic left heart catheterization, cannulation of femoral veins is less commonly performed during surgery and anesthesia in adults. Primary concerns include the risks of deep vein thrombus and cannula-related sepsis and, in trauma patients, the possibility of traumatic injuries to the abdominal venous system. I often use femoral vein cannulation during major surgery in infants and children but rarely insert the line into the thoracic venous system.

EQUIPMENT NEEDED

Sterile gloves
Antiseptic solution
Intravenous infusion
Central venous cannula tray (2-ml syringe, 25-gauge needle, 1% lidocaine, 22-gauge needle, 5-ml syringe, 18-gauge or 20-gauge intravenous cannula, J-wire, central venous cannula of appropriate length, 3-0 nonabsorbable suture on a cutting needle)
Usual monitoring devices
Resuscitation drugs and equipment

PREPARATION AND POSITIONING

Position the patient supine on the operating room table. Cleanse the skin on the lower abdomen and upper thigh on the side of intended venous cannulation with antiseptic solution (Fig. 15–28). Inject 1% lidocaine into the skin 1 cm medial to the femoral pulse and 1 cm distal to the inguinal ligament.

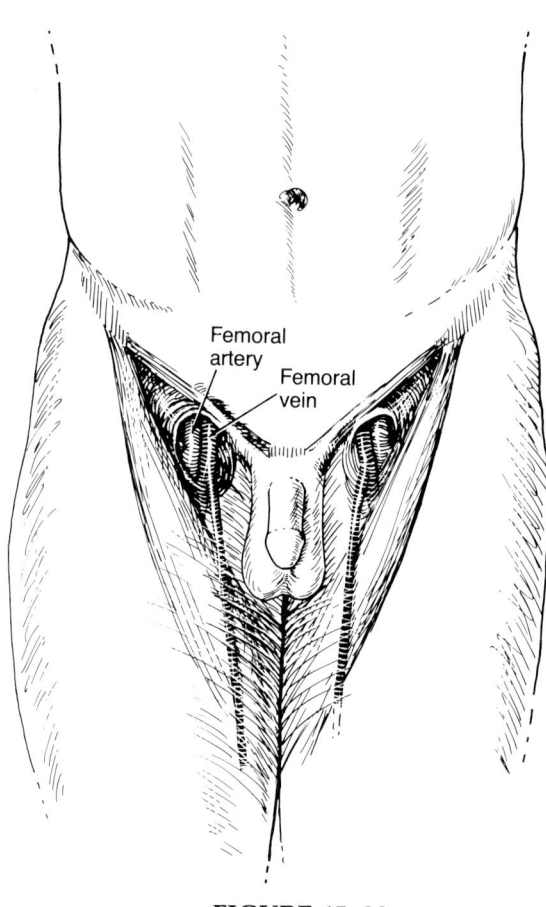

FIGURE 15–28

CANNULATION OF FEMORAL VEIN

Advance the 18-gauge (or 20-gauge in children) intravenous cannula through the skin wheal until dark venous blood is aspirated into the syringe (Fig. 15–29). As soon as the vein is entered, slide the cannula off the needle and into the vein. Remove the needle. (During periods when the hub of the venous cannula is exposed to air, it is wise to cover the hub with your gloved thumb to avoid air entrainment and subsequent air embolism.) Reattach the syringe to the cannula. If free flow of *venous* blood is obtained, remove the syringe and pass the J-wire through the short cannula up the femoral vein into the external iliac vein (Fig. 15–30). Remove the short cannula (Fig. 15–31), and incise the skin with the scalpel (Fig. 15–32). Pass the longer, 14-gauge to 20-gauge central cannula over the wire into the femoral and external iliac vein (Fig. 15–33). Remove the wire and connect the cannula (after all air has been aspirated from it) to an intravenous infusion or transducer tubing (Fig. 15–34). Secure the central cannula to the skin with one or two 3-0 nylon sutures.

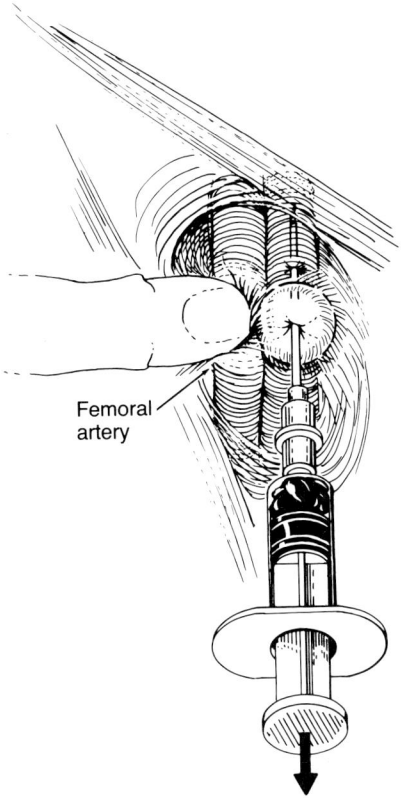

FIGURE 15–29

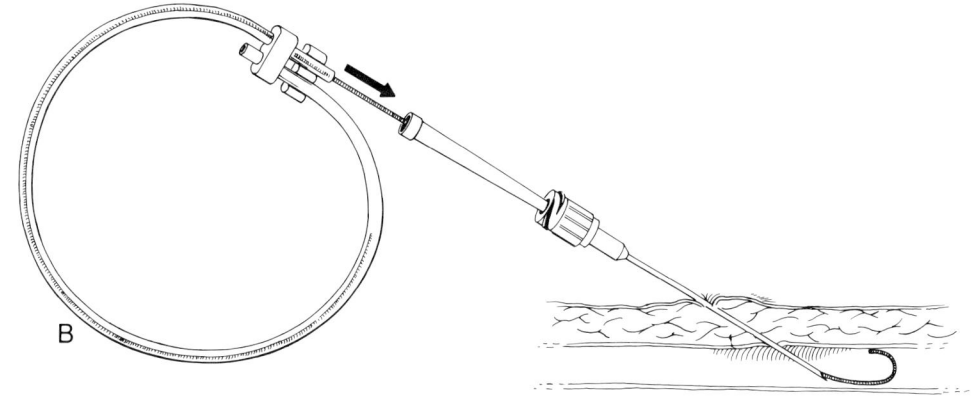

FIGURE 15–30

In children, I normally perform femoral venous cannulation after induction of general anesthesia. The insertion site is closer to the femoral pulse and inguinal ligament than in adults, and I normally use smaller diameter (infants, 20 gauge; small children, 18 gauge) and shorter central venous cannulae.

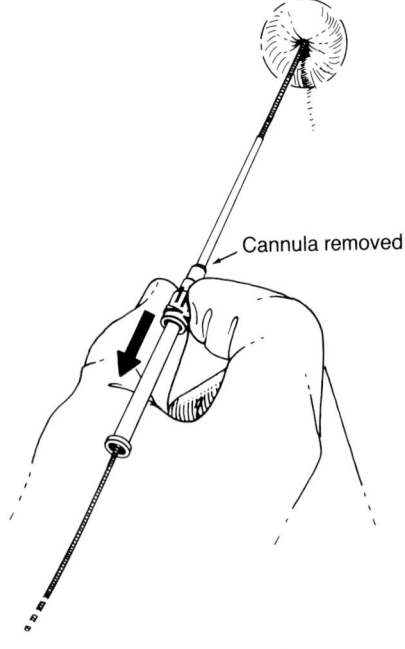

FIGURE 15–31

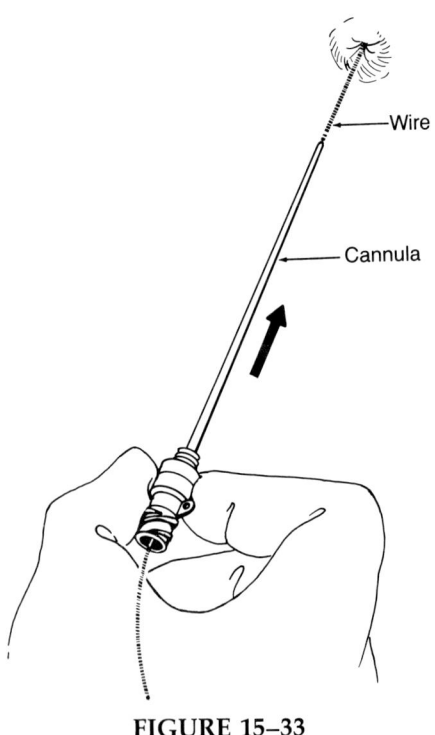

FIGURE 15–33

FIGURE 15–32

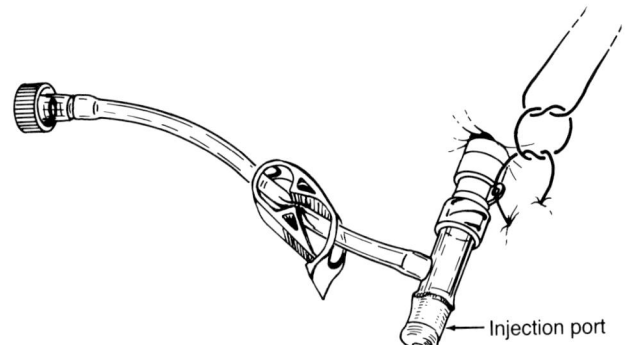

FIGURE 15–34

References

GENERAL

Burri C, Ahnefeld FW: The Caval Catheter. Berlin, Springer-Verlag, 1978

Heavner JE, Flindes C, McMahon DJ, Bernigan T, Badgwell JM: Technical Manual of Anesthesiology, pp 57–67. New York, Raven Press, 1989

Risk C, Rudo N, Fulltrich, Otto CW: Central venous pressure monitoring. In Blitt CD (ed): Monitoring in Anesthesia and Critical Care Medicine, pp 121–165. New York, Churchill Livingstone, 1985

Seldinger SI: Catheter replacement of needle in percutaneous arteriography: A new technique. Acta Radiol 39:368–376, 1953

INTERNAL JUGULAR VEIN CANNULATION

Daily PO, Griepp RB, Shumway NE: Percutaneous internal jugular vein cannulation. Arch Surg 101:534–536, 1970

Jernigan WR, Gardner WC, Mahr NN, Milburn JL: Use of the internal jugular vein for placement of central venous catheter. Surg Gynecol Obstet 130:520–524, 1970

Metz S, Horrow JC, Balcar I: A controlled comparison of techniques for locating the internal jugular vein using ultrasonography. Anesth Analg 63:673–679, 1984

Oda M, Fukushima Y, Hirota T, Tanaka A, Aono M, Sato T: The paracarotid approach for internal jugular vein catheterization. Anaesthesia 36:896–900, 1981

EXTERNAL JUGULAR VEIN CANNULATION

Blitt CD, Carlson GL, Wright WA, Otto CW: J-wire versus straight wire for central venous system cannulation via the external jugular vein. Anesth Analg 61:536–537, 1982

Blitt CD, Wright WA, Petty WC, Webster TA: Central venous cannulation via the external jugular vein: A technique employing the J-wire. JAMA 229:817–818, 1974

Gravenstein JS, Paulus DA: Clinical Monitoring Practice, 2nd ed, pp 122–123. Philadelphia, JB Lippincott, 1987

SUBCLAVIAN VEIN CANNULATION

Borja AR: Current status of infraclavicular subclavian vein catheterization. Ann Thorac Surg 13:615–624, 1972

Linus DA, Mucha P Jr, van Heerden JA: Subclavian vein: A golden route. Mayo Clin Proc 55:315–321, 1980

BASILIC VEIN CANNULATION

Kellner GA, Smart JF: Percutaneous placement of catheters to monitor "central venous pressure." Anesthesiology 36:515–516, 1972

Webre DR, Arens JF: Use of cephalic and basilic veins for introduction of central venous catheters. Anesthesiology 38:389–392, 1973

FEMORAL VEIN CANNULATION

Burri C, Ahnefeld FW: The Caval Catheter, p 30. Berlin, Springer-Verlag, 1978

Hohn AR, Lamert EC: Continuous venous catheterization in children. JAMA 197:658–660, 1966

16

Intravascular Electrocardiography

It is often useful to accurately position the tip of a central venous cannula during anesthesia and surgery. For example, the distal tips of both ventriculoatrial shunts inserted for treatment of hydrocephalus and central venous cannulae inserted for aspiration of venous air emboli need to be positioned near the junction of the right atrium and superior vena cava. In both of these circumstances, intravascular electrocardiography can be helpful. The technique relies on the characteristic electrocardiographic waveforms that may be obtained as the cannula tip moves within the thoracic venous system.

Technique

EQUIPMENT NEEDED

Central venous cannula supplies (see Chapter 15)
22-gauge or smaller spinal needle
Electrocardiographic wire lead with alligator clip
Electrocardiographic monitor
3% saline solution
Usual monitoring devices
Resuscitation drugs and equipment

PREPARATIONS

I usually disconnect the electrocardiographic monitor from wall current (allowing the monitor to run on battery power), hoping to reduce the risk of microshock injury (but recognize that this may be an unnecessary precaution). Fill the cannula to be monitored with a saline solution (I prefer 3% saline over 0.9% saline for the former's superior conductivity) and place the cannula in the superior vena cava (see Chapter 15). Make sure that there is a rubber injection port on the proximal end of the central venous cannula.

Insert a sterile spinal needle with its stylet in place through the rubber injection port. Connect the cannula to the electrocardiographic monitor by attaching a sterile alligator clip to the spinal needle. Recording from the caval cannula may substitute for either the left arm or the precordial (V) lead (Fig. 16–1). Place the remaining

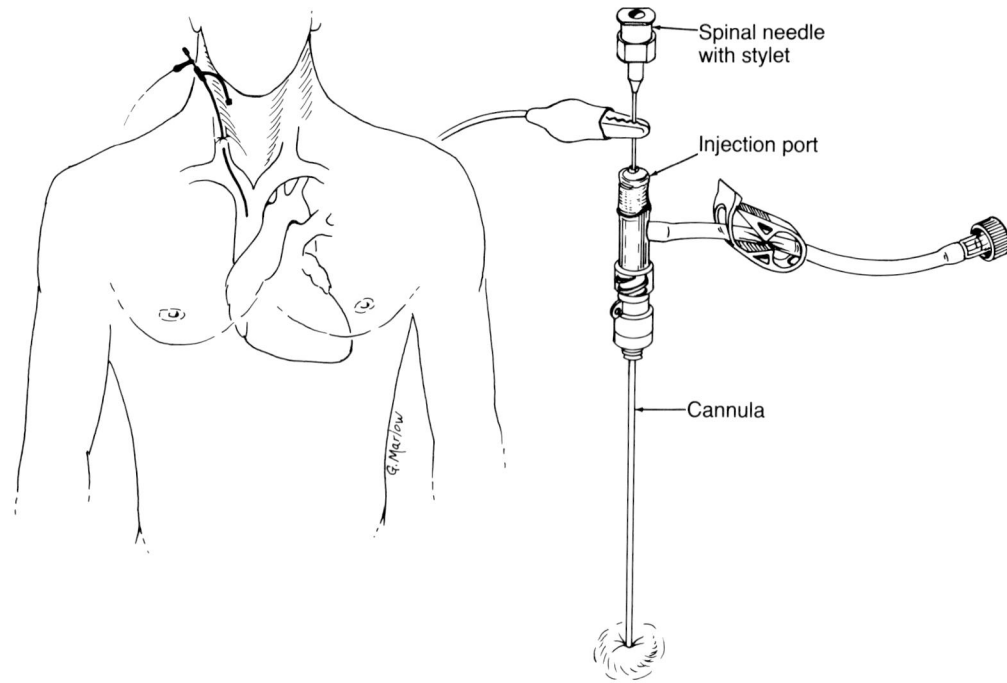

FIGURE 16–1

leads in their customary positions. Display either lead I (if the left arm electrode is used) or the precordial lead (if the precordial electrode is selected) on the electrocardiographic monitor.

ADVANCEMENT OF CANNULA INTO POSITION

With the cannula in the superior vena cava (but relatively far from the heart) P and QRS waves should be down-going (Fig. 16–2). As the cannula advances toward the cavoatrial junction, the P and QRS waves become larger (Fig. 16–3). When the cannula enters the right atrium, the P wave becomes biphasic (Fig. 16–4). As the cannula passes into the right ventricle, the QRS wave changes polarity and becomes larger (Fig. 16–5).

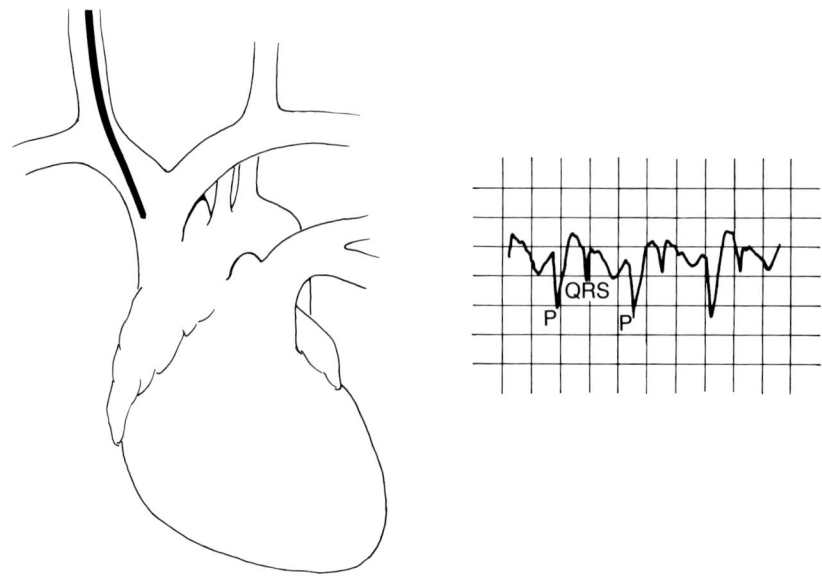

FIGURE 16–2

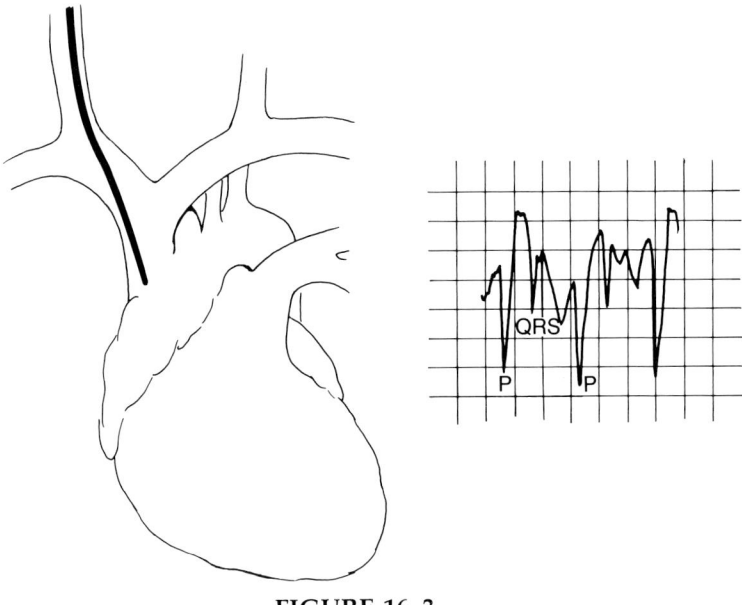

FIGURE 16-3

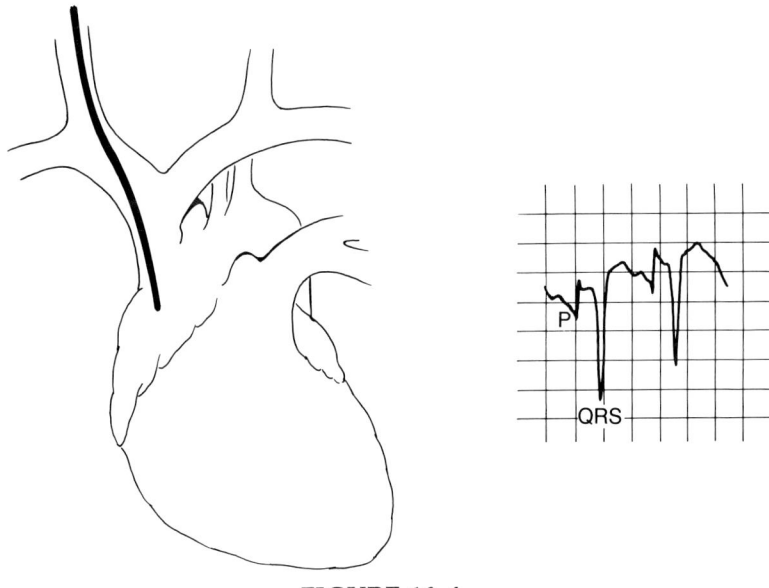

FIGURE 16-4

In the case of ventriculoatrial shunts, positioning the tip near the midpoint of the right atrium offers the maximum capacity for growth before the shunt will need replacement. Moreover, oscillation of the tip within the right atrium may help prevent its occlusion by thrombi. For patients undergoing surgery in the sitting position, the cannula should be positioned so that the P wave is maximally biphasic for optimal aspiration of venous air emboli.

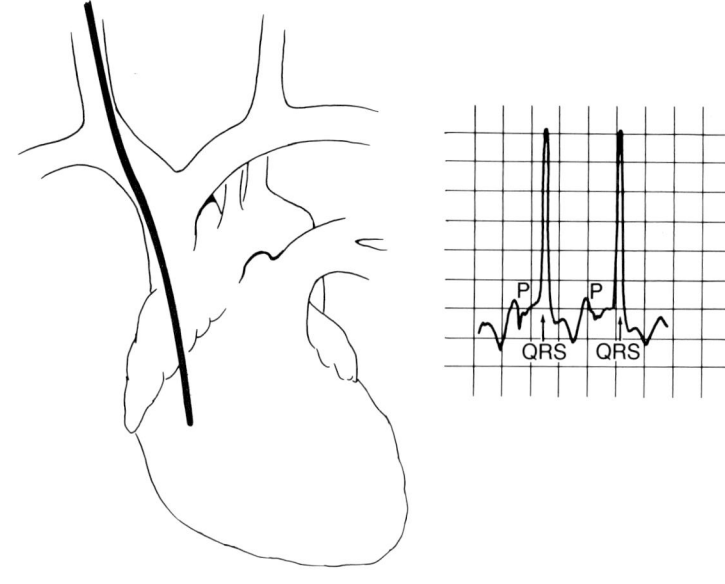

FIGURE 16-5

References

Bunegin L, Albin MS, Helsel PE, Hoffman A, Hung T-K: Positioning the right atrial catheter: A model for reappraisal. Anesthesiology 55:343–348, 1981

Martin JT: Neuroanesthetic adjuncts for patients in the sitting position: III. Intravascular electrocardiography. Anesth Analg 49:793–805, 1970

Michenfelder JD: Central venous catheters in the management of air embolism: Whether as well as where. Anesthesiology 55:339–341, 1981

Robertson JT, Schick RW, Morgan F, Matson DD: Accurate placement of ventriculoatrial shunt for hydrocephalus under electrocardiographic control. J Neurosurg 18:255–257, 1961

17

Pulmonary Artery Catheterization

Although pulmonary artery catheterization is a common monitoring technique used for many elective surgical procedures (e.g., myocardial revascularization and aortic reconstruction), its relative risks and benefits remain the subject of debate. Indeed, a recent editorial in *Chest* entitled "Death by Pulmonary Artery Flow-directed Catheter" suggested a moratorium on pulmonary artery catheterization in the setting of acute myocardial infarction until a well-controlled study can demonstrate improved outcome. Careful consideration should be given as to whether this form of monitoring is truly needed in each individual case. Nonetheless, it seems clear that the information available from the thermodilution pulmonary arterial catheter improves the management of certain high-risk patients.

Indications

Perioperative pulmonary artery catheterization is used to monitor fluid resuscitation and oxygen delivery in major trauma or other critical illness, in patients with cardiac failure (either by history or anticipated) and pulmonary edema of unclear etiology, when intraoperative aortic cross-clamping is anticipated (controversial), and in adult patients undergoing cardiac surgery with cardiopulmonary bypass (controversial).

Risks

The risks of pulmonary artery catheterization include the following:

Arrhythmias
Bleeding and bruising
Misapplication/misinterpretation of data
Carotid puncture (internal jugular approach)
Pneumothorax (subclavian or internal jugular approach)
Cardiac valvular damage
Pulmonary artery infarction or hemorrhage (especially with pulmonary hypertension)
Infection
Thrombosis
Dislodgement of transvenous pacemaker wires
Precipitation of heart block
Knotting of catheter

Insertion Sites

The initial step in pulmonary artery catheterization is the insertion of an introducer/sheath apparatus into an appropriate central venous site (see Chapter 15). Gaining central venous access is more likely to cause an acute complication during pulmonary artery catheterization than any subsequent step of the procedure.

In anesthesia practice, the most commonly used and convenient site for insertion of a pulmonary artery catheter is the right internal jugular vein. The right internal jugular vein lies in a direct line with the superior vena cava, and perhaps for this anatomic reason seems to be the approach from which catheters may be placed expeditiously. Other sites (in order of decreasing preference) include left internal jugular vein, left subclavian vein, right subclavian vein, right or left external jugular vein, right or left basilic vein, and right or left femoral vein. During cardiac surgery, catheters inserted into sites other than the right internal jugular vein have an unfortunate tendency to occlude and malfunction when self-retaining sternal retractors are in place.

Technique

EQUIPMENT NEEDED

Sterile gown and gloves
Antiseptic solution
Sheath introducer tray (5 ml lidocaine 1%, 2 or more syringes, 25-gauge and 22-gauge needles, J-wire, 18-gauge or 16-gauge IV cannula (that permits passage of J-wire))
Pulmonary artery catheter
Transducer/flush assembly for pulmonary artery (distal) channel
Transducer/flush assembly, intravenous infusion, syringe of heparinized saline for (proximal) right atrial (central venous) channel
Intravenous infusion (or syringe of heparinized saline) for right ventricular channel
Injectate coil and 10-ml syringe for cardiac output measurements
Cardiac output computer
Means for placing patient in Trendelenburg position (e.g., "shock blocks")
Usual monitoring devices
Resuscitation drugs and equipment

An assistant is needed during this procedure.

I advocate donning a sterile surgical gown in addition to sterile gloves during the insertion of pulmonary arterial catheters. Gowns are readily available, the cost is low, the time expended in donning a gown is minimal, and the likelihood of contaminating the rather expensive pulmonary artery catheter is reduced.

PASSAGE OF J-WIRE

Attach the electrocardiographic electrodes, blood pressure cuff (and, usually, invasive intra-arterial pressure monitor), and pulse oximeter probe for monitoring during the procedure.

After preparing and draping the insertion site, injecting local anesthetic, and locating the vein of choice with a finder needle, place an intravenous cannula (large enough to permit passage of the J-wire) in a central vein. There should be no question as to whether this cannula is located within the central vein and not, for example, within the carotid artery. Test for proper placement by aspirating blood from the putative central venous cannula and comparing its color to that of an arterial sample (which should be brighter red) drawn concurrently by an assistant. If doubt remains, connect the cannula to a length of intravenous extension tubing, which may be used as a crude manometer to confirm that the blood pressure is less than 20 cm H_2O. Alternatively, send a blood sample from the putative central venous site for blood gas analysis.

Pass a J-wire through the intravenous cannula into the central vein and withdraw the intravenous cannula over the wire. Take care not to lose the J-wire (i.e., by advancing it so far into the patient that it cannot be retrieved). The J-wire never need be advanced more than half its length into the patient.

With the J-wire in place (Fig. 17–1), inject additional local anesthetic and lance the skin with a scalpel to facilitate insertion of the dilator and introducer sheath (Fig. 17–2). When making an incision in the skin of the neck (in particular), direct the blade of the knife parallel to the natural skin folds (Langer lines) so that the patient will not have an unnecessarily large scar.

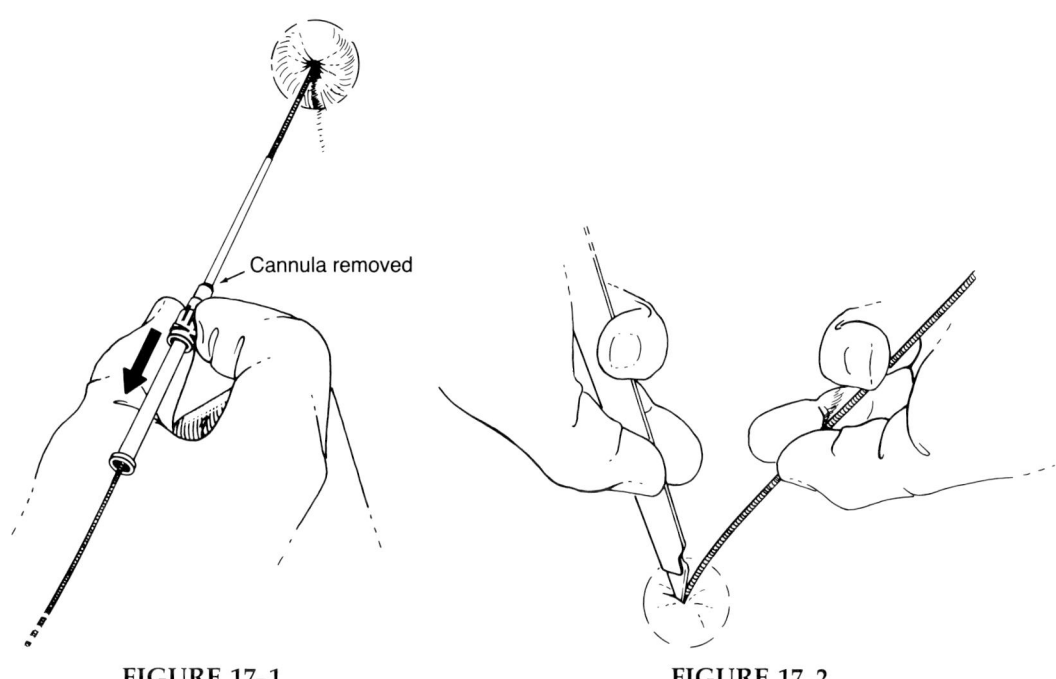

FIGURE 17–1   FIGURE 17–2

INSERTION OF INTRODUCER SHEATH

Insert the dilator through the sheath/introducer (with the side port attached) (Fig. 17–3). This creates a closed system, avoids the possibility of an air embolus during inspiration, and reduces blood loss. Advance the dilator and sheath over the J-wire into the vein (Fig. 17–4). Often the dilator and sheath can be more readily advanced if they are also gently rotated as they are advanced.

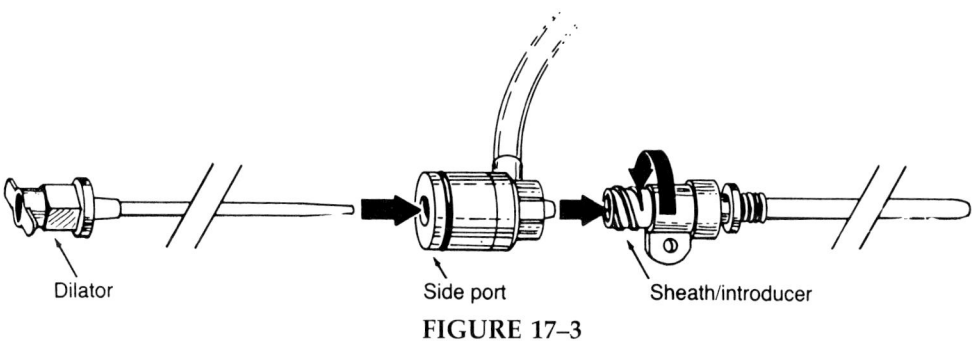

FIGURE 17–3

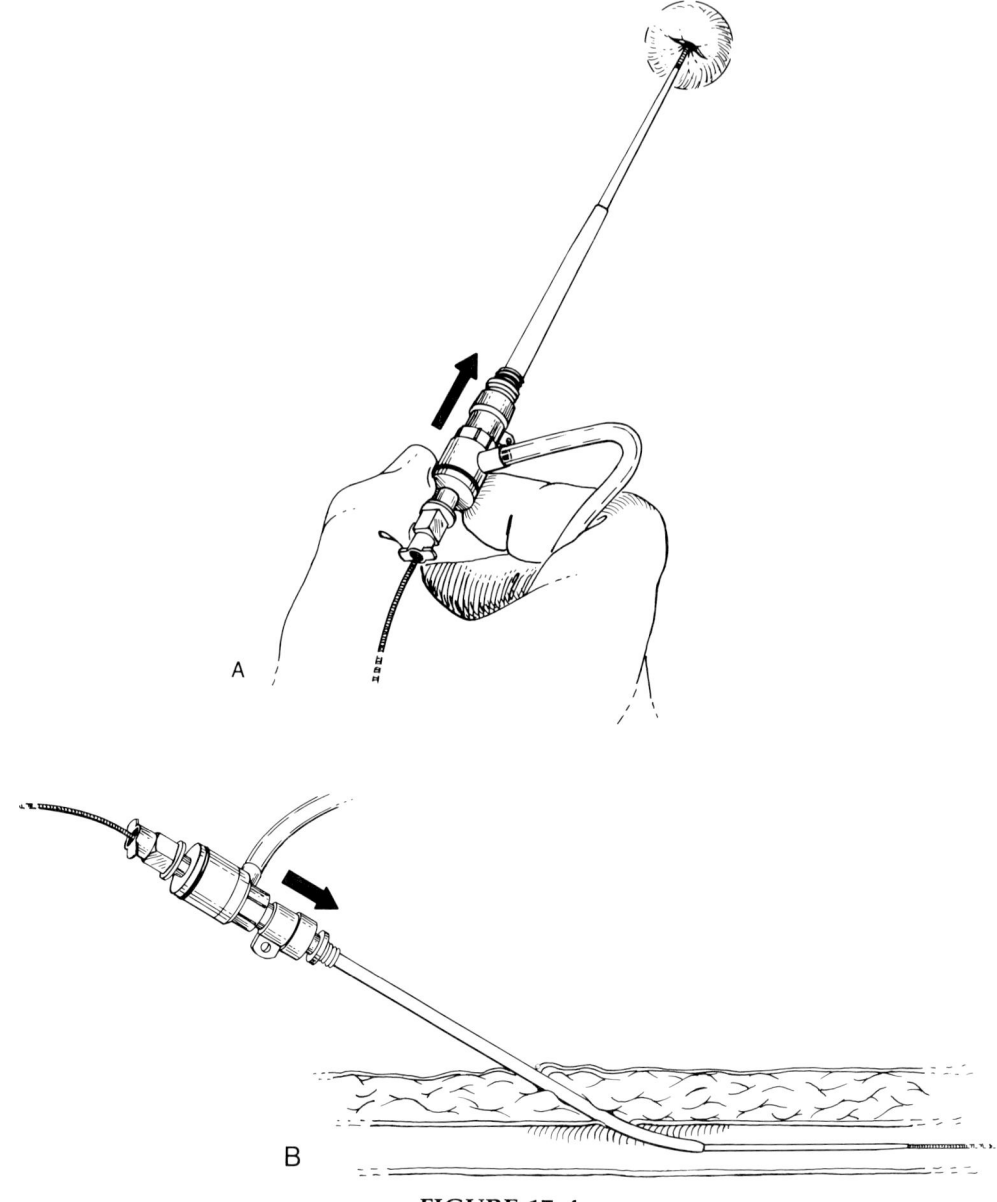

FIGURE 17-4

Occasionally, the skin nick will be insufficiently large to permit advancing the dilator and sheath. When difficulty is encountered, it makes sense not to continue making vain, painful (to the patient and all observers) attempts to advance the dilator and sheath; rather, it is time to enlarge the skin nick. Failure to do so may result in fraying the tip either of the dilator or the sheath, necessitating an additional tray for another sheath/dilator assembly and needlessly tormenting an awake patient.

Once the dilator and sheath have been inserted into the vein, remove the dilator and wire (Fig. 17-5). The side port must be quickly attached to the sheath if this has not been done previously. Hand the side port extension to the assistant (with the syringe attached for aspiration of all air from the sheath and side port), and have the assistant connect it to an appropriate intravenous infusion line (Fig. 17-6). Sew the sheath/side port apparatus to the underlying skin with 3-0 nylon suture.

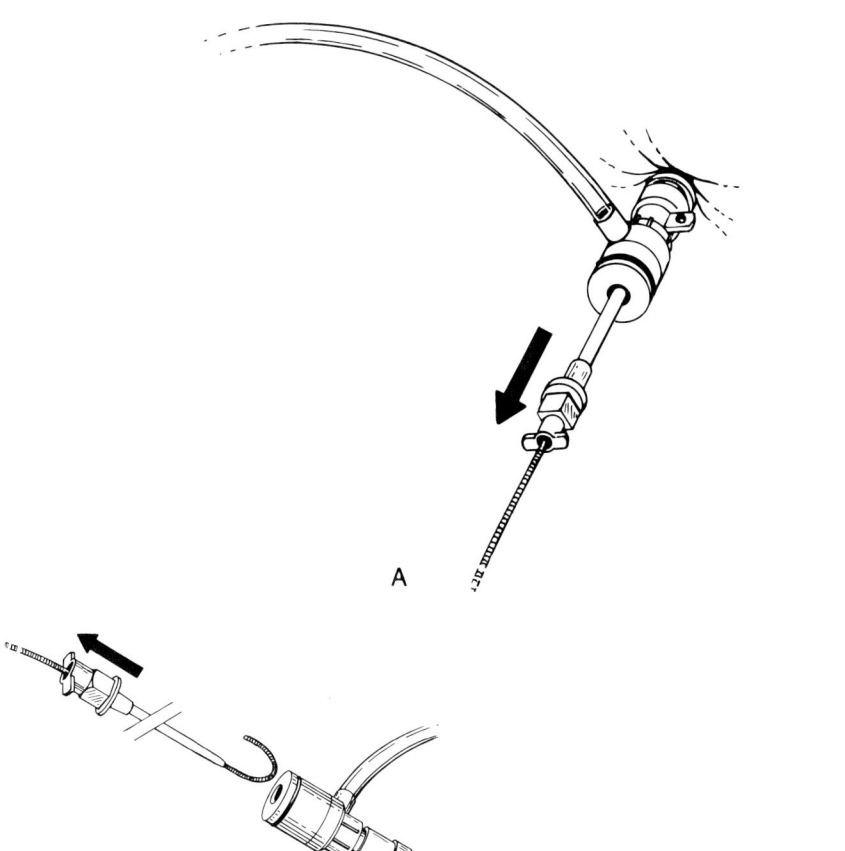

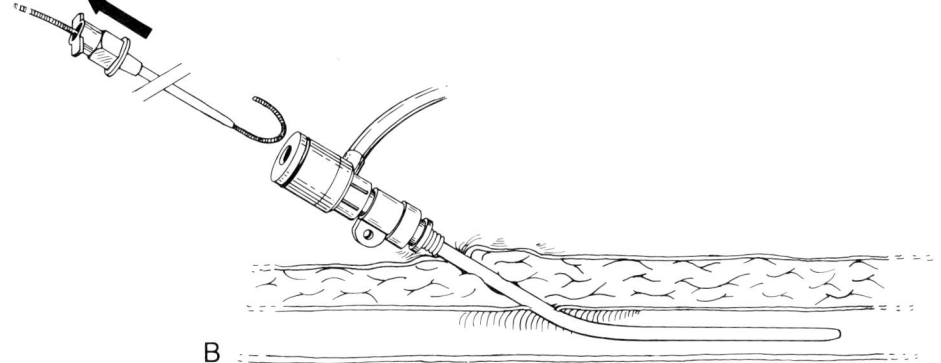

FIGURE 17–5

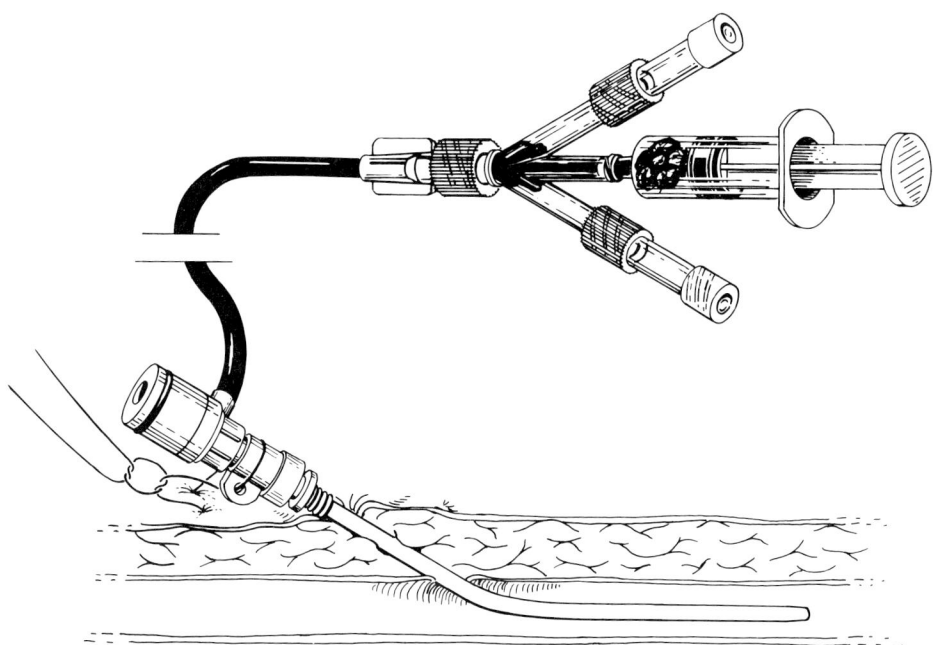

FIGURE 17–6

PREPARATION OF PULMONARY ARTERY CATHETER

Have the assistant uncover the pulmonary artery catheter in a sterile fashion (Fig. 17–7). Hand the proximal ends of the catheter to the assistant to flush all air from the several channels of the catheter. Have the assistant flush the distal pulmonary artery port with heparinized saline and connect it to a functioning, properly "zeroed" and tested transducer. Likewise, the assistant should flush the proximal central venous (or right atrial) channel and connect it to a syringe of heparinized saline, an intravenous infusion, or a transducer. Air in the infusion/right ventricular (or pacing wire channel) should be flushed out with a syringe of heparinized saline or with an intravenous infusion. *Air must be cleared from all channels of the catheter before it is inserted into the patient.*

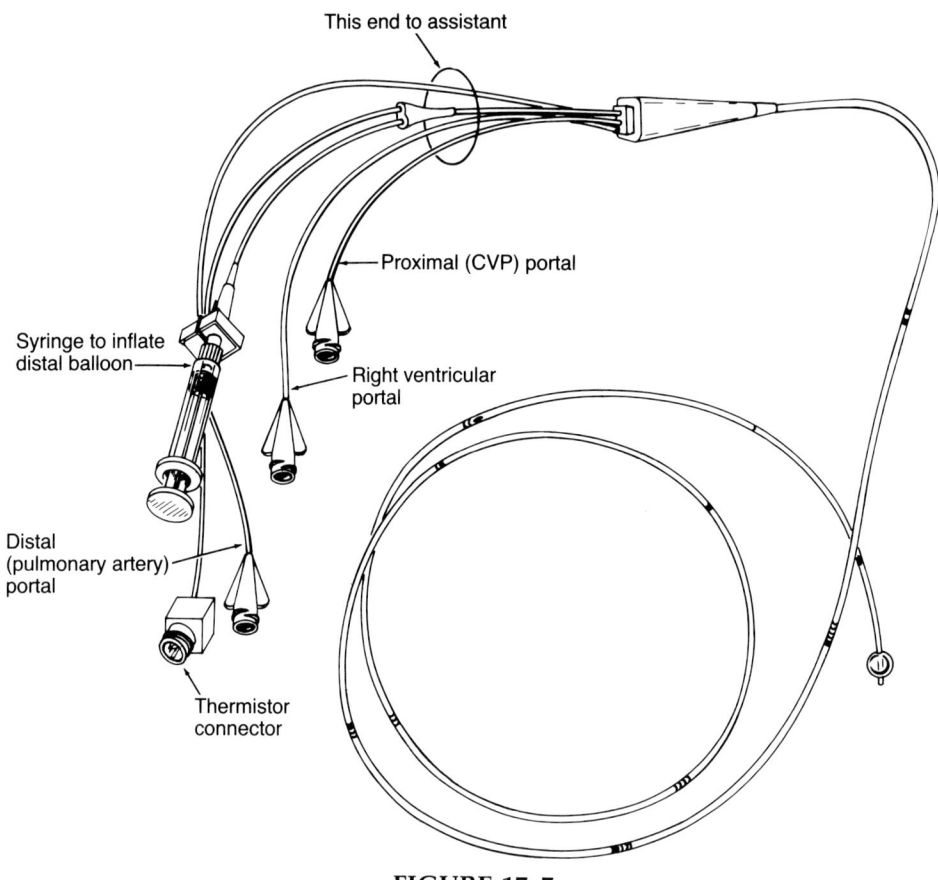

FIGURE 17–7

Pass the catheter through the sterility shield (Fig. 17–8), and have the assistant check the distal balloon by injecting 1.0 to 1.5 ml of air (the appropriate volume will be specified in the catheter's package insert). Have the assistant connect the pulmonary artery thermistor to the cardiac output computer. If the thermistor, connecting cable, and display are functional, operating room temperature will be displayed on the cardiac output computer.

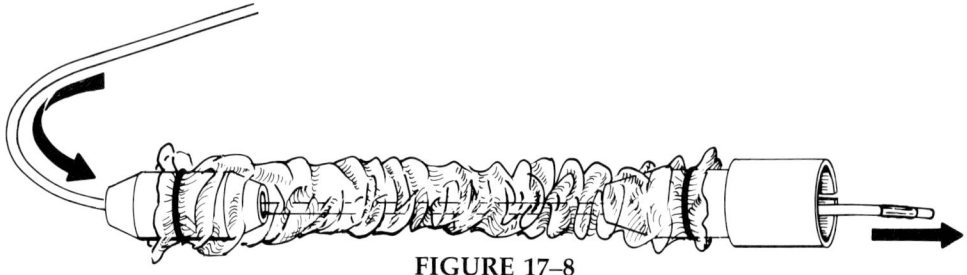

FIGURE 17–8

FLOATING OF CATHETER INTO THE PULMONARY ARTERY

With the balloon deflated and all air flushed from the catheter, insert the catheter 20 cm into the introducer sheath. A central venous pressure waveform should be displayed on the oscilloscope as transduced (through the distal channel) from the tip of the catheter (Fig. 17–9). The thermistor should measure the patient's body temperature.

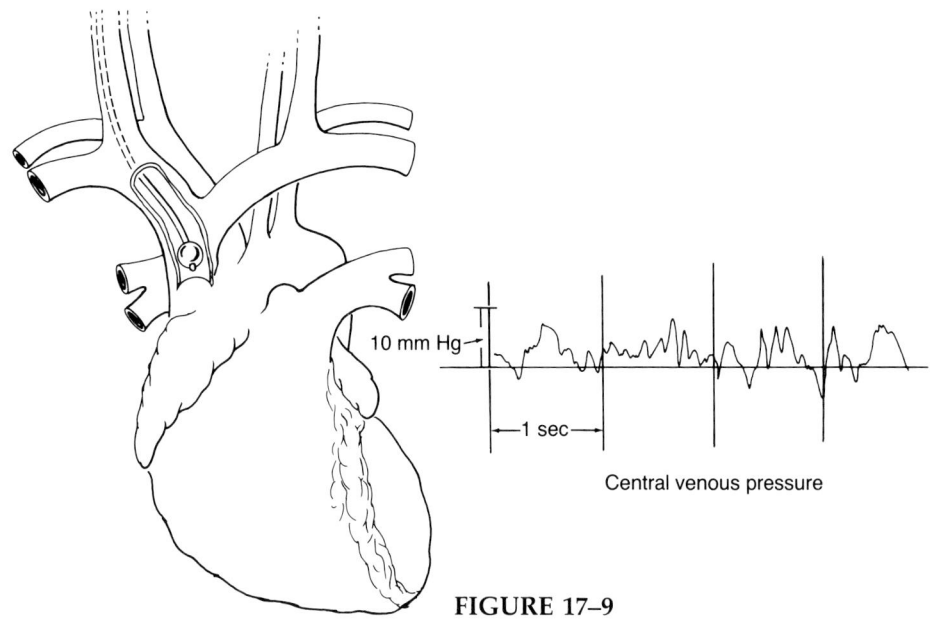

FIGURE 17–9

Have the assistant inflate the balloon. Advance the catheter through the introducer sheath while continuously observing the oscilloscope display. A central venous pressure tracing (which varies during inspiration and expiration) will be displayed until the tip of the catheter enters the right ventricle.

Usually, the catheter must be advanced 30 to 35 cm (using the right internal jugular vein approach) before right ventricular pressures and waveforms are first seen (Fig. 17–10). Arrhythmias (usually premature ventricular beats) are often elicited by the catheter while its tip remains within the right ventricle.

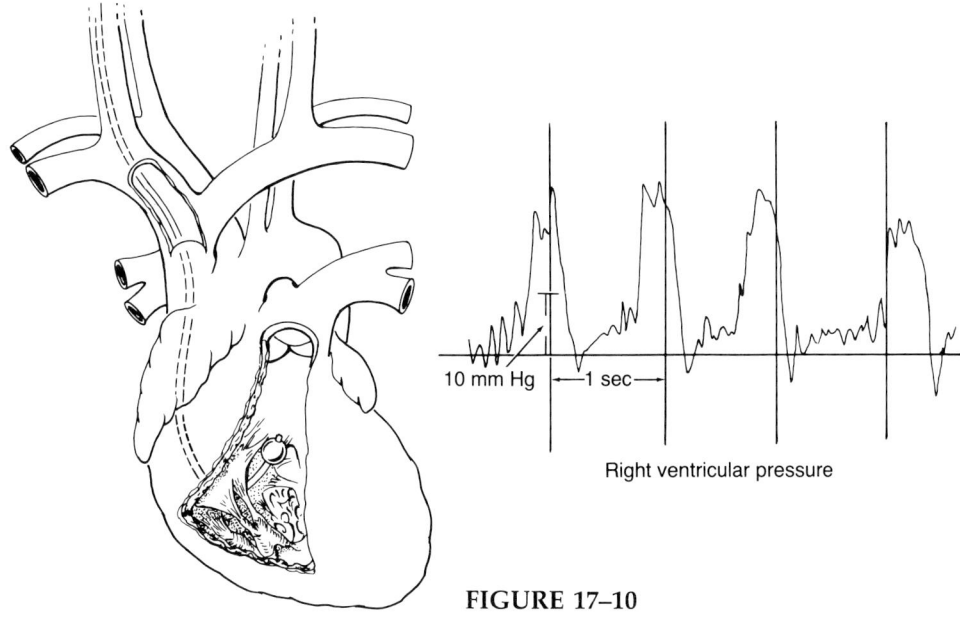

FIGURE 17–10

Five to 10 cm farther, the catheter will cross the pulmonary valve. A pulmonary artery pressure waveform will be seen on the oscilloscope display (Fig. 17–11). The catheter may be safely left in this position for measurement of cardiac output by thermodilution or may be advanced 5 to 10 cm farther into the "wedged" or "occlusion" position, in which an approximation of left atrial pressure can be measured (Fig. 17–12).

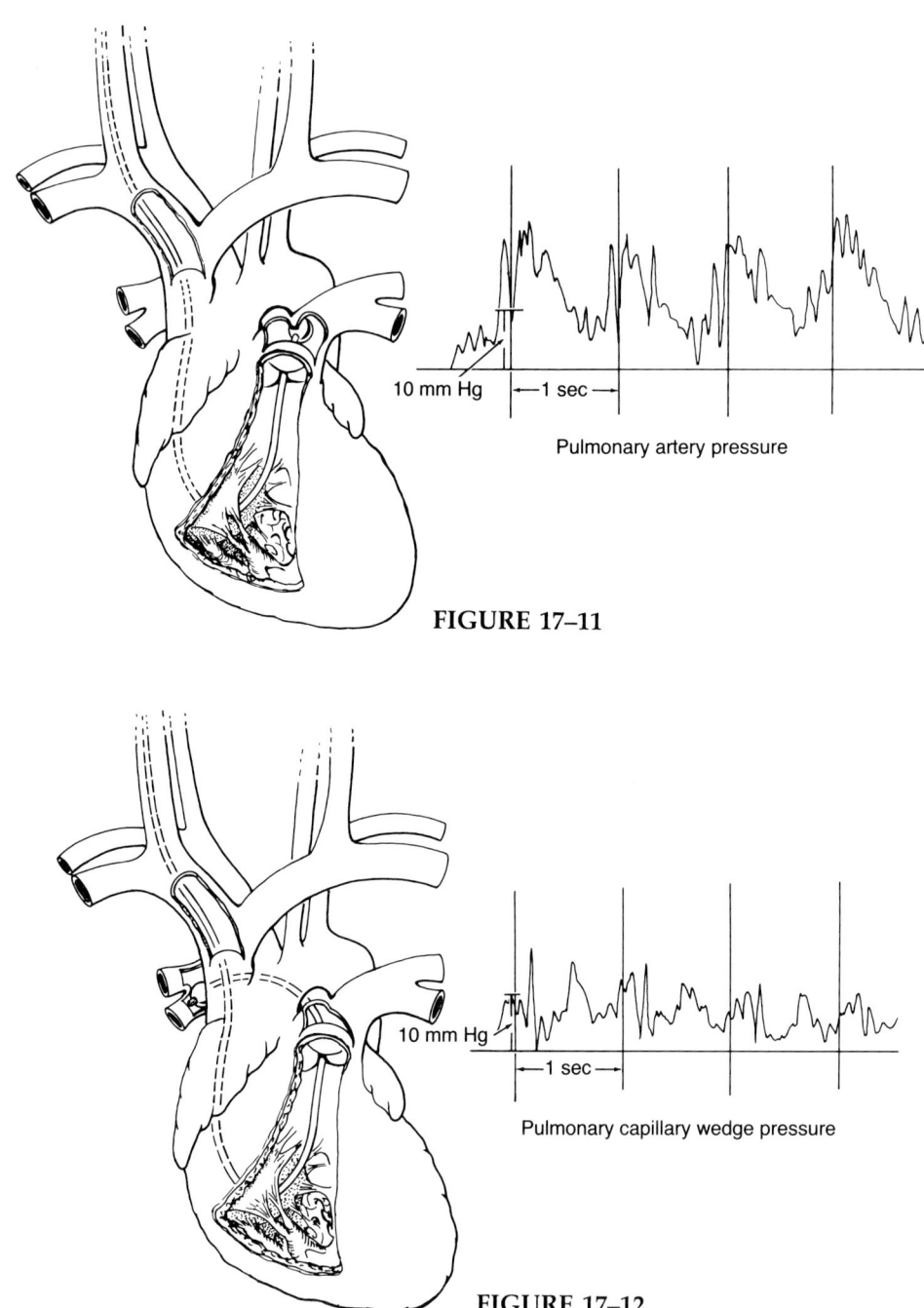

FIGURE 17–11

FIGURE 17–12

After advancing the catheter beyond the pulmonary valve into a "wedged" position, have the assistant deflate the balloon. If a pulmonary artery pressure tracing does not reappear on the oscilloscope display, withdraw the catheter (with the balloon deflated) until a pulmonary artery pressure tracing is obtained.

Advance the sterile sheath over the catheter and attach it to the introducer assembly (Fig. 17–13). Secure the sheath to the catheter with an adhesive strip (packaged with the sheath in the introducer tray) to prevent the sheath from sliding. When the sheath has been secured to the catheter, the "sterile" portion of the catheter can be distinguished from the "contaminated" part. In the absence of the sterility sheath, the catheter cannot be safely advanced (if that should be required) subsequently. Finally, apply a sterile dressing to the insertion site.

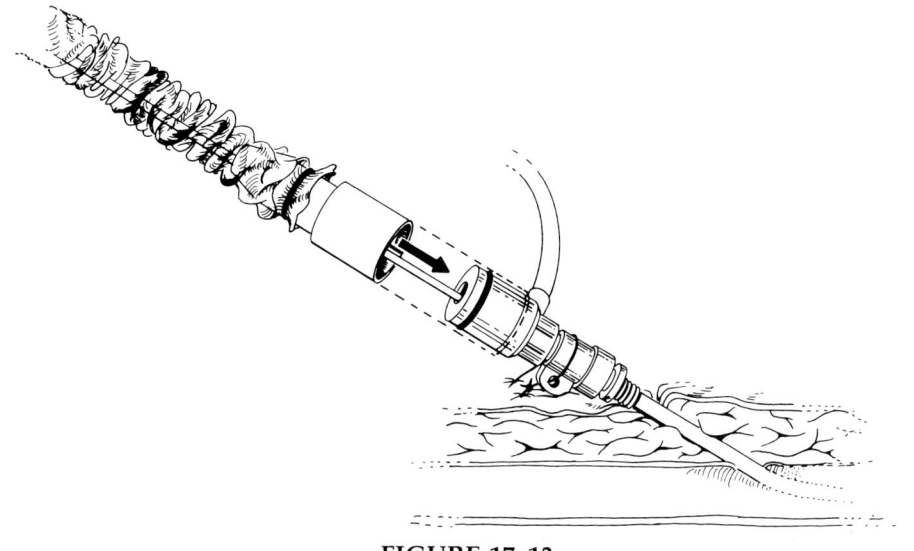

FIGURE 17–13

Difficult Catheter Placements

Common "Mechanical" Problems

Inability to place catheter in pulmonary artery:
  Burst balloon
  Transducer failure
  Improperly turned stopcock
  Excessive balloon inflation
  Hypovolemia
Inability to obtain appropriate cardiac output measurements:
  Thermistor failure
  Cable failure or disconnection (very common)
  Improper programming of cardiac output computer

When difficulty is encountered in passing the catheter into the right atrium, it may be helpful to rotate the patient (using the controls on the operating room table) so that his right side is lower than his left. Make sure that the catheter's natural curve is directed into the right side of the heart, not out the brachiocephalic vein. If the cause of the difficulty is inadequate venous return and cardiac output, sometimes success can be had by a 5-ml/kg transfusion of intravenous fluid or by asking the patient to take a deep breath (the decrease in intrathoracic pressure will momentarily increase venous return).

When the tip of the catheter cannot be passed across the pulmonary valve, sometimes it may be helpful *not* to maximally inflate the balloon. By inflating the balloon with a volume just barely sufficient to inflate it, rather than the "maximal volume," the smaller balloon may more readily cross the valve. Once again, asking the patient to take a deep breath may be helpful. When these maneuvers do not work, fluoroscopy may be helpful to guide placement of the catheter.

Uses

Measurements

Pulmonary artery pressure (systolic, diastolic, mean, occlusion, wedge)
Cardiac output
Oxygen delivery
Right ventricular end-systolic and end-diastolic volume and ejection fraction (available with certain catheters)
Mixed-venous oxygen saturation

Other Uses

Pacing the heart (pacing electrodes are incorporated in some catheters; other catheters allow transvenous wires to be passed through the right ventricular port)
Aspiration of air emboli (limited capacity)
Characterization of arrhythmias (e.g., cannon *a* wave on central venous pressure waveform with junctional rhythm)
Monitoring mitral valve function (*v* wave on wedge tracing)

MEASUREMENT OF CARDIAC OUTPUT BY THERMODILUTION

Measurement of cardiac output by thermodilution is, I believe, the most useful feature of pulmonary artery catheterization. Thermodilution cardiac output measurement uses a "washout" technique. I recommend using a closed system for cooling dextrose solution before injecting it through the right atrial (proximal) port.

To record an accurate cardiac output, both thermistor probes (injectate and pulmonary arterial) must be connected and functioning, the cardiac output computer must be activated (by pressing the "start" button), the proper constant must be chosen for calculation, and the correct volume of fluid must be injected. Each pulmonary artery catheter type *and* injectate volume (i.e., 5 or 10 ml) will require a specific constant to be entered in the computer. The value will be given in the package insert of the pulmonary artery catheter.

SUGGESTIONS FOR MORE EFFECTIVE USE

Measure pulmonary wedge pressure at end expiration. Determine cardiac output at end expiration (*do not* disconnect the respirator).

References

Pearson KS, Gomez MN, Moyers JR, Carter JG, Tinker JH: A cost/benefit analysis of randomized invasive monitoring for patients undergoing cardiac surgery. Anesth Analg 69:336–341, 1989
Robin ED: Death by pulmonary artery flow-directed catheter. Chest 92:727–731, 1987
Shah KB, Rao TLK, Laughlin S, El-Etr AA: A review of pulmonary artery catheterization in 6245 patients. Anesthesiology 61:271–275, 1984
Shoemaker WC, Kram HB, Appel PL: Therapy of shock based on pathophysiology, monitoring, and outcome prediction. Crit Care Med 18:S19–S25, 1990
Sprung CL: The Pulmonary Artery Catheter: Methodology and Clinical Applications. Baltimore, University Park Press, 1983
Vender JS: Invasive cardiac monitoring. Crit Care Clin 4:455–478, 1988
Whittemore AD, Clowes AW, Hechtman HB, Mannick JA: Aortic aneurysm repair reduced operative mortality associated with maintenance of optimal cardiac performance. Ann Surg 192:414–421, 1980

18

Arterial Cannulation

Over the past decade, peripheral arterial cannulation has become remarkably commonplace in the practice of anesthesia and critical care medicine. The risks are low for the usual 1 to 2 days of monitoring most often required for elective surgical cases but increase in patients who are in shock or who will require the cannula to remain in place for more than 2 days.

The indications for arterial cannulation include hemodynamic instability (either present or anticipated), cardiopulmonary bypass, and need for frequent blood sampling (particularly blood gas sampling). Risks of the procedure include bleeding and/or bruising, arterial occlusion (common), infection (uncommon), digital or extremity ischemia (uncommon), and cerebral emboli (probably uncommon).

Site Selection

In adults and children presenting for elective surgery, the site most often selected for cannulation is the radial artery at the wrist. If only one wrist will be easily accessible during the anesthetic, then that wrist is the preferred site for cannulation. Alternatively, the nondominant wrist should be selected. If during intrathoracic vascular surgery the aorta will be clamped near the left subclavian artery (e.g., for thoracic aortic aneurysm resection), cannulation of the right radial artery will be necessary.

Some practitioners routinely perform the Allen test to determine whether collateral flow through the ulnar artery is normal prior to radial artery cannulation. No studies demonstrate that complications from radial arterial cannulation are more likely when the Allen test is abnormal. In general, the risk of thrombosis seems related to the size of the cannula (smaller is better) and inversely related to the flow (higher flow is better) through the cannulated vessel.

During head and neck surgery and in neurosurgery, when the anesthetist is often positioned nearer to the patient's feet than to his head, cannulation of the dorsalis pedis artery should be considered. This is also a preferred site in children. The practitioner, however, should remember that systolic arterial blood pressure measured in the dorsalis pedis tends to be higher than that measured in the radial artery.

During cardiac surgery, radial artery cannulae are most often used. However, sterile cannulation of the femoral arteries (from the operative field by the surgeon) has the advantage of providing a ready portal through which an intra-aortic balloon counterpulsation device may be inserted. Finally, when radial cannulation is difficult, brachial arterial cannulation is often easily accomplished. In my institution there have been no serious complications after brachial artery cannulation in any hemodynamically stable patient undergoing elective cardiac surgery. Brachial artery pressures more accurately track aortic pressures (than radial artery pressures) after hypothermic cardiopulmonary bypass in adults.

Withdrawal of Arterial Sample

Remember that to obtain an undiluted (by flush solution) blood sample, a volume equal to three times the "dead space" between cannula tip and stopcock should be withdrawn before the arterial sample is withdrawn. I recommend that the aspirated blood and flush solution be reinfused into the patient through a *venous* cannula, rather than back through the arterial line because of the potential risk of cerebral embolism from "bolus" flushing of the arterial line.

Flushing of Arterial Line

Excessive flushing of arterial cannulae may carry the risk of cerebral arterial embolization, if the minute bubbles (which are ubiquitous, even with careful technique) are propelled retrograde into the central arterial circulation by a "blast" of saline flush solution. A continuous-flow flush device should always be used in adult patients. However, in small children, careful *slow* flushing with a small (1 to 3 ml) syringe may be preferable. A rapid bolus of as little as 3 ml has been shown to cause retrograde flow from the radial artery into the central circulation of an adult.

Technique

EQUIPMENT NEEDED

Sterile gloves
Antiseptic solution
2-ml syringe of 1% lidocaine (25-gauge needle)
10-ml syringe of heparinized saline (2 units heparin/ml of 0.9% saline)
Arterial extension tubing with stopcock
Arm board or arm rest
Rolled towel or a stack of gauze sponges
20-gauge 2-inch intravenous cannulae (substitute 22-gauge or 24-gauge in children)
Adhesive tape (both narrow and wide)
Tincture of benzoin (optional)
3-0 nylon suture on Keith needle (optional)

PREPARATION AND POSITIONING

Position the hand and wrist dorsiflexed over a rolled towel. This position tends to stretch the radial artery and reduce its ability to "wander" during attempts at cannulation. I usually loosely tape the patient's hand (across the fingers) and distal forearm to the arm board.

INJECTION OF LOCAL ANESTHETIC

Cleanse the overlying skin with antiseptic solution. Locate the artery by palpation proximal to the proximal wrist crease, lateral to the tendon of flexor carpi radialis (Fig. 18–1).

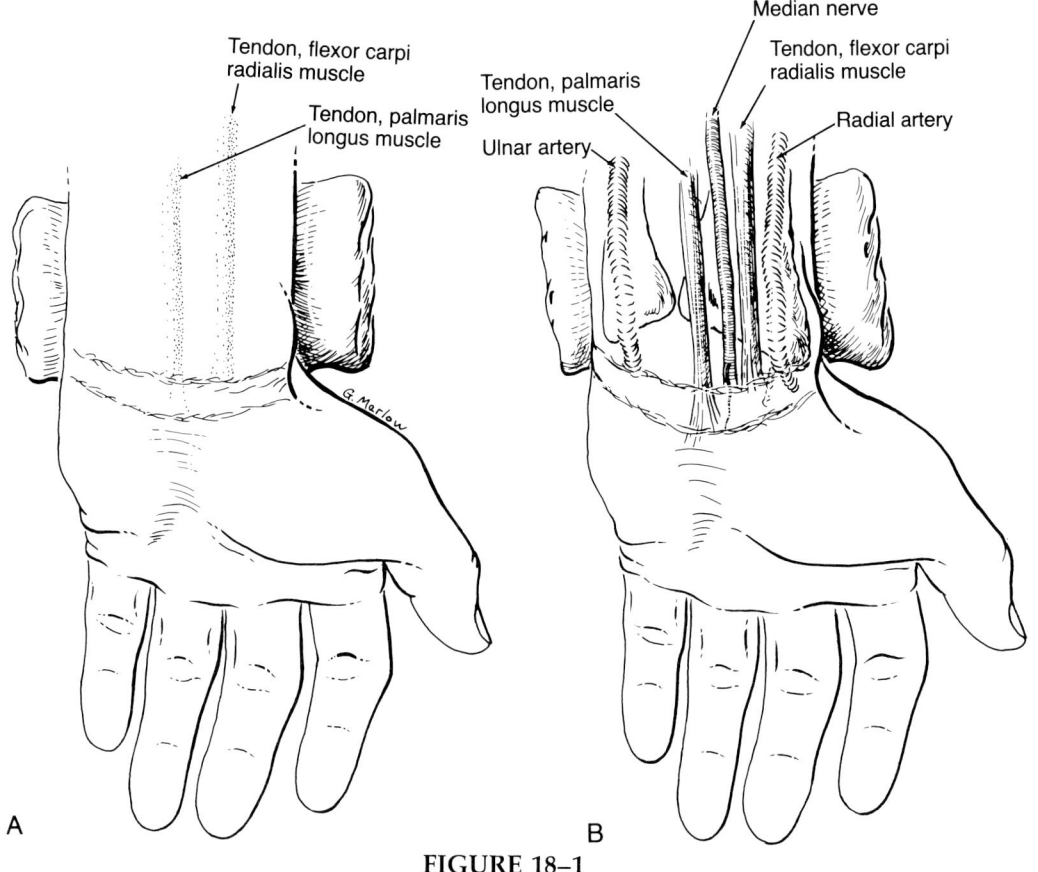

FIGURE 18–1

Inject 1% lidocaine in the skin at the site of intended puncture (Fig. 18–2). Some recommend that skin puncture be accomplished with an 18-gauge needle to avoid fraying the tip of the cannula. I believe that this is an unnecessary step.

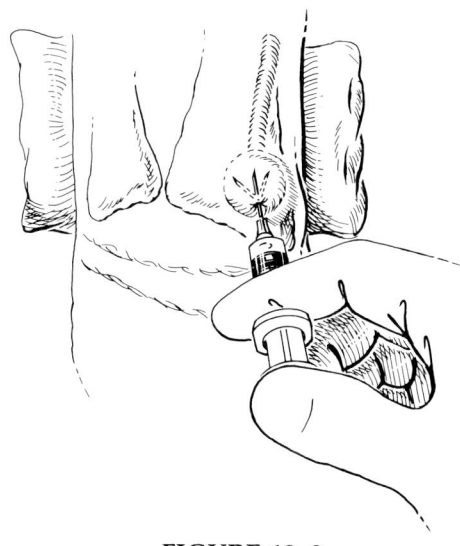

FIGURE 18–2

INSERTION OF CANNULA

Advance the needle and cannula through the skin at an angle of 30° to 45° along the line of travel of the artery, attempting to enter the artery within 1 cm of the puncture site (Fig. 18–3).

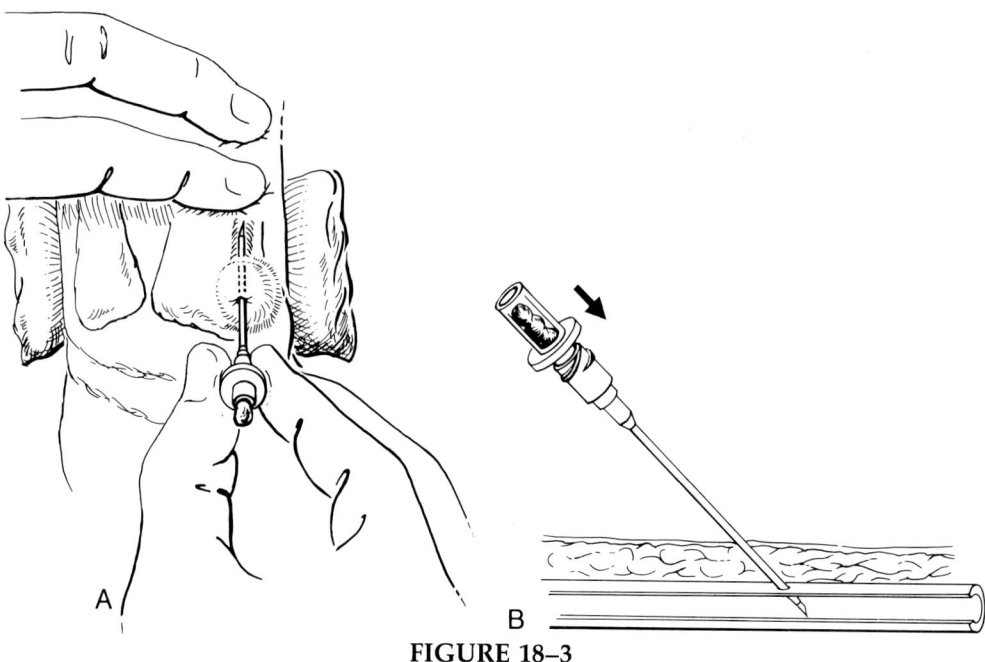

FIGURE 18–3

When blood "flashes" back into the hub of the needle, reduce the angle of entry of the needle and cannula, advance the needle and cannula an additional millimeter, then advance the cannula over the needle into the artery (Fig. 18–4). Finally, remove the needle from the cannula, compress the artery proximal to the cannula to reduce blood loss, and connect the cannula to the transducer tubing (Fig. 18–5).

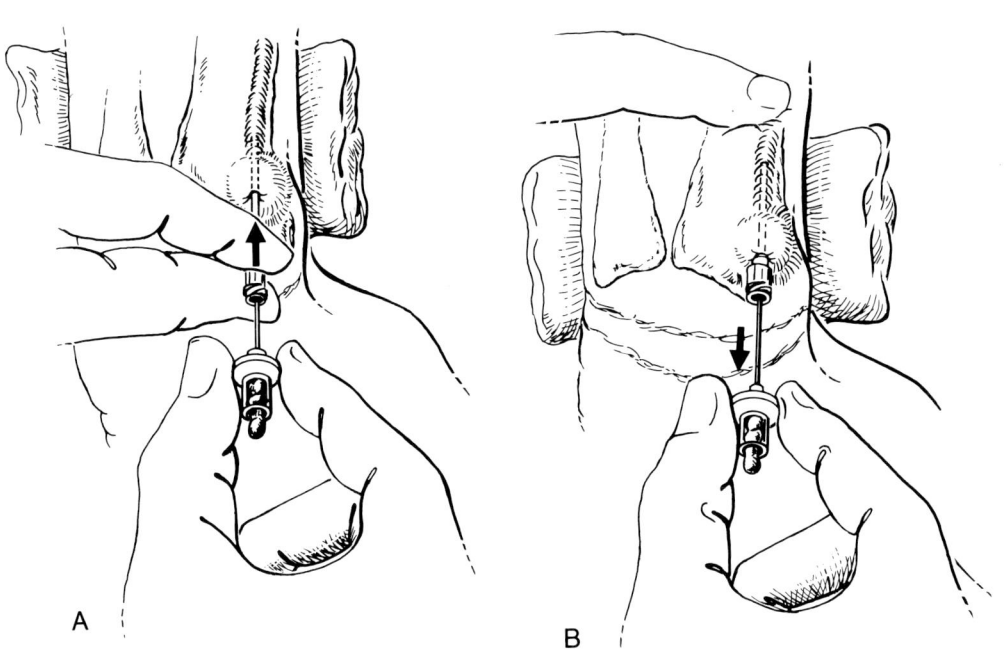

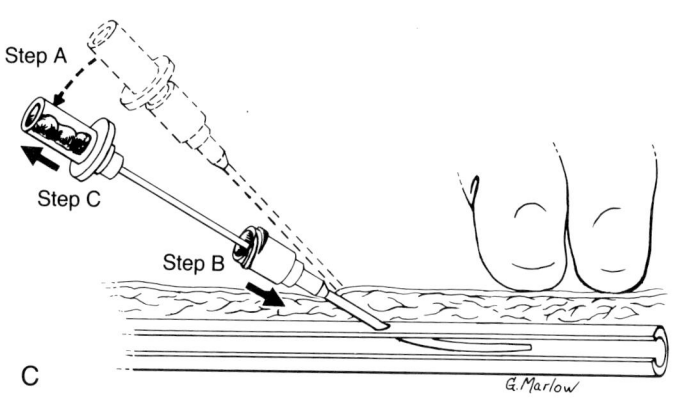

FIGURE 18–4

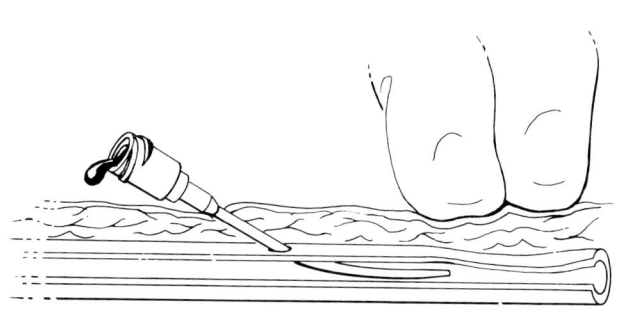

FIGURE 18–5

TRANSFIXATION TECHNIQUE

Alternatively, when blood "flashes" back, advance the needle farther (until the operator is sure that the tip of the cannula has "transfixed" the artery from front to back) (Fig. 18–6), withdraw the needle, then slowly withdraw the cannula until arterial blood begins to spurt from the distal tip of the cannula (Fig. 18–7). At this point, advance the cannula into the artery (Fig. 18–8).

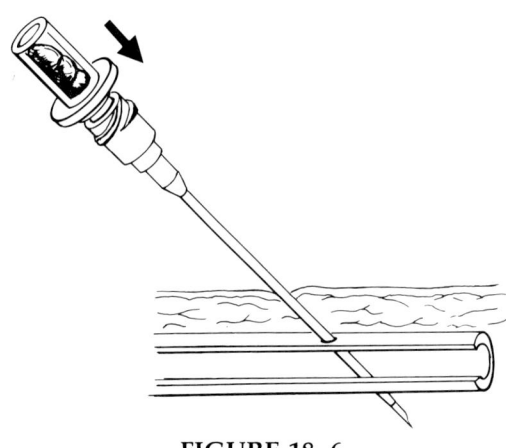

FIGURE 18–6

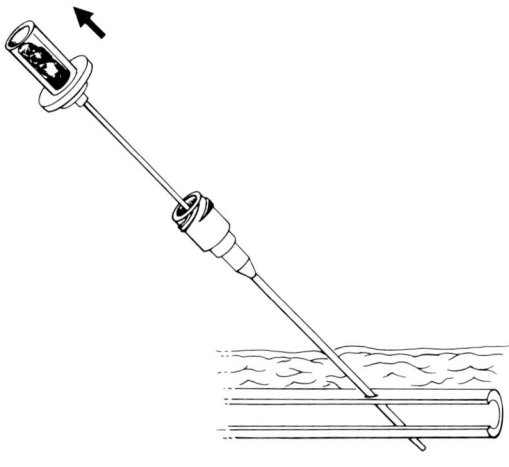

FIGURE 18–7

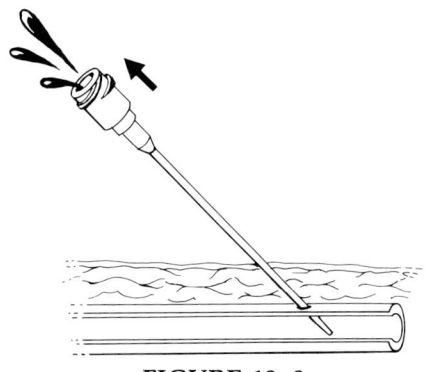

FIGURE 18–8

GUIDE WIRES

Sometimes, despite free, pulsatile flow of arterial blood from an arterial cannula, it cannot be advanced into the artery. In these rare instances, a guide wire can sometimes be passed through the cannula into the artery, permitting the cannula to be passed over the wire beyond the point of obstruction within the artery.

FLUSHING AND SECURING OF CANNULA

Following a successful cannulation, connect the arterial cannula either to an extension tube with a stopcock (all previously filled with heparinized saline) or to a high-pressure transducer line (also previously filled with heparinized saline) (Fig. 18–9). Flushing the cannula with heparinized saline will prevent it from clotting.

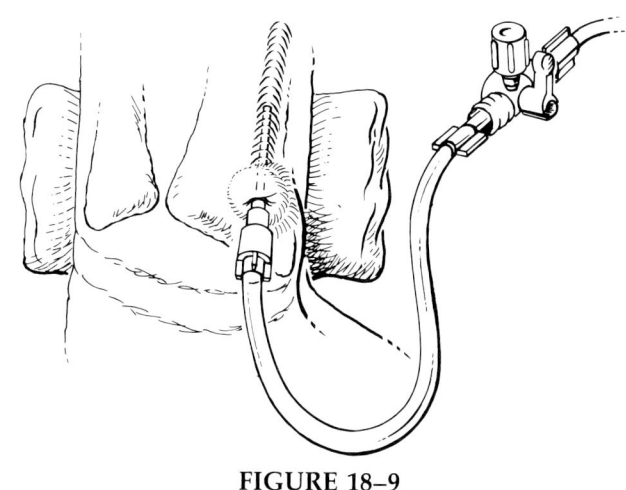

FIGURE 18–9

The cannula should be secured with adhesive tape, after application of tincture of benzoin to the skin (Fig. 18–10). In most cases, it is unnecessary to suture a properly taped arterial line in place. The taping should reflect a high degree of paranoia on the part of the operator (Fig. 18–11). Anticipate that the patient's arm may be suspended aloft by the arterial transducer tubing (I have seen it)!

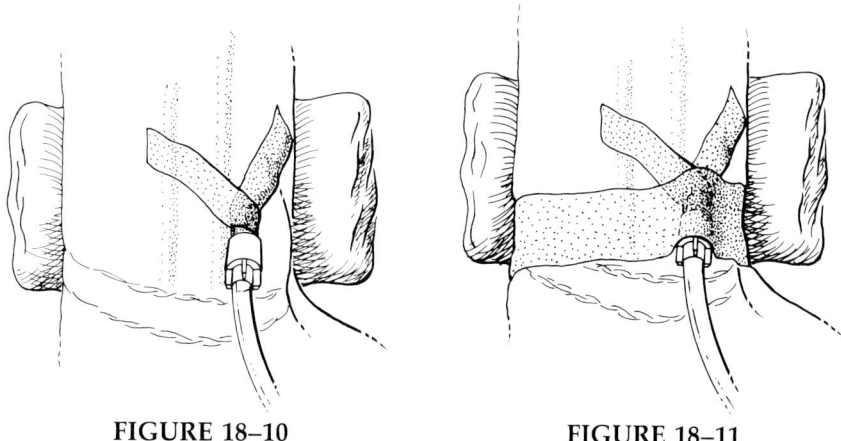

FIGURE 18–10   FIGURE 18–11

I often tape the patient's hand and wrist to a short arm board to prevent wrist flexion and kinking of the arterial cannula. This is an especially important maneuver if the arm in which the arterial cannula has been inserted must be tucked by the patient's side during surgery.

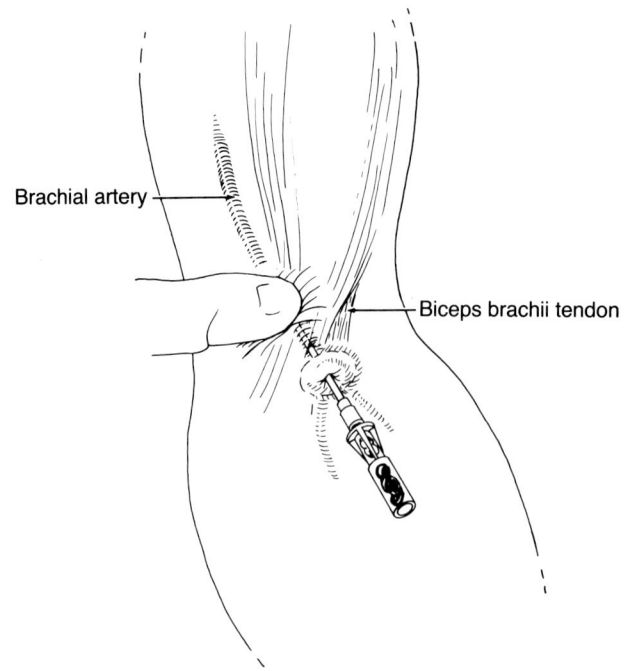

FIGURE 18–12

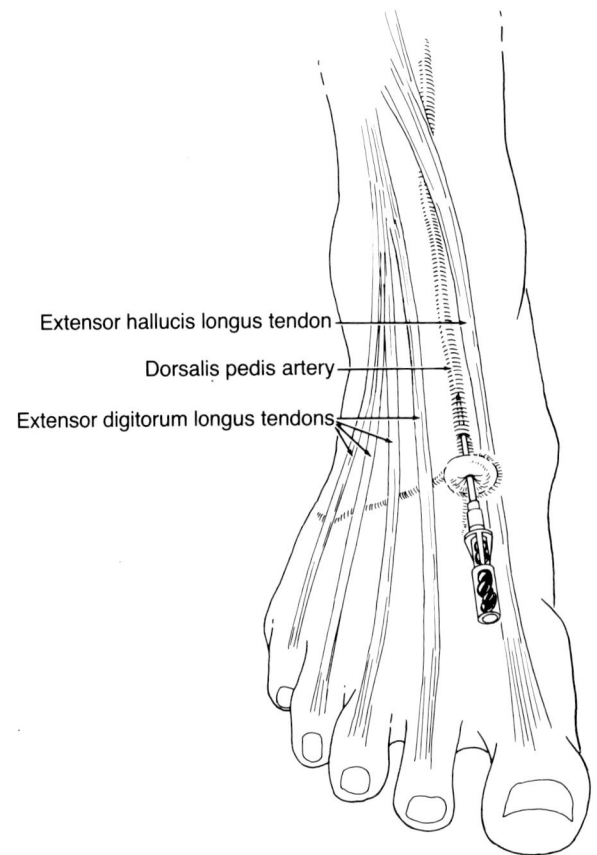

FIGURE 18–13

Alternatives to Radial Artery Cannulation

BRACHIAL ARTERY CANNULATION

The brachial artery lies medial to the tendon of biceps and lateral to pronator teres in the antecubital fossa. It may be cannulated just proximal to the skin crease of the antecubital fossa (Fig. 18–12). The arm should be extended at the elbow; otherwise, a similar technique to that used for radial arterial cannulation may be employed.

DORSALIS PEDIS CANNULATION

The dorsalis pedis lies medial to extensor digitorum longus and lateral and deep to the extensor hallucis longus. It is easily cannulated at the level of the metatarsals (Fig. 18–13).

FEMORAL ARTERY CANNULATION

The femoral artery is usually cannulated 1 to 2 cm distal to the inguinal ligament (Fig. 18–14). The technique resembles that of internal jugular vein cannulation. The artery is initially cannulated with a 2-inch venous cannula, which is replaced (over a J-wire) with an 18-gauge 6-inch pediatric central venous cannula.

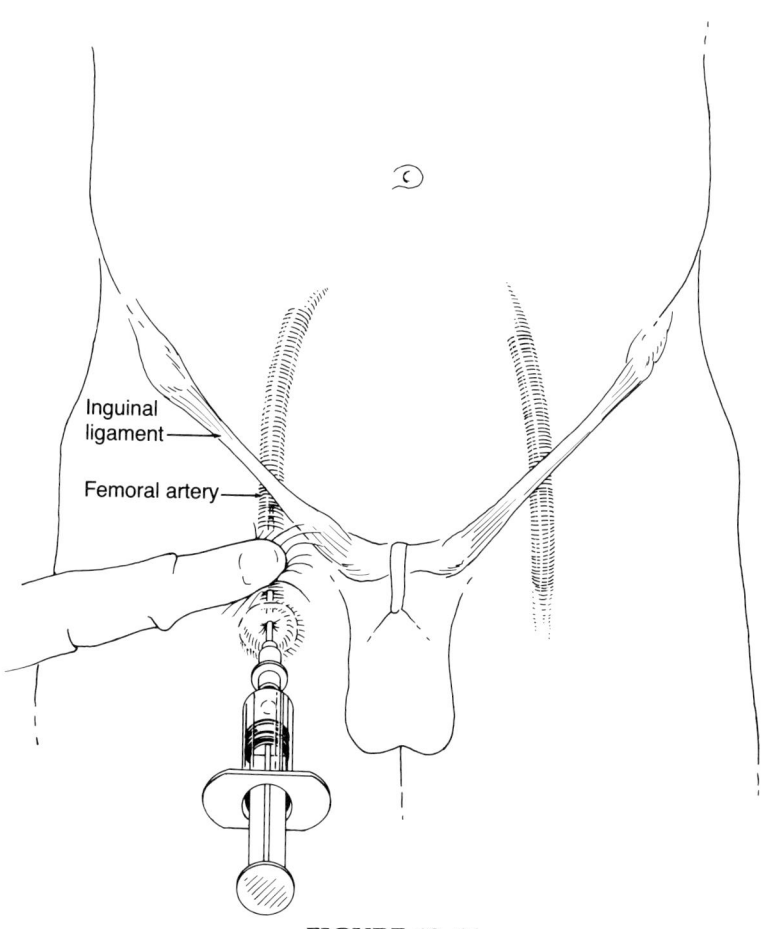

FIGURE 18–14

References

Bazaral MG, Welch M, Golding LAR, Badwar K: Comparison of brachial and radial arterial pressures in patients undergoing coronary artery bypass surgery. Anesthesiology 73:38–45, 1990

Bedford RF: Invasive blood pressure monitoring. In Blitt CD (ed): Monitoring in Anesthesia and Critical Care Medicine, pp 41–85. New York, Churchill Livingstone, 1985

Bedford RF: Radial arterial function following percutaneous cannulation with 18- and 20-gauge catheters. Anesthesiology 47:37–39, 1977

Heavner JE, Flinders C, McMahon DJ, Branigan T, Badgwell JM: Technical Manual of Anesthesiology: An Introduction, pp 57–67. New York, Raven Press, 1989

Lowenstein E, Little JW III, Lo HH: Prevention of cerebral embolization from flushing radial-artery cannulas. N Engl J Med 285:1414–1415, 1971

Slogoff S, Keats AS, Arlund C: On the safety of radial artery cannulation. Anesthesiology 59:42–47, 1983

19

Suture Techniques

Few things are more likely to produce snickering on the part of surgeons than surgical knot tying by anesthetists. Fortunately, expertise in the technique is quickly acquired and easily maintained with a minimal degree of practice.

When passing suture material through the skin, separate the entrance and exit wounds of the needle by large rather than small distances. Small "bites" are more likely to result in skin necrosis than large "bites." Use nonabsorbable and nonreactive (I recommend nylon) rather than absorbable (e.g., cat gut) or reactive (e.g., silk) suture material, particularly when securing cannulae to the skin of the neck. Nonabsorbable, nonreactive suture materials produce less skin reaction and smaller scars than other suture materials. To prevent slippage, use an adequate number of half-hitches in the knot. Nylon suture material requires at least four half-hitches to produce a secure knot; silk, on the other hand, requires only three half-hitches.

Types of Knots

Suture material can be tied using either a one-handed or a two-handed technique, starting with either the dominant or nondominant hand. In this chapter I will describe how to tie a square knot using only the left hand and how to tie a square knot with both hands. Surgeons will often use a two-handed knot technique preferentially when the success of an operation depends on the security of a particular knot. For most situations in anesthesia, either technique may be used safely.

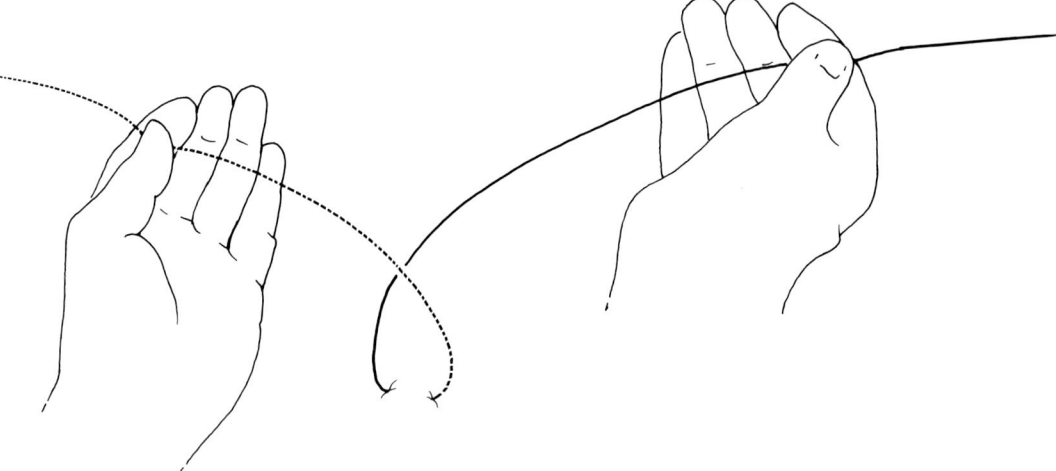

FIGURE 19–1

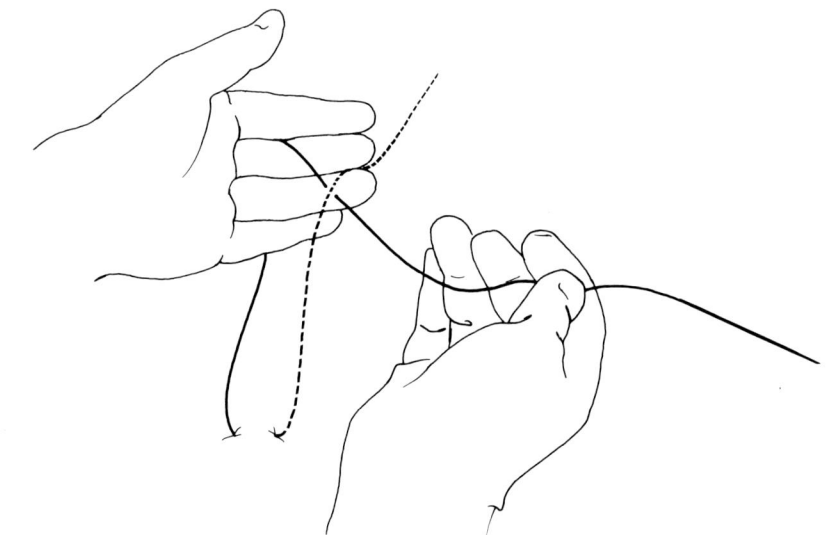

FIGURE 19–2

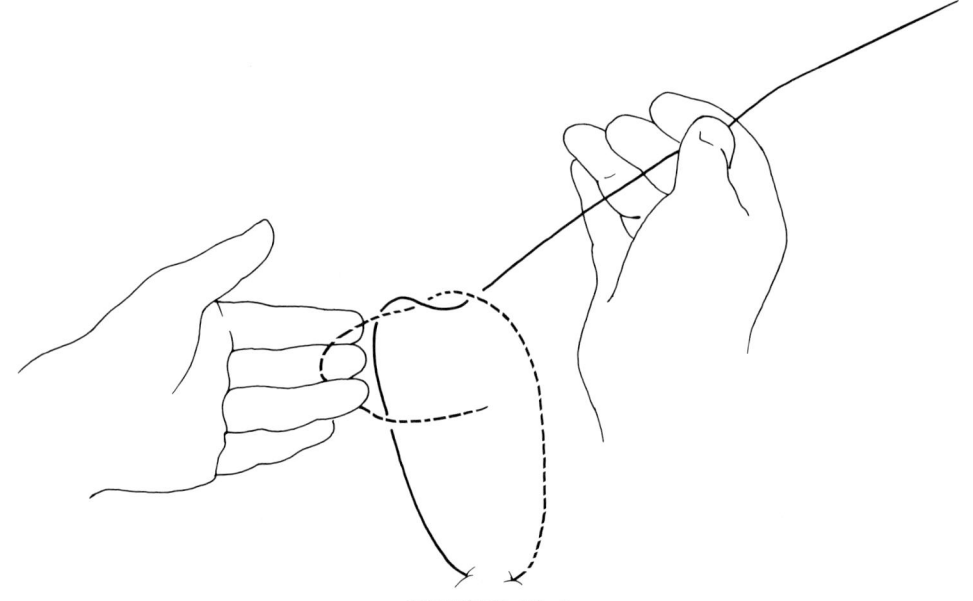

FIGURE 19–3

Tying a Square Knot with the Left Hand

Insert the needle through the skin. Pull the suture material through the skin and around the vascular cannula (Fig. 19–1). Hold the end of the suture material attached to the needle with the right hand, and lay it over the middle finger of the left hand (Fig. 19–2). Cross the two ends and pull the shorter end through the loop (formed by the crossing of the two ends) with the middle and ring fingers of the left hand (Fig. 19–3). Tighten the knot until it lies flat by pulling on the shorter end.

Cross the two ends of the suture material over the index finger of the left hand (Fig. 19–4). Use the index finger of the left hand to "reach around" the taut longer end (held by the right hand) and drag the shorter end through the loop (Fig. 19–5). Tighten the knot until it lies flat by pulling on the shorter end. Repeat both steps at least twice (when using a nylon suture).

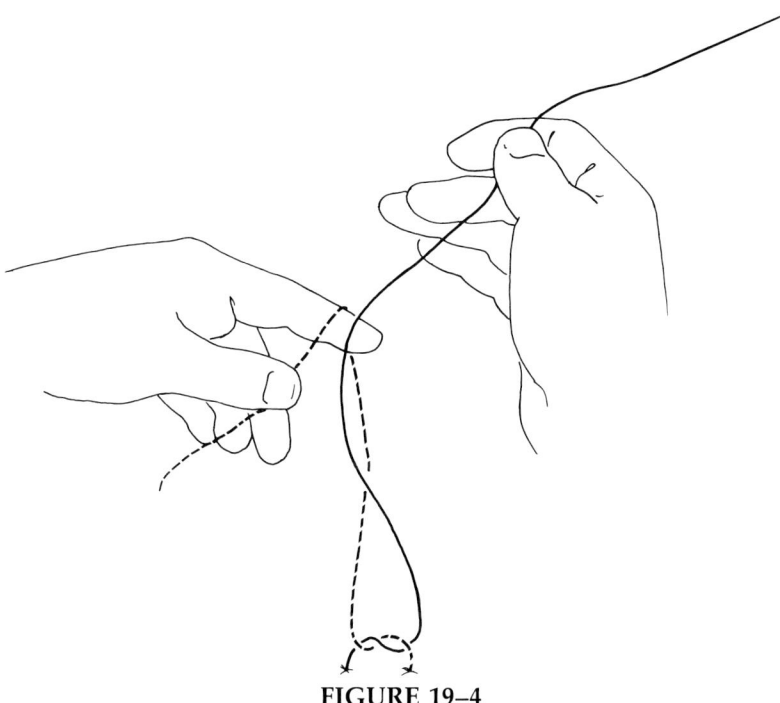

FIGURE 19–4

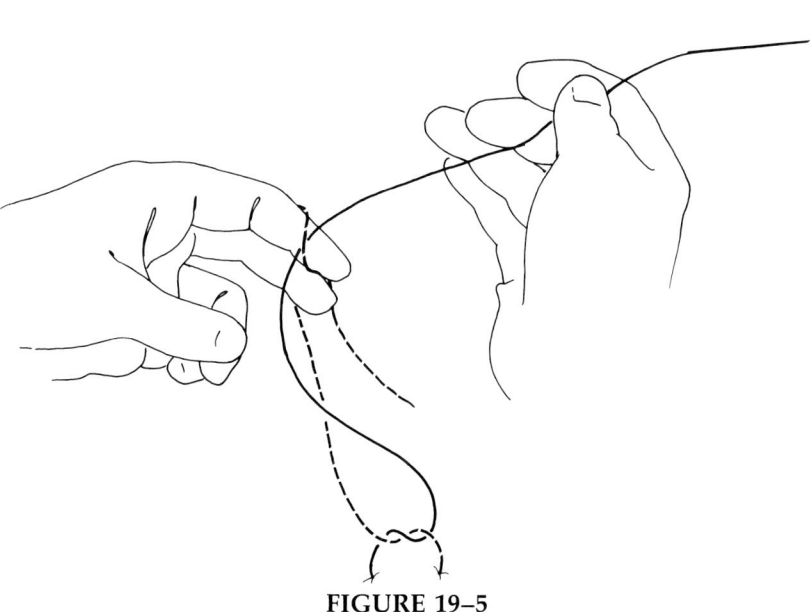

FIGURE 19–5

Tying a Square Knot with Both Hands

Insert the needle through the skin. Pull the suture material through the skin and around the vascular cannula (Fig. 19–6). Grasp one end of the suture material with the right hand and cross the other end over it with the left hand, forming a loop over the right thumb (Fig. 19–7). Slide the right index finger through the loop and lay the left-hand end of the suture material over the right index finger (Fig. 19–8). Grasp the end of the suture material being held by the left hand between the thumb and index finger of the right hand and push it through the loop (Fig. 19–9). Tighten the knot until it lies flat by pulling on both ends.

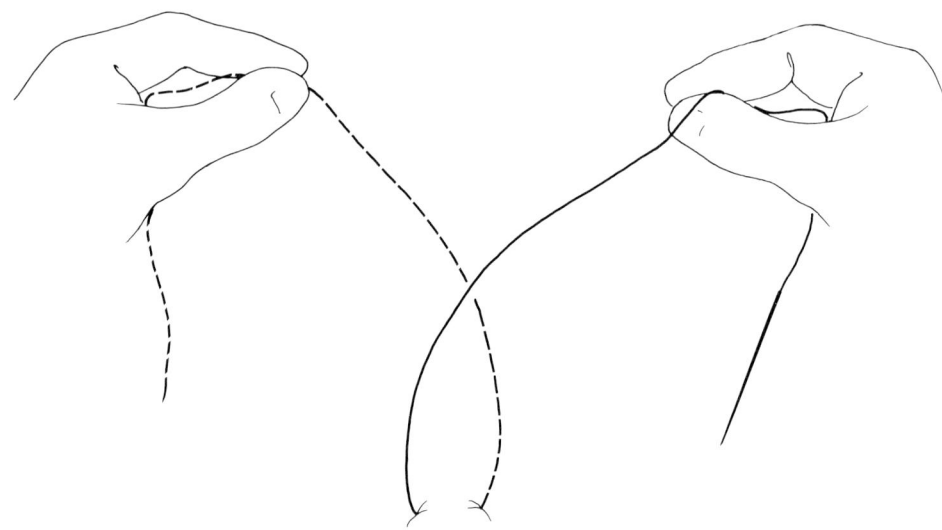

FIGURE 19–6

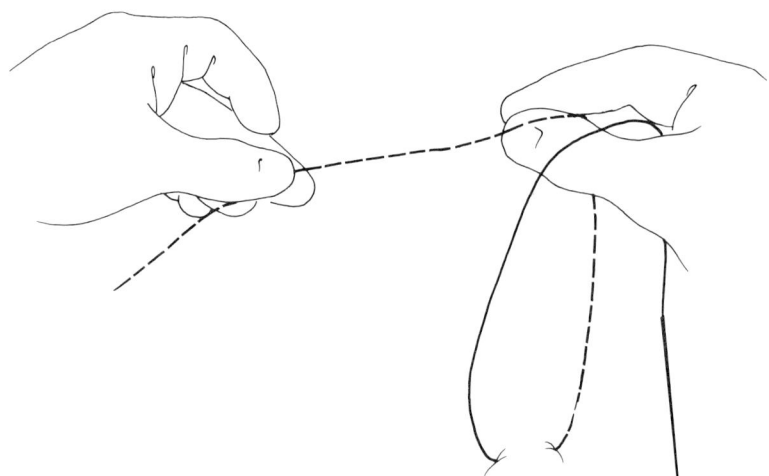

FIGURE 19–7

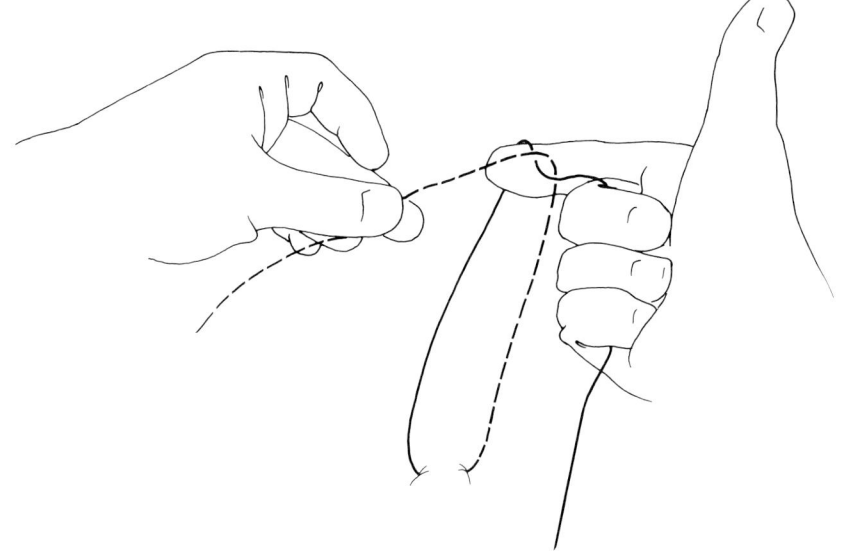

FIGURE 19–8

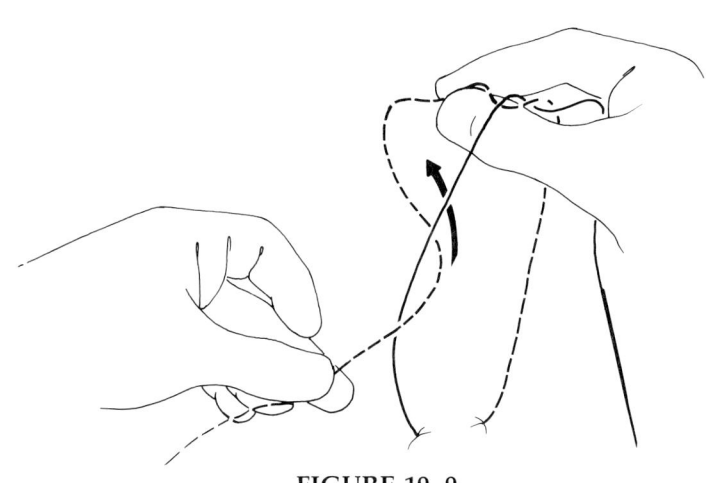

FIGURE 19–9

Grasp the free end of the suture material with the left hand. Form a loop over the right index finger with the two strands (Fig. 19–10). Grasp the end of the suture material being held by the left hand between the index finger and thumb of the right hand and pull it through the loop (opposite to the direction of the first half-hitch) (Fig. 19–11). Grasp the free end with the left hand. Tighten the knot until it lies flat by pulling on both ends. Note that the operator's hands will pull in alternate directions on alternate half-hitches to ensure that the knot is tied (Fig. 19–12). Repeat steps 1 and 2 at least twice (when using a nylon suture). Trim the ends from the knot.

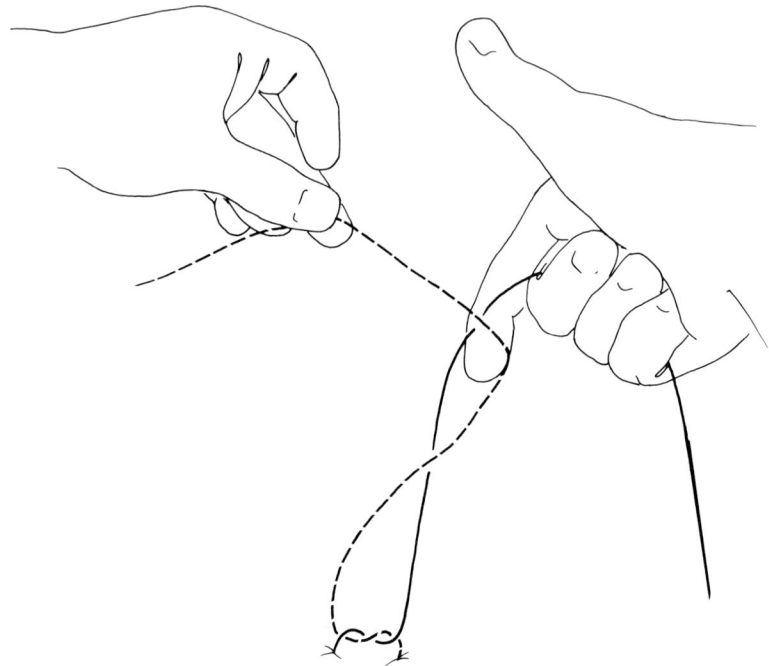

FIGURE 19–10

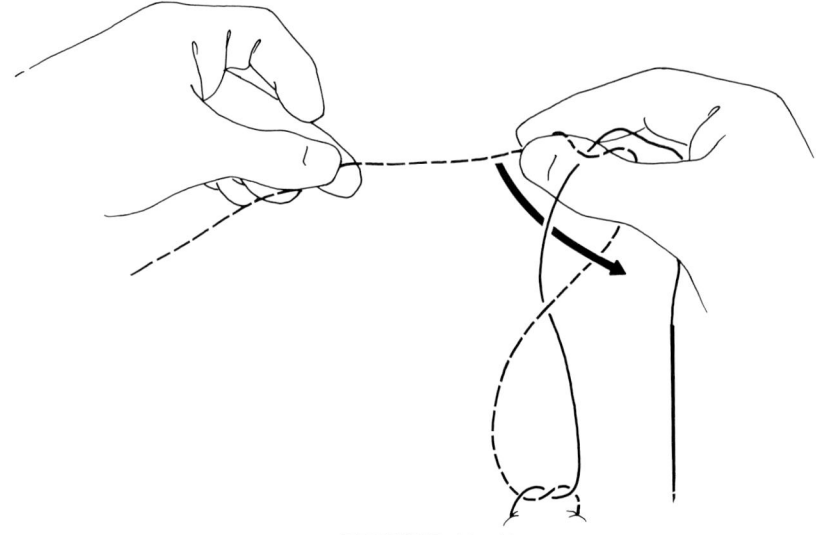

FIGURE 19–11

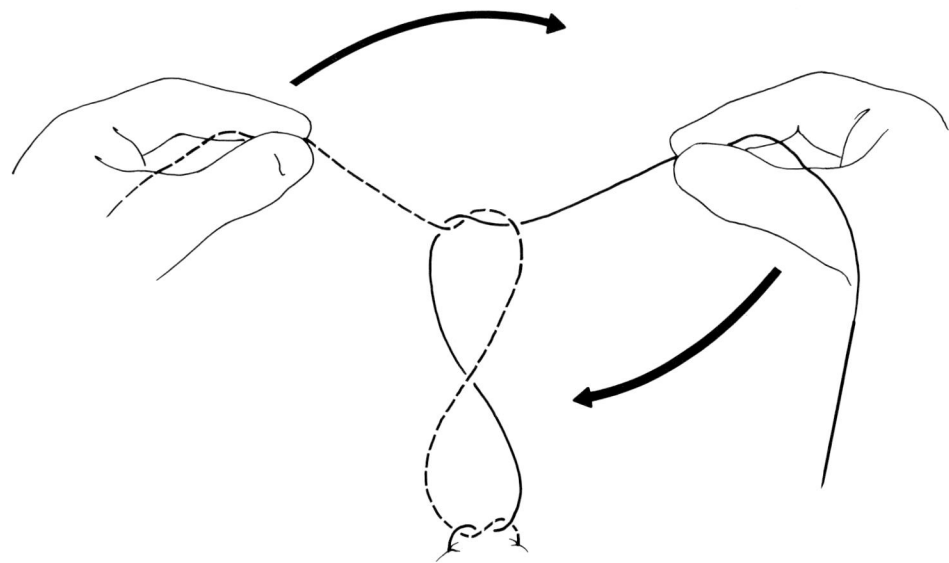

FIGURE 19–12

III

REGIONAL ANESTHESIA

20

Local Infiltration of Anesthetic

The simplest form of regional anesthesia consists of injection of local anesthetic in the skin. Surprisingly, many physicians show limited expertise with this technique.

Technique

EQUIPMENT NEEDED

Sterile gloves
Local anesthetic
22-gauge needle
Syringe of appropriate size

PROCEDURE

Concentrated local anesthetics should not be used for local infiltration. Epinephrine should be added only if necessary, since epinephrine-containing local anesthetics cause more pain than plain local anesthetic solutions when they are injected subcutaneously. I commonly use lidocaine 0.5% to 1.0% or bupivacaine 0.25%, which are concentrations below those required for major nerve blocks.

For maximal patient comfort, use the smallest possible needle. Inject the local anesthetic as the needle is advanced so that subsequent needle insertions are made through areas of skin already anesthetized. Do not insert the needle ahead of the anesthetic solution through unanesthetized skin (Fig. 20–1).

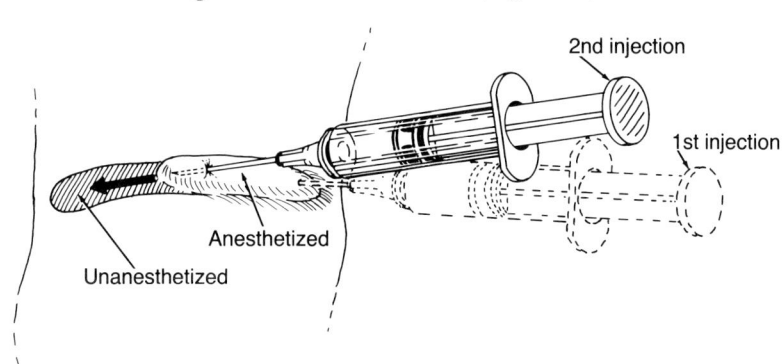

FIGURE 20–1

There is usually no need to aspirate through the needle before infiltration of small amounts of dilute local anesthetic. Even if the needle tip were to be located within a vein, the dose of local anesthetic injected would be insufficient to cause serious side effects. Repeated aspirations serve only to prolong the duration of the injection.

21

Intravenous Regional Anesthesia

Intravenous regional anesthesia (or Bier block) is a convenient means for reliably producing distal anesthesia of the upper or lower extremity for surgery that will last no longer than about an hour. The technique is commonly regarded as "foolproof." As with many other "foolproof" techniques, there are numerous ways to make the technique unsuccessful. Probably the two most common are (1) to exsanguinate the extremity inadequately prior to injecting the local anesthetic and (2) to apply and/or inflate the tourniquet inadequately prior to injecting the local anesthetic. The former will lead to inadequate filling of the vasculature with local anesthetic solution and dilution of the anesthetic by blood. The latter will lead to unexpected loss of local anesthetic solution and (often) to toxic central nervous system side effects.

Intravenous regional anesthesia is poorly suited for patients who may suffer pain or harm during application of the Esmarch bandage. Thus, it should be avoided in patients with infections or multiple fractures in the extremity to be blocked.

Technique

EQUIPMENT NEEDED

Sterile gloves
Antiseptic solution
50-ml syringe
50 ml lidocaine (or prilocaine) 0.5%
Intravenous infusion cannula with T-piece or "heparin-lock" adapter
Esmarch bandage
Double pneumatic tourniquet
Venous tourniquet
Usual monitoring devices
Resuscitation drugs and equipment

PREPARATION AND POSITIONING

Insert an intravenous cannula in the nonoperative arm. Attach the electrocardiographic leads, blood pressure cuff, and pulse oximeter probe for monitoring during the procedure. Position the patient supine on the operating room table. Apply a venous tourniquet to the extremity to be anesthetized (Fig. 21–1). Cleanse the skin of the hand (or foot, as appropriate) with antiseptic solution, inject local anesthesia in the skin, and insert an intravenous cannula with a T-piece or "heparin-lock" connector. Place the cannula in as distal a vein as possible. Avoid antecubital veins, for example, for intravenous regional anesthesia for hand surgery (Fig. 21–2). Tape the cannula in place and apply the double pneumatic tourniquet to the upper arm (or lower leg, as appropriate).

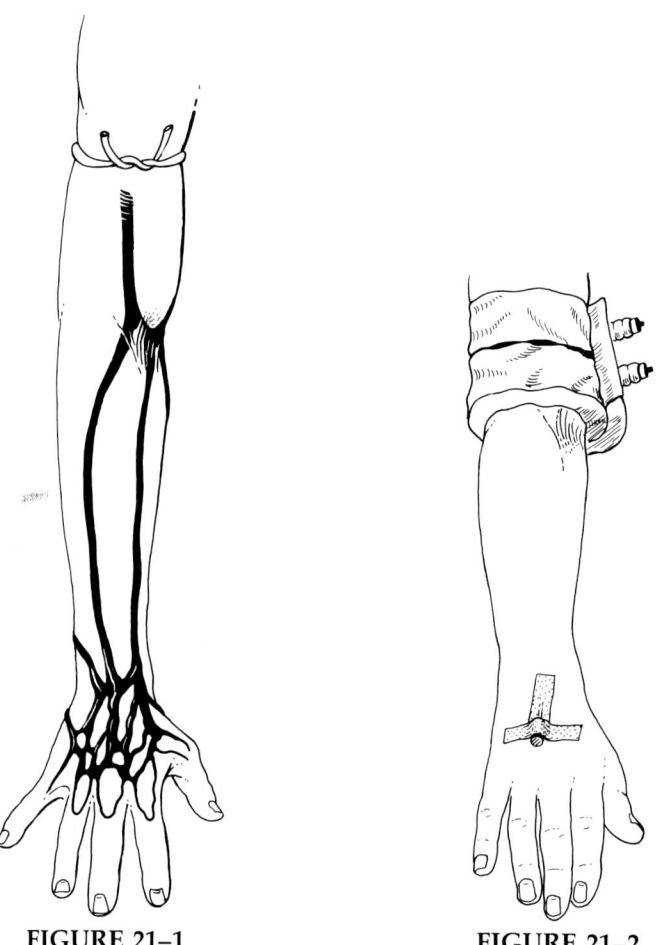

FIGURE 21–1   FIGURE 21–2

Hold the extremity to be anesthetized in an elevated position for at least a minute, and then wrap an Esmarch bandage tightly (Fig. 21–3), starting at the most distal point of the extremity and proceeding proximally up to and overlapping the double tourniquet (Fig. 21–4). Wrap the bandage carefully and smoothly to maximally exsanguinate the extremity. After fully wrapping the extremity with the bandage, inflate the distal pneumatic tourniquet to no less than 300 mm Hg on the arm (or 350 mm Hg on the leg) (Fig. 21–5). Higher tourniquet pressures may be necessary in hypertensive patients or obese patients with large upper extremities. After the distal tourniquet has been fully inflated, inflate the proximal tourniquet and remove the Esmarch bandage (Fig. 21–6). Deflate the distal tourniquet and prepare to inject the local anesthetic through the intravenous catheter.

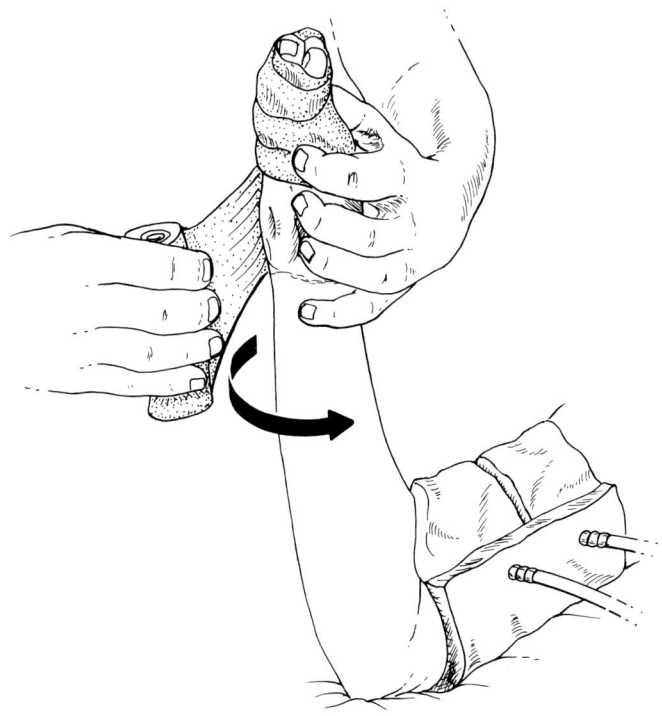

FIGURE 21–3

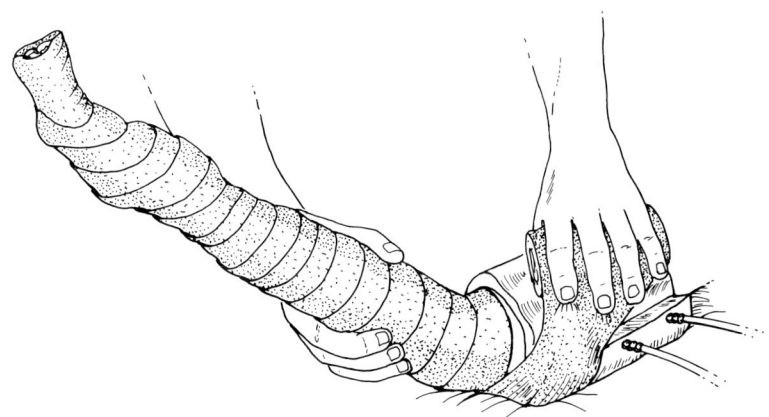

FIGURE 21–4

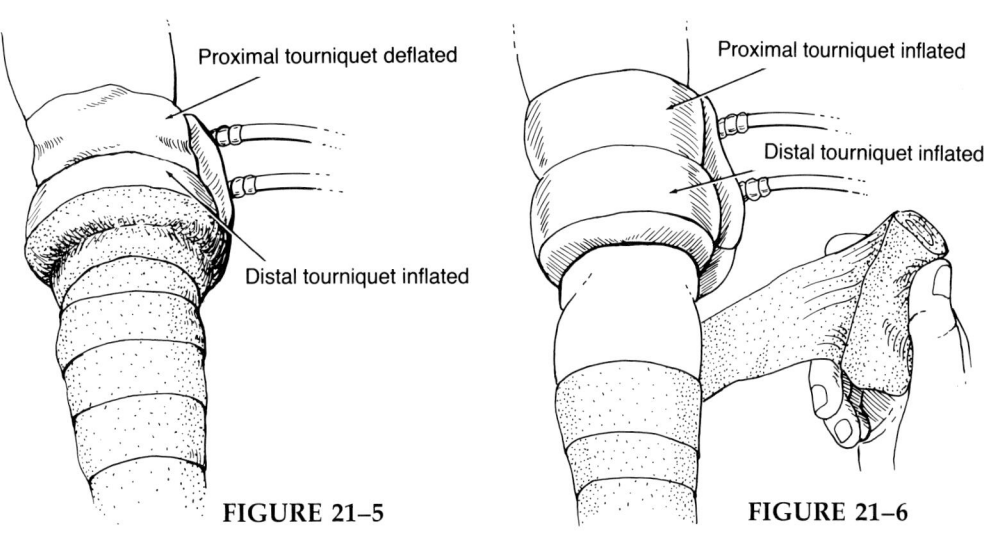

FIGURE 21–5

FIGURE 21–6

Since the dose of local anesthetic to be injected is sufficient to cause severe central nervous system side effects (if it were to be given as an intravenous bolus), it is imperative that the pneumatic tourniquets be fully inflated *before* the local anesthetic is injected.

INJECTION OF ANESTHETIC

In the arm, I inject 40 to 50 ml of 0.5% lidocaine (or prilocaine). In the leg I inject 50 to 70 ml of 0.5% lidocaine (or prilocaine). When the surgery will take place on the hand or fingers, I usually place a small, secondary venous tourniquet around the wrist before injecting the first half of the local anesthetic solution (Fig. 21–7), in an attempt to ensure that the local anesthetic adequately fills the distal veins in the region of the surgery. I then release the secondary tourniquet before injecting the second half of the solution (Fig. 21–8). The anesthesia takes effect within minutes; thus skin preparation by the surgeon should proceed as soon as the local anesthetic has been injected.

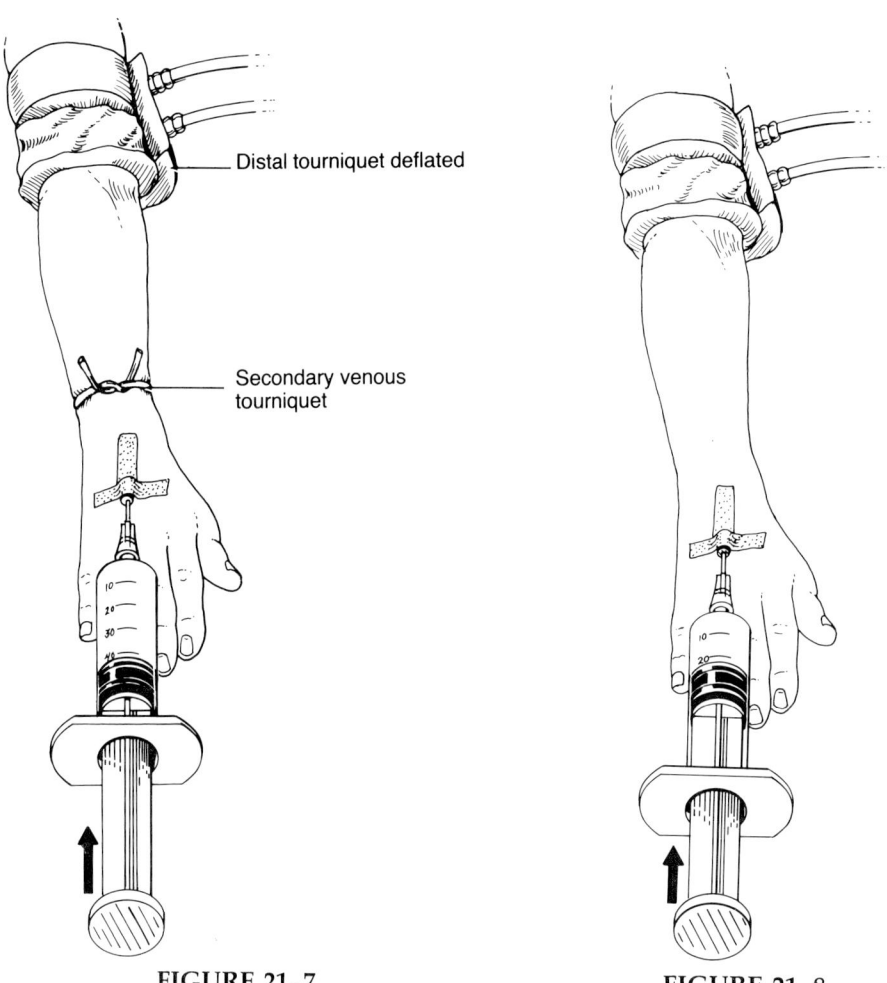

FIGURE 21–7   FIGURE 21–8

INFLATION AND DEFLATION OF TOURNIQUET

If the patient should experience tourniquet discomfort during the anesthesia, inflate the distal tourniquet (which should now overlie an anesthetized area of the extremity). The proximal tourniquet may be deflated after the distal tourniquet is *fully* inflated. I have found that this will usually relieve symptoms of tourniquet pain provided that the procedure lasts no longer than about an hour.

When time comes to release the tourniquet at the completion of surgery, if the surgery has been accomplished in less than 30 minutes I usually deflate the tourniquet briefly (seconds), then reinflate it (attempting to limit the bolus of local anesthetic brought into the circulation) before finally deflating it 2 to 3 minutes later. On the other hand, if the surgery has persisted longer than 30 minutes, I usually just deflate the tourniquet completely and leave it deflated.

References

Grice SC, Morell RC, Balestrieri FJ, Stump DA, Howard G: Intravenous regional anesthesia: Evaluation and prevention of leakage under the tourniquet. Anesthesiology 65:316–320, 1986

Holmes CM: Intravenous regional analgesia. Lancet 1:245–247, 1963

Lillie PE, Glynn CJ, Fenwick DG: Site of action of intravenous regional anesthesia. Anesthesiology 61:507–510, 1984

Sukhani R, Garcia CJ, Munhall RJ, Winnie AP, Rodvold KA: Lidocaine disposition following intravenous regional anesthesia with different tourniquet deflation techniques. Anesth Analg 68:633–637, 1989

22

Digital Nerve Block

Fingers and toes are easily and effectively anesthetized by injection of local anesthetic solutions near the four digital nerves, which course in pairs on either side of the digits. Digital blocks of the hand are commonly used in emergency departments for repair of lacerations. In anesthetic practice, I have found digital blocks useful for reinforcing nascent brachial plexus blocks that are progressing more slowly than I would prefer. Digital blocks can be used for postoperative analgesia in children or others who choose general over regional anesthesia for surgery of the fingers or toes.

Digital block should not be performed with epinephrine-containing local anesthetic solutions because of the risk of digital ischemia.

Technique

EQUIPMENT NEEDED

Sterile gloves
Antiseptic solution
5-ml syringe
25-gauge needle
Local anesthetic (*without epinephrine*)
Usual monitoring devices
Resuscitation drugs and equipment

PROCEDURE

Cleanse the skin of the hand or foot. Inject local anesthetic in the web space between the digit to be blocked and its nearest (lateral) neighbor at the level of the metacarpal (or metatarsal) heads. Advance a 25-gauge needle through the skin wheal (Fig. 22-1). Inject 1 to 2 ml of local anesthetic while continuing to advance the needle in a dorsal to palmar direction, around the proximal phalanx.

Repeat the local anesthetic injection on the other side of the digit.

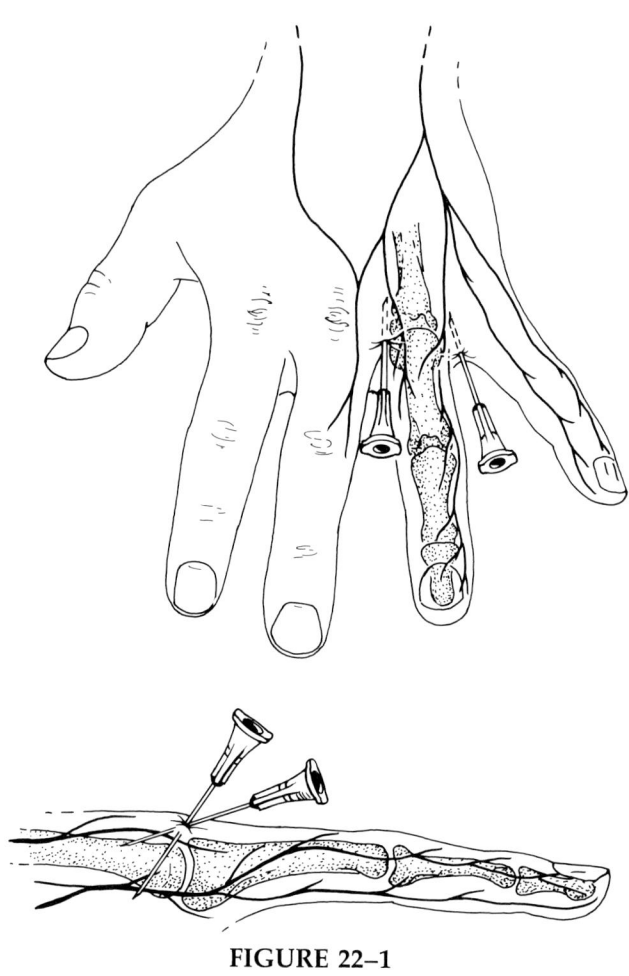

FIGURE 22-1

References

Adriani J: Labat's Regional Anesthesia, ed 4, pp 524–526. St. Louis, Warren H. Green, 1985

Eriksson E: Digital nerve block. In Eriksson E (ed): Illustrated Handbook in Local Anaesthesia, ed 2, p 50. London, Edward Arnold, 1979

Moore DC: Regional Block, ed 4, pp 304–306. Springfield, IL, Charles C Thomas, 1965

Scott DB: Techniques of Regional Anaesthesia, pp 114–115. Norwalk, CT, Appleton & Lange, 1989

23

Upper Extremity Nerve Blocks

Brachial Plexus Block

Brachial plexus block is suitable for nearly all upper extremity surgical procedures. The three most popular approaches to the plexus—axillary, supraclavicular, and interscalene—have a typical distribution of blocked and unblocked nerves following instillation of local anesthetic. Thus, through the choice of technique, the anesthetist can tailor the anesthetic to the operative site. By careful selection of the local anesthetic, the anesthetist can provide anesthesia of whatever duration (<8 hours) the surgeon anticipates will be required. One should choose the best approach to the plexus by the site of surgery rather than by uniformly selecting a "favorite" technique (e.g., axillary block) for all cases. A nerve distribution diagram is provided to assist in the selection of technique (Fig. 23–1).

For all three approaches, I recommend using a blunt "B-bevel" needle attached through an intravenous extension tubing to the syringe of local anesthetic. This arrangement allows the operator to concentrate on maintaining an immobile needle after eliciting paresthesia, while the assistant concentrates on aspiration, test dosing, and injection of the local anesthetic. Likewise, for all major (i.e., other than digital nerve) upper extremity blocks, I recommend that an intravenous infusion be started (if one is not present) and that the electrocardiogram, blood pressure, and arterial oxygen saturation be monitored continuously.

Each technique has been described in numerous variations. I will limit this discussion to what I believe to be simple and effective approaches to each block. Points of controversy and alternative techniques are covered in much greater detail in several of the references.

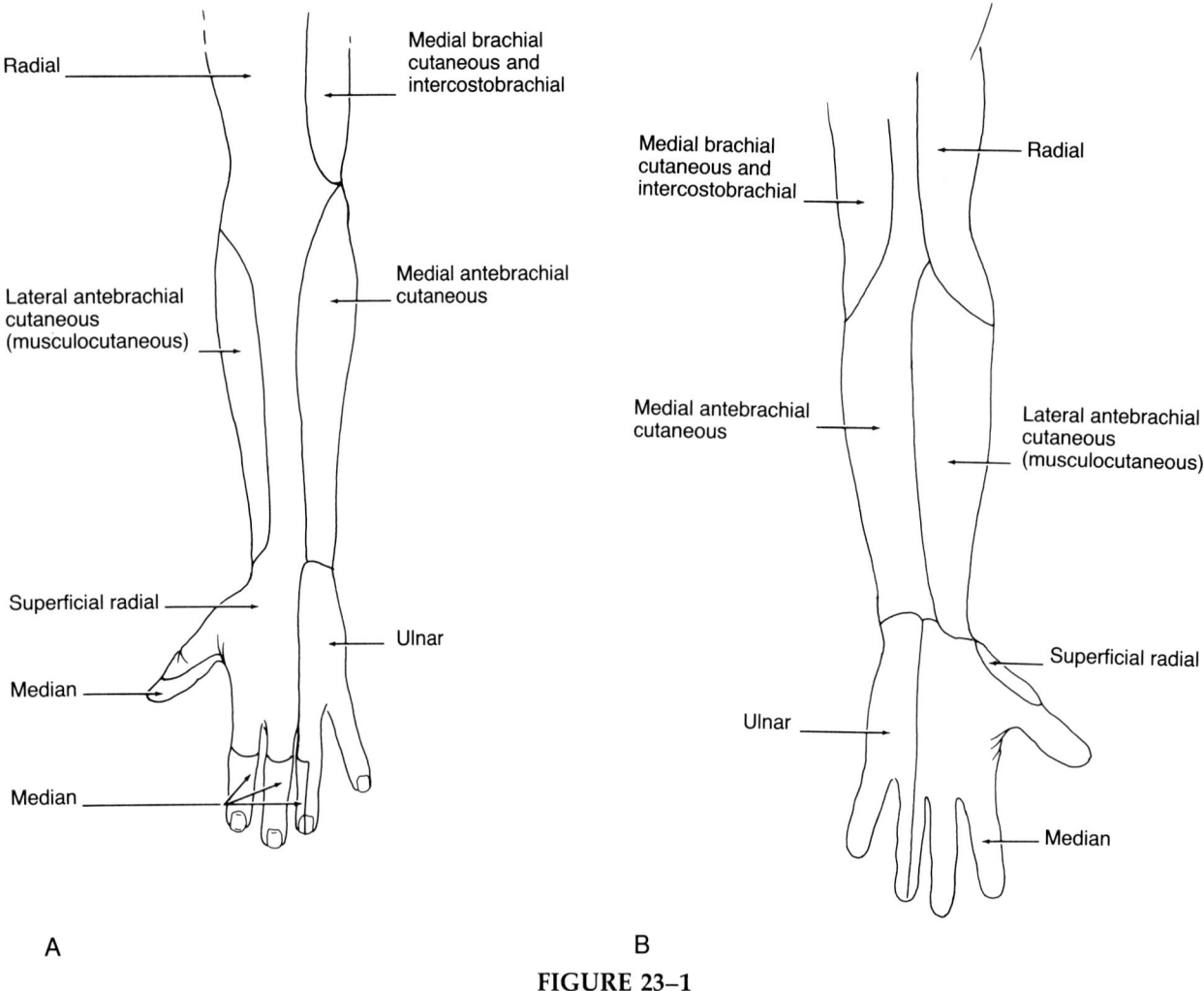

FIGURE 23-1

LOCAL ANESTHETICS

Although a wide variety of local anesthetics have been and can be used for brachial plexus block, I recommend only two of them. Mepivacaine 1.5% can be used for cases in which regional anesthesia is required for 3 hours or less and in which postoperative pain relief is not sought. Thus, mepivacaine is used for most outpatient surgery. For anesthesia of longer duration, I recommend bupivacaine 0.5%. Bupivacaine can also be used in cases in which prolonged postoperative analgesia is desired. I routinely *add* epinephrine (1:400,000) to plain solutions of either mepivacaine or bupivacaine before injecting these drugs for brachial plexus blocks.

EQUIPMENT NEEDED

Sterile gloves
Antiseptic solution
Local anesthetic of choice
Epinephrine
Tuberculin syringe (to measure epinephrine)
Blunt ("B-bevel") needle

Extension tubing
20-ml syringes
Usual monitoring devices
Resuscitation drugs and equipment

AXILLARY APPROACH

The axillary approach to the brachial plexus is an easy and effective technique for providing anesthesia for surgery on the hand and distal forearm. Whether or not full anesthesia of median, ulnar, and radial nerves usually follows a *single* injection of local anesthetic in the axilla remains controversial. Septa separating the nerves within the axillary fascial sheath have been demonstrated in cadaver dissections. Nonetheless, many clinicians advocate a single (large) injection technique. I prefer a conservative approach, in which at least two injections are made to minimize the possibility of an incomplete block.

Accidental intravenous (or intra-arterial) injection of local anesthetic is always a possibility during axillary block. Other complications (axillary hematoma, neuritis) other than unblocked nerves are uncommon.

The most commonly missed nerves during axillary block include the medial brachial cutaneous nerve (which exits the neurovascular fascial sheath proximal to the site of local anesthetic injection), the intercostobrachial nerve (which is not a branch of the brachial plexus), the lateral cutaneous nerve of the forearm (the sensory continuation of the musculocutaneous nerve), and the radial nerve (Fig. 23–2). The first two of these may be blocked by infiltration of 5 ml of local anesthetic in a fanwise fashion into the skin overlying the pulse of the axillary artery. The intercostobrachial and medial brachial cutaneous nerves must be blocked if a pneumatic tourniquet will be placed on the upper arm. The musculocutaneous nerve may be blocked by local anesthetic injection in the axilla, or its sensory branch can be anesthetized selectively in the antecubital fossa. The radial nerve may be blocked by local anesthetic injection in the antecubital fossa or by instillation of local anesthetic at the wrist. These supplementary blocks are described separately.

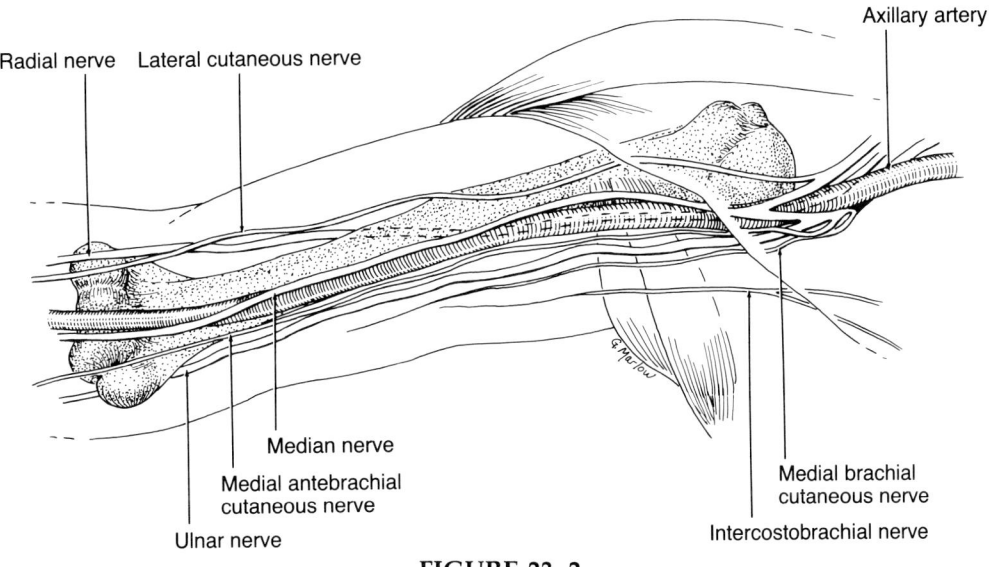

FIGURE 23–2

Preparation and Positioning

Position the patient supine with the arm abducted at 60° to 90° at the shoulder (extreme abduction is *not* helpful), flexed at the elbow, and externally rotated (Fig. 23–3). Cleanse the axilla with antiseptic solution. Inject local anesthetic in the skin overlying the pulse of the axillary artery. Flush local anesthetic solution through the extension tubing and the "B-bevel" needle.

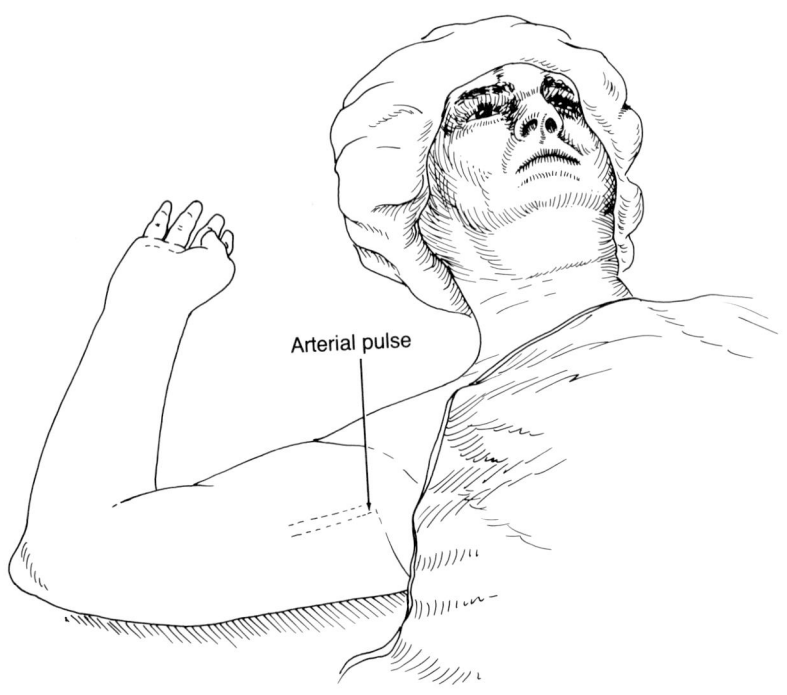

FIGURE 23–3

Needle Insertion

Insert the blunt "B-bevel" needle through the local anesthetic wheal, aiming the "B-bevel" needle superior to the axillary pulse (Fig. 23–4). Have the assistant attempt aspiration with the syringe so that if the needle tip enters the axillary artery or vein, it will be quickly detected. A "pop" may be felt as the needle passes through the fascia surrounding the axillary artery and the brachial plexus. The hope is that a brief paresthesia will be produced in the distribution of the median nerve. Paresthesia must be plainly described in advance as an "electrical shock" or "like hitting your funny bone"; otherwise the patient may misinterpret local discomfort as paresthesia. Some experienced anesthetists use the characteristic feel of the needle passing through the axillary facial sheath as a marker for correct needle placement.

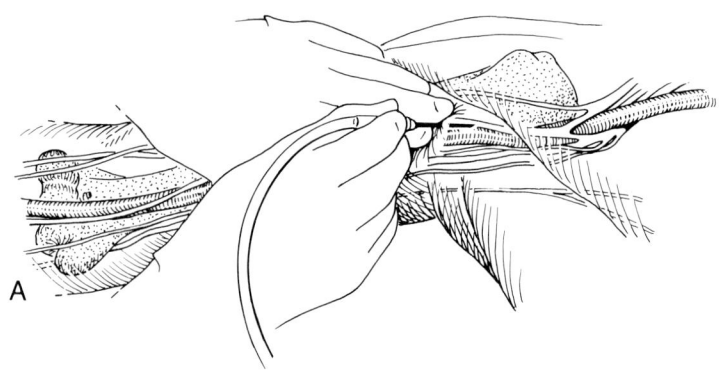

FIGURE 23–4A

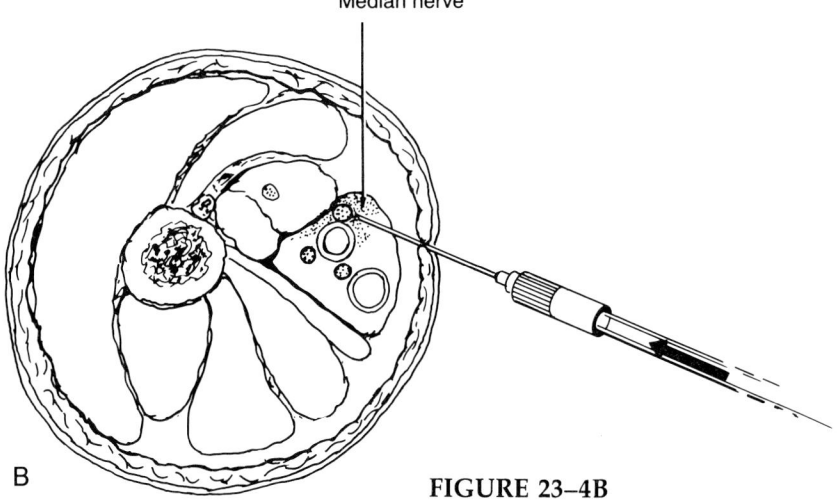

FIGURE 23-4B

Test Dose of Local Anesthetic

When a paresthesia (to the hand or lower arm) is identified by the patient, inject 5 ml of local anesthetic (after aspiration has confirmed that the needle tip is not within a blood vessel). A full 45 to 60 seconds should pass after the first 5-ml injection to be certain that the injection has not entered a blood vessel. Signs of intravenous injection will include tinnitus, circumoral numbness, metallic tastes (all a consequence of the local anesthetic), tachycardia, and hypertension (the latter two are consequences of the added epinephrine). Patients on β-adrenergic receptor blockers may demonstrate hypertension and reflex bradycardia (or no change in heart rate at all) following intravenous injection of an epinephrine-containing test dose.

If there are no signs of intravascular injection, inject half the intended total local anesthetic dose in 5-ml increments. The anesthetist should pause after each 5-ml injection and check by aspiration to be sure that the needle tip has not migrated into a blood vessel.

Second Injection

Next, redirect the needle inferiorly, aiming at or below the axillary arterial pulse (Fig. 23-5). If a second paresthesia is obtained in the radial or ulnar nerve distribu-

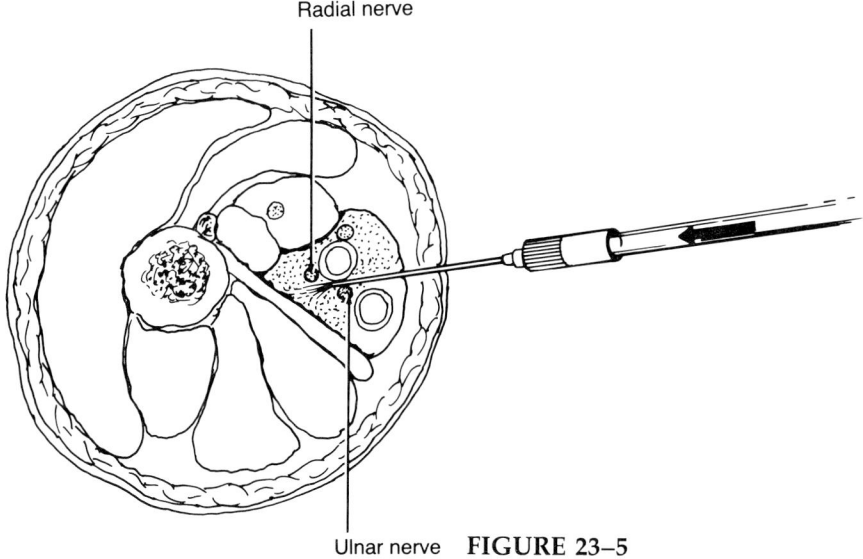

FIGURE 23-5

tion, inject local anesthetic (after test dosing) as described previously. Alternatively, if the axillary artery or vein is penetrated, advance the needle until its tip lies just behind the posterior wall of the artery (i.e., blood can no longer be aspirated from the needle), then inject half the remaining anesthetic in 5-ml increments (Fig. 23–6). Next, withdraw the needle until its tip lies just anterior to the anterior wall of the vessel (i.e., blood can no longer be aspirated from the needle, but the needle is still within the axillary fascial sheath). Here, inject the remaining anesthetic in 5-ml increments. The total local anesthetic volume is usually about 0.6 ml/kg.

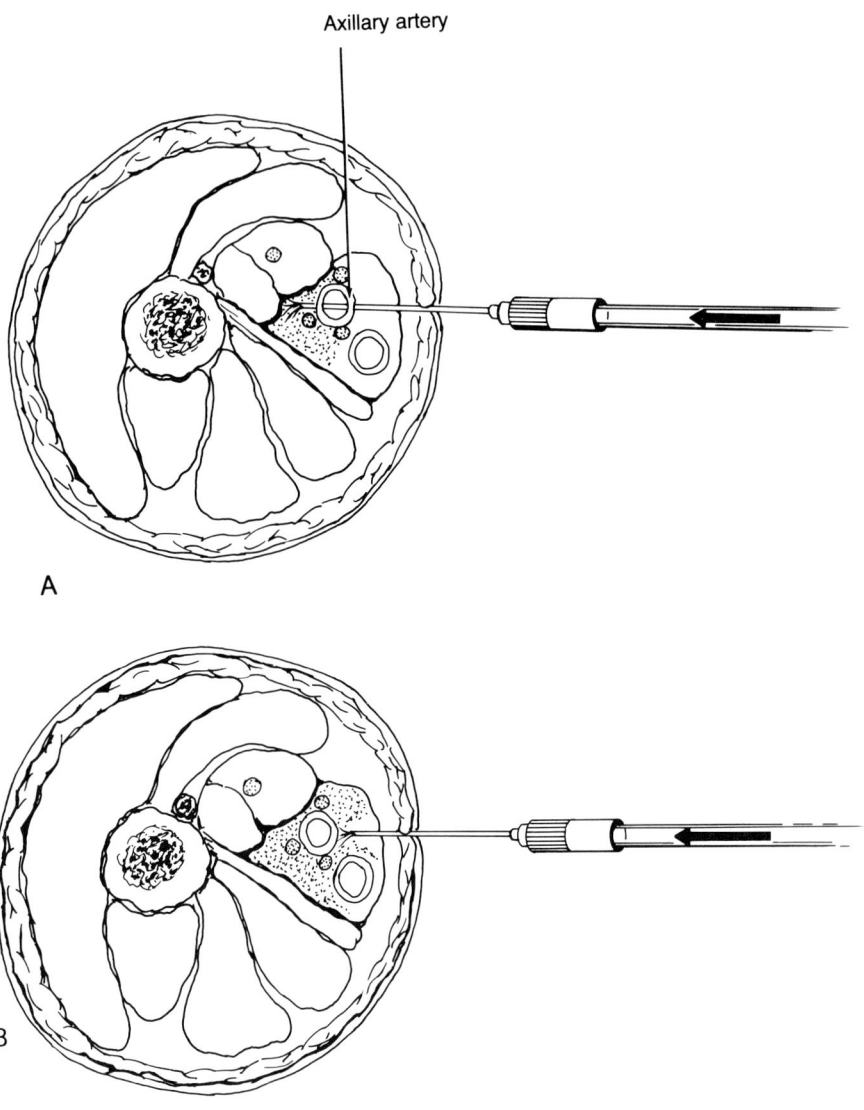

FIGURE 23–6

Transarterial vs. Paresthesia Technique

In many cases, the artery (or less commonly, the vein) will be entered before any paresthesia is obtained. I accept axillary arterial puncture as a sure sign that the axillary fascial sheath has been entered and inject the local anesthetic (half on either side of the blood vessel). Although I do *not* regard arterial puncture as a failure, I prefer to produce a brief paresthesia in the nerve distribution of the intended surgery, before injecting local anesthetic, if possible.

SUPRACLAVICULAR APPROACH

The supraclavicular approach to the brachial plexus has several important advantages and one equally important disadvantage over the axillary and interscalene approaches. Of the three techniques, the supraclavicular approach is the least likely to produce incomplete anesthesia. The anatomy is simple, and the onset of anesthesia is faster than with either the axillary or interscalene blocks. On the other hand, this is the only approach to the brachial plexus that carries a significant risk of a *surgical* complication (i.e., pneumothorax). Even in experienced hands the risk of pneumothorax is probably at least 1%. Admittedly, the pneumothoraces produced usually are small, usually do not present with significant hemodynamic or respiratory distress, and usually do not require tube thoracostomy drainage (most often they will be absorbed spontaneously). Nonetheless, the fear of pneumothorax deters many clinicians from using what I believe to be the most versatile technique for brachial plexus blockade. The supraclavicular approach is ideally suited for surgery of the upper arm, forearm, or hand and is a superior choice to axillary block for any operation at the level of or proximal to the antecubital fossa.

Preparation and Positioning

Position the patient supine with his head turned to the side opposite the site of intended needle puncture. Wash the skin of the neck and shoulder with antiseptic solution.

Palpate the "interscalene groove" between the anterior and middle scalene muscles, just posterior to the posterior border of the sternocleidomastoid muscle. Trace the interscalene groove caudad toward the clavicle (Fig. 23–7). The subclavian arterial pulse can usually be palpated in the interscalene groove behind the clavicle. The brachial plexus lies immediately posterior to the subclavian artery as the plexus courses over the first rib and dives under the clavicle on its way to the axilla. Sometimes, the first rib itself can be palpated behind the clavicle. "Stretch" the plexus by having the patient "reach" for the knee on the side of the block.

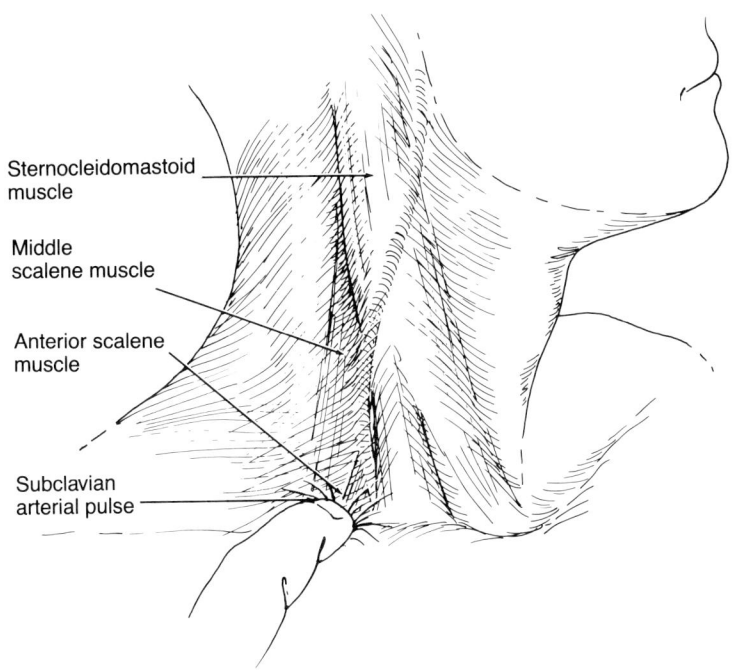

FIGURE 23–7

Needle Insertion

Inject local anesthetic in the skin posterior to the palpating finger (which should remain on the subclavian artery pulse) in the interscalene groove.

Advance the blunt ("B-bevel") needle caudad (aimed at the feet) through the skin wheal, so that it passes just dorsad to the subclavian artery pulse (Fig. 23–8). Usually a paresthesia will be encountered on the first or second pass. If not, the needle will often touch the first rib at a depth of 1.0 to 1.5 cm. In that event, the course of the first rib must be visualized so that the needle tip can be "walked"

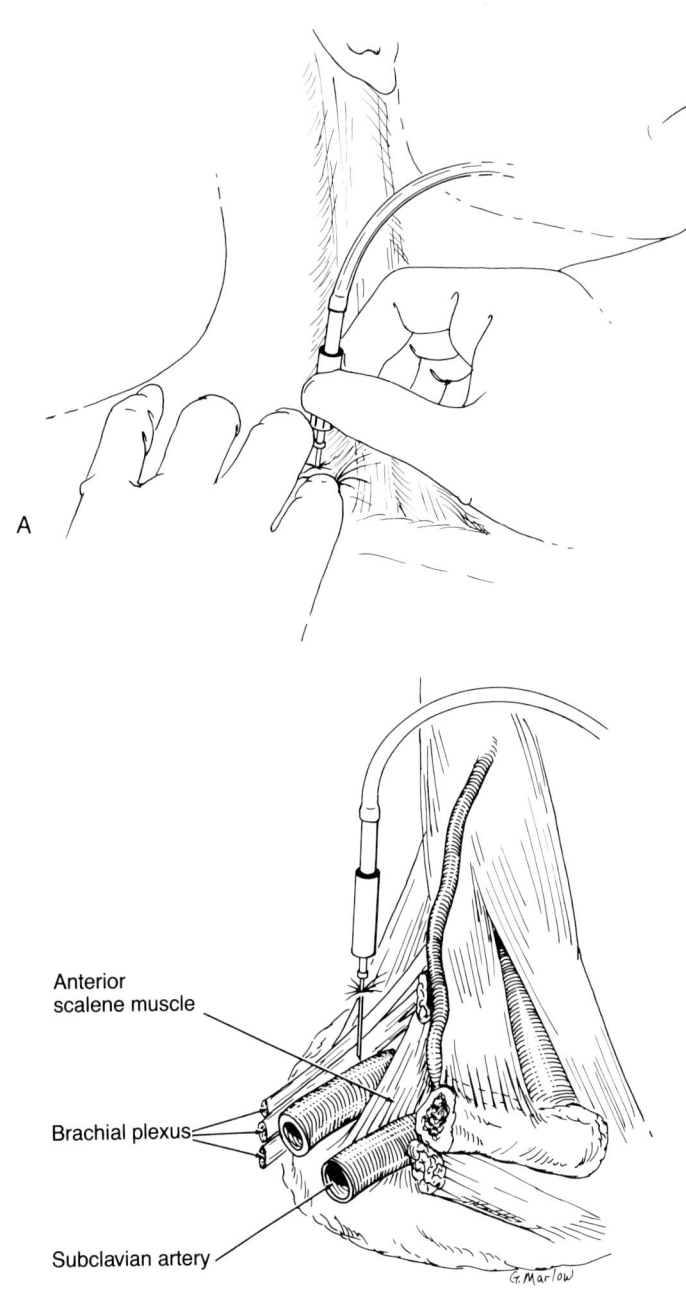

FIGURE 23–8

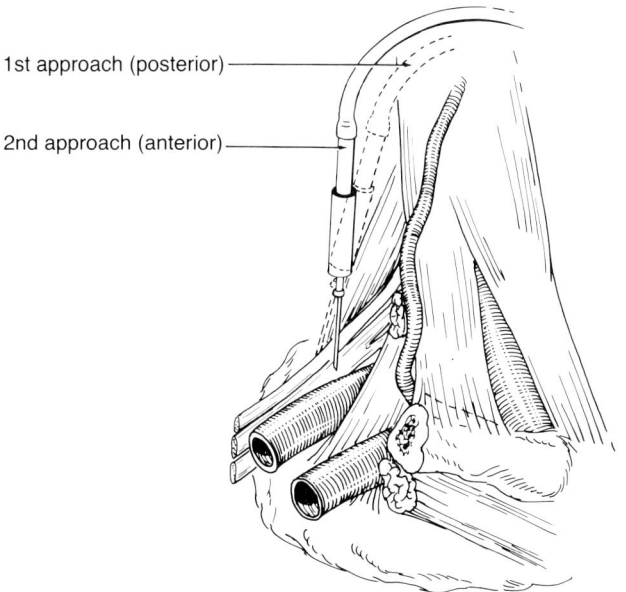

FIGURE 23–9

along the rib in the direction of the brachial plexus (Fig. 23–9). The needle must be withdrawn nearly to the skin before each pass. Usually, the needle should be advanced in a mostly anterior but slightly medial direction. It is important not to "walk" off the rib and to remember that the plexus is superficial. A pneumothorax may result if the needle tip enters the cupola of the lung (which lies inferior and both medial and lateral to the first rib). Any paresthesia felt in the arm below the shoulder indicates correct needle placement.

Injection of Local Anesthetic

Unlike axillary and interscalene blocks, supraclavicular block carries a low risk of accidental intravascular injection of local anesthetic. Nevertheless, the initial 5-ml injection should be preceded by aspiration and followed by close observation of the patient to be certain that the needle tip has not migrated into the subclavian artery.

When the first few milliliters of anesthetic is injected, the patient will often complain of an "aching," "pressure" sensation, which would lead one to suspect an intraneural injection if it had been elicited during attempted axillary block. These usually worrisome sensations nearly always occur during successful supraclavicular blocks. Subsequent injections (after the first 5 ml) up to the 25 to 35 ml required to produce complete blockade usually are not accompanied by pressure paresthesias. The minimum volume of local anesthetic required for the supraclavicular approach is less than that required for axillary or interscalene approaches. I usually administer between 0.3 and 0.5 ml/kg.

Onset of Anesthesia

The onset of anesthesia from supraclavicular block can be extremely rapid. On occasion I have seen a completely anesthetic, immobile arm less than 10 minutes following supraclavicular injection of bupivacaine. Onset of anesthesia is rarely as rapid when using either of the other two approaches. Nonetheless, the onset of anesthesia should be carefully monitored so that supplementation, if necessary, can be administered without delay.

INTERSCALENE APPROACH

The interscalene approach is the technique of choice for providing regional anesthesia of the upper arm and shoulder through brachial plexus blockade. Conversely, it is the least desirable technique of the three brachial plexus approaches for surgery on the hand. The interscalene approach has a set of unique complications. Misdirected needles near the spine can result in local anesthetic injected into carotid or vertebral arteries or the epidural or subarachnoid spaces. Successful anesthesia will always be accompanied by signs of the Horner syndrome (ptosis, miosis, anhydrosis, scleral injection, ipsilateral flushing of the face) and usually by phrenic nerve block. Thus the interscalene approach should be avoided in patients who will not tolerate unilateral diaphragmatic paralysis. Concurrent bilateral interscalene blocks are not recommended!

Preparation and Positioning

Position the patient supine with the head turned to the side opposite the site of intended needle puncture. Cleanse the skin of the neck and shoulder with antiseptic solution. Depress the shoulder inferiorly by asking the patient to "reach for the knee." Identify the "interscalene groove," located between the anterior and middle scalene muscles (posterior to the sternocleidomastoid muscle) (Fig. 23–10). Identify the Chassaignac tubercle (the transverse process of the sixth cervical vertebra) by *gentle* palpation. The Chassaignac tubercle, the most prominent cervical transverse process, is at approximately the same level as the cricoid cartilage. Vigorous palpation of this bone is most uncomfortable.

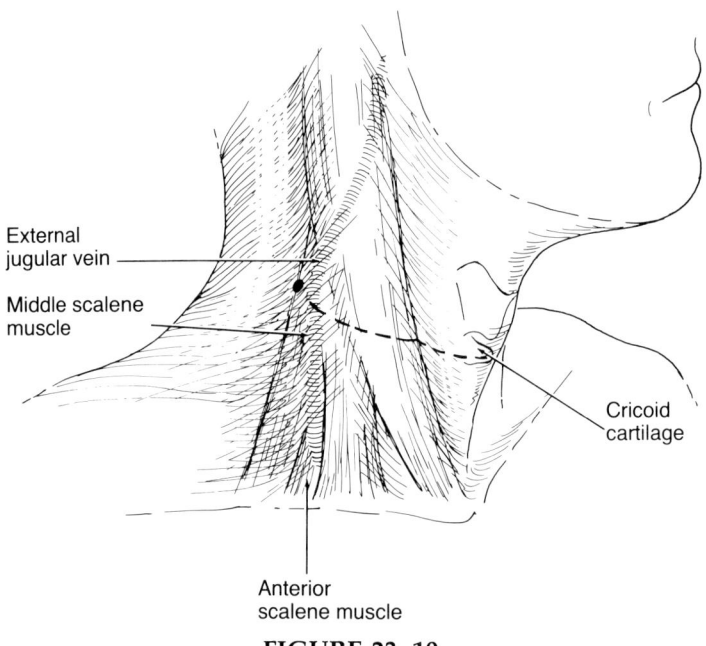

FIGURE 23–10

Needle Insertion

Inject local anesthetic in the skin overlying the interscalene groove, superior to the Chassaignac tubercle. Often this will coincide with the site where the external jugular vein crosses the interscalene groove (Fig. 23–11). Insert the blunt tip ("B-bevel") needle through the skin wheal, and aim it caudally, medially, and along the axis of the interscalene groove, toward the superior surface of the Chassaignac tubercle.

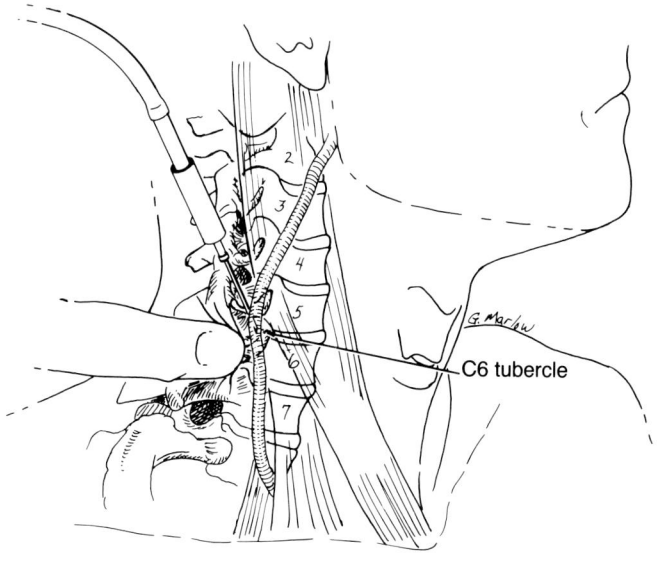

FIGURE 23–11

Do not aim the needle superiorly or directly medially, because of the increased risk of passing the needle between the transverse processes into such aberrant locations as the vertebral artery or spinal canal. The natural, downward "aim" of the intervertebral foramina makes an inferiorly directed needle a safer option.

Paresthesias below the shoulder indicate correct placement of the needle. Do not be tempted to accept a paresthesia to the top of the shoulder or to the back. The dorsal scapular nerve exits from the brachial plexus very proximally (near the site of attempted interscalene block). I (sadly) have on occasion injected local anesthetic after producing a paresthesia to the shoulder, resulting in a splendid, dense anesthesia of the dorsal scapular nerve but no block of the brachial plexus.

Injection of Local Anesthetic

When an acceptable paresthesia is obtained, and only if careful aspiration has yielded neither cerebrospinal fluid nor blood, inject a 5-ml test dose of local anesthetic. While the test dose is small and will produce only brief symptoms if the solution is injected accidentally into a vein, if the solution is injected into either the vertebral or carotid arteries (either artery may be entered by accident during interscalene block), less than 1 ml of local anesthetic may be sufficient to produce a seizure. Moreover, 5 ml of local anesthetic injected into the cervical cerebrospinal fluid will usually produce total spinal anesthesia. Finally, in the rare circumstance that the needle has been placed in the cervical epidural space, test doses and aspiration will demonstrate no (immediate) adverse responses. Unfortunately, only 5 to 7 ml of local anesthetic is required to produce solid cervical epidural anesthesia. Thus when a volume of local anesthetic appropriate for interscalene block is injected in the cervical epidural space, a "total" epidural anesthesia will be likely.

The total volume of local anesthetic necessary to achieve full anesthesia in an adult is usually about 0.6 ml/kg, in common with axillary block. The most commonly unblocked regions following attempted interscalene block are served by C8 and T1. Following injection of local anesthetic, the onset of anesthesia should be carefully monitored so that supplementation (if required) can be provided in a timely fashion. If the C8 and T1 nerve roots remain unblocked and anesthesia in the ulnar distribution is required for hand surgery, supplementation is easily accomplished by ulnar nerve block at the elbow or wrist. If surgery is on the forearm, anesthesia of the medial antebrachial cutaneous nerve, also a product of C8 and T1 nerve roots, must be obtained.

Block of the Musculocutaneous Nerve and Its Branches

Owing to the very proximal emergence of the musculocutaneous nerve from the lateral cord of the brachial plexus, an otherwise complete axillary block may occasionally leave this nerve unanesthetized. The musculocutaneous nerve supplies the biceps, coracobrachialis, and brachioradialis muscles; thus, block of the musculocutaneous nerve prevents flexion of the forearm at the elbow. The lateral cutaneous nerve of the forearm, the sensory continuation of the musculocutaneous nerve, supplies the sensory innervation of the skin on the radial side of the forearm. Depending on the intended duration of the surgery, inject either 1.5% mepivacaine with 1:400,000 epinephrine or 0.5% bupivacaine with 1:400,000 epinephrine.

Supplemental anesthesia of the musculocutaneous nerve can be accomplished proximally by injection of local anesthetic into the coracobrachialis muscle in the axilla. Alternatively, the lateral cutaneous nerve of the forearm can be anesthetized using a technique nearly identical to that for radial nerve block.

EQUIPMENT NEEDED

Sterile gloves
Antiseptic solution
Local anesthetic of choice
Epinephrine
Tuberculin syringe (to measure epinephrine)
5-ml syringe
22-gauge needle
25-gauge needle
Usual monitoring devices
Resuscitation drugs and equipment

MUSCULOCUTANEOUS NERVE BLOCK

Cleanse the axilla with antiseptic solution. Identify the coracobrachialis muscle, which is caudad and adjacent to the biceps muscle. Inject local anesthetic in the skin overlying the coracobrachialis muscle (Fig. 23–12). Advance a 22-gauge needle through the skin wheal and inject 5 ml of local anesthetic in a fanwise fashion into the muscle.

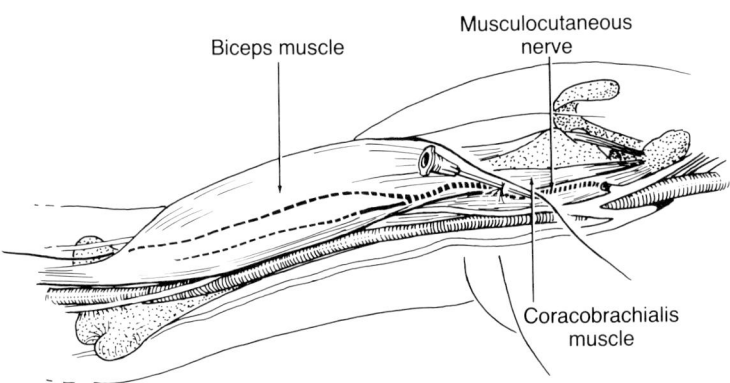

FIGURE 23–12

LATERAL CUTANEOUS NERVE BLOCK

Cleanse the skin of the antecubital fossa with antiseptic solution. Inject local anesthetic in the skin overlying the cleft between the tendon of biceps and the origin of brachioradialis.

The lateral cutaneous nerve of the forearm lies medial to the radial nerve in the cleft between the tendon of biceps and the origin of the brachioradialis. Insert a 22-gauge needle through the skin wheal lateral to the biceps tendon in the intercondylar line (Fig. 23–13). Both radial and musculocutaneous nerves are relatively superficial at this point; thus, needle insertions should be no deeper than 1 cm and directed toward the lateral epicondyle. A paresthesia in the distribution of either the radial nerve or the lateral cutaneous nerve of the forearm indicates the correct location of the needle tip. After aspiration, inject 5 ml of local anesthetic.

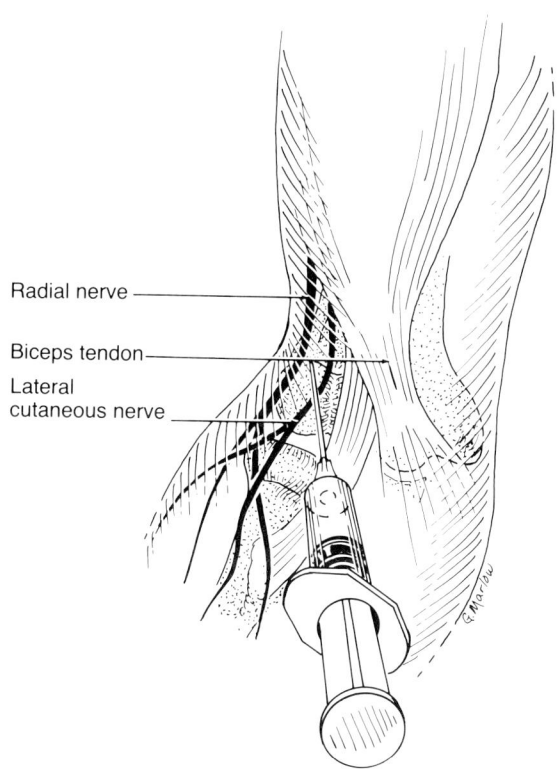

FIGURE 23–13

Nerve Blocks at the Elbow

Although blocks of the median, ulnar, and radial nerves at the elbow may be used for complete anesthesia of the hand, these blocks (and blocks of the lateral cutaneous nerve of the forearm) are most useful for supplementation of brachial plexus anesthesia. Most orthopedists, neurosurgeons, and plastic surgeons prefer to use the pneumatic tourniquet placed on the upper arm during hand surgery, for which nerve blocks at the elbow will provide inadequate anesthesia.

Some anesthesiologists avoid ulnar block at the elbow, fearing that any postoperative paresthesias (or subsequent ulnar nerve injuries) will be blamed on the nerve block procedure. I see no reason not to use ulnar nerve blocks when they are clearly indicated—usually to supplement incomplete brachial plexus anesthesia.

I recommend use of the same local anesthetics for nerve blocks at the elbow that I use for brachial plexus block (either mepivacaine 1.5% with 1:400,000 epinephrine for shorter procedures or bupivacaine 0.5% with 1:400,000 epinephrine for longer procedures).

EQUIPMENT NEEDED

Gloves
Antiseptic solution
Local anesthetic of choice
Epinephrine
Tuberculin syringe (to measure epinephrine)
22-gauge needle
25-gauge needle
Usual monitoring devices
Resuscitation drugs and equipment

ULNAR NERVE BLOCK

Position the patient supine on the operating room table. Cleanse the skin of the elbow with antiseptic solution. Flex the patient's arm at the elbow at about 90°. Bring the arm over and across the patient's chest. Advance the needle through the skin between the medial epicondyle of the humerus and the olecranon process of the ulna seeking a brief paresthesia to the little finger (Fig. 23–14).

After eliciting a paresthesia (to the little or ring finger), slowly inject less than 1 ml of local anesthetic. If the paresthesia recurs during the initial injection, withdraw the needle by a few millimeters and reinject a second test dose. When no paresthesia is obtained during injection of the test dose, inject the remainder of the anesthetic for a total dose of 5 ml.

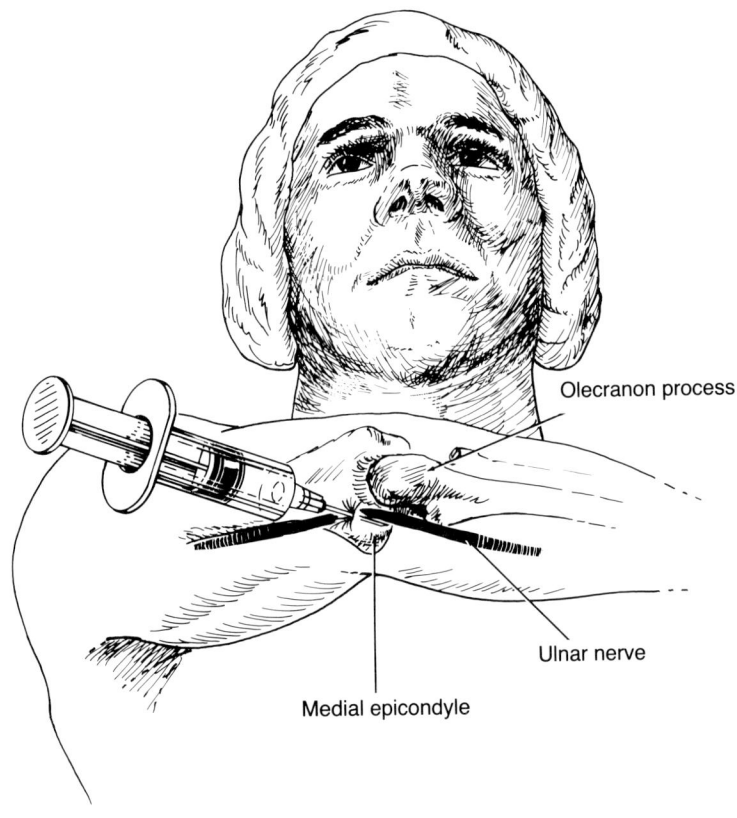

FIGURE 23–14

MEDIAN NERVE BLOCK

Position the patient supine on the operating room table. Cleanse the skin of the antecubital fossa with antiseptic solution. Palpate the brachial artery. The tendon of the biceps lies lateral to the artery; the insertion of the pronator teres lies medial to the artery. Create a skin wheal of local anesthetic medial to the pulse of the brachial artery, proximal to the elbow crease. Advance the needle medial to the brachial pulse, "popping" through the lacertus fibrosus (bicipital aponeurosis) (Fig. 23–15).

When a paresthesia is obtained (felt in the index or middle finger), the needle should be gently aspirated (given the close proximity of the brachial artery) and a small test dose (<1 ml) of local anesthetic injected.

If the paresthesia does not recur during injection of the test dose, the remainder of the 5 ml of local anesthetic should be injected. If the paresthesia recurs during injection, the needle should be withdrawn 1 mm and a second test dose given, as described for ulnar nerve block, before injecting the full local anesthetic dose (5 ml).

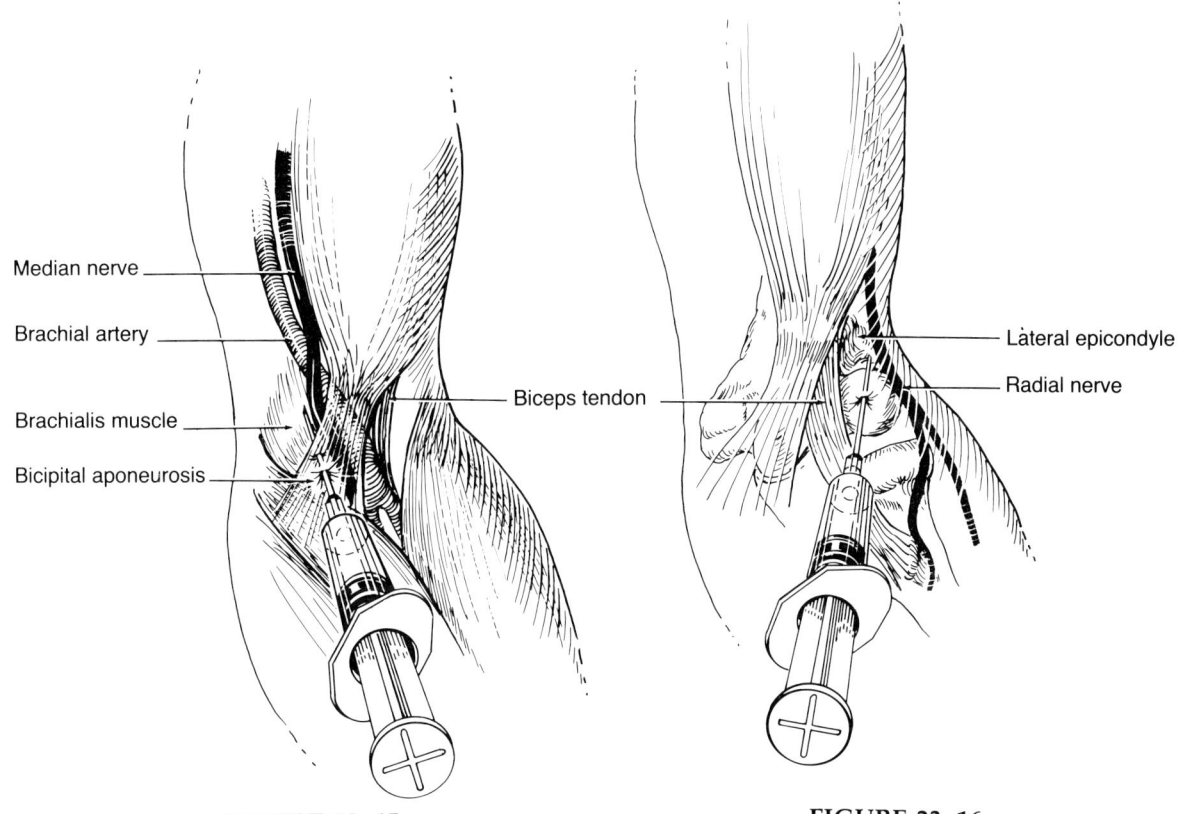

FIGURE 23–15   FIGURE 23–16

RADIAL NERVE BLOCK

Position the patient supine on the operating room table. Cleanse the skin of the antecubital fossa with antiseptic solution. Palpate the lateral border of the biceps tendon and the medial border of the brachioradialis muscle. Create a skin wheal of local anesthetic proximal to the elbow crease in the fossa between the biceps and brachioradialis.

Advance the needle in the midline of the fossa toward the lateral epicondyle of the humerus (Fig. 23–16). If the bone is contacted before a paresthesia is obtained, the needle should be redirected in a more lateral fashion.

When a paresthesia is obtained (usually to the back of the hand), aspiration, test dosing, and local anesthetic injection (5 ml) should proceed as described for median and ulnar blocks. If no paresthesia is obtained, 5 ml of local anesthetic may be injected fanwise as the needle is withdrawn from the lateral epicondyle.

Nerve Blocks at the Wrist

Blocks of the median, radial, and ulnar nerves at the wrist are useful techniques for emergency department work and for supplementation of a nearly complete brachial plexus block in which the local anesthetic has "overlooked" one of the three nerves (or has "overlooked" nerve roots or trunks that terminate in an unblocked nerve) (Fig. 23–17). These blocks can also be used to speed the onset of what is anticipated to be a completely successful brachial plexus block so that surgery can begin sooner. These blocks are usually not suitable for providing complete anesthesia for hand surgery owing to the use of the pneumatic tourniquet by most surgeons and to innervation of the deep structures of the hand by branches of the radial nerve's main trunk in the forearm.

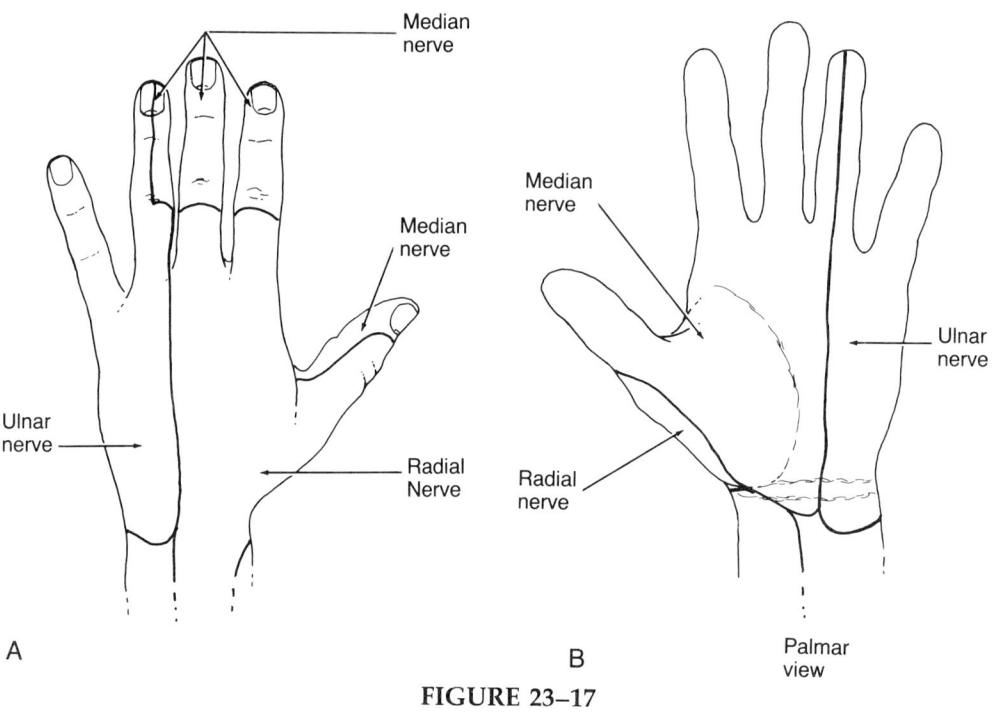

FIGURE 23–17

I recommend the same local anesthetics that I use for brachial plexus block (either mepivacaine 1.5% with 1:400,000 epinephrine for procedures lasting 3 hours or less or bupivacaine 0.5% with 1:400,000 epinephrine for procedures lasting more than 3 hours) for median and ulnar nerve blocks. I block the radial nerve with local anesthetic solutions one half as concentrated as those for the other two nerves.

EQUIPMENT NEEDED

Sterile gloves
Antiseptic solution
Local anesthetic of choice
Epinephrine
Tuberculin syringe (to measure epinephrine)
10-ml syringe and needles
25-gauge, 22-gauge needles
Usual monitoring devices
Resuscitation drugs and equipment

MEDIAN NERVE BLOCK

Position the patient supine on the operating room table with the operative wrist's palmar surface uppermost. Cleanse the skin of the wrist and hand with antiseptic solution.

Have the patient forcibly extend his fingers so that the tendon of the palmaris longus (this muscle is absent in 10% to 20% of normal persons) and of the flexor carpi radialis may be palpated. The median nerve lies between these two structures (but closer to the palmaris longus), passing beneath the deep transverse carpal ligament into the carpal tunnel (schematized in Fig. 23–18).

Create a skin wheal of local anesthetic between the two tendons in line with the styloid process of the ulna. If the palmaris longus is absent, inject the local anesthetic at the midpoint of the most proximal wrist crease, in line with the styloid process.

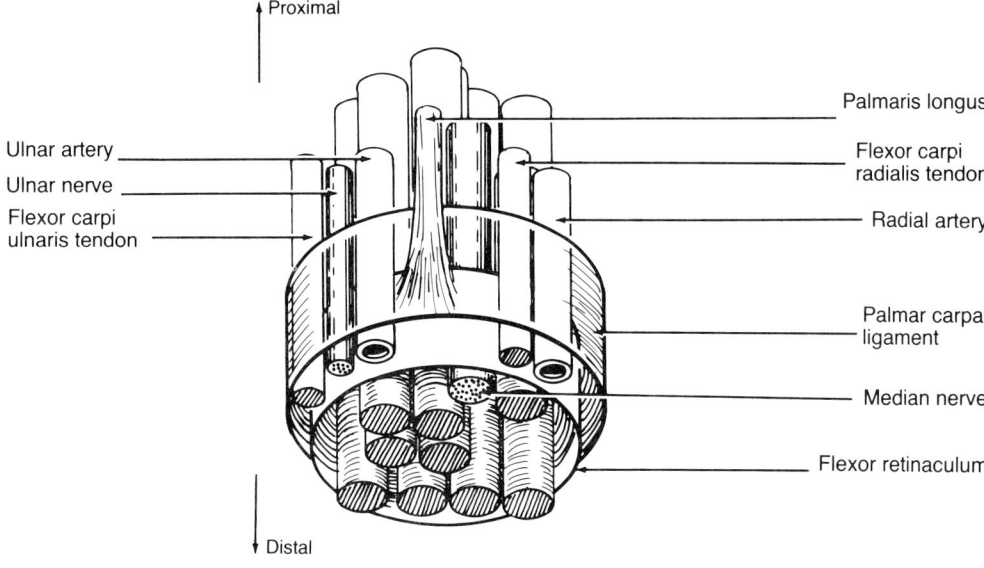

FIGURE 23–18

Advance a 22-gauge needle through the skin wheal lateral to the palmaris longus tendon (or just radial to the midline if the tendon is absent) 0.5 to 0.75 cm until the needle is felt to "pop" through the deep transverse carpal ligament (Fig. 23-19).

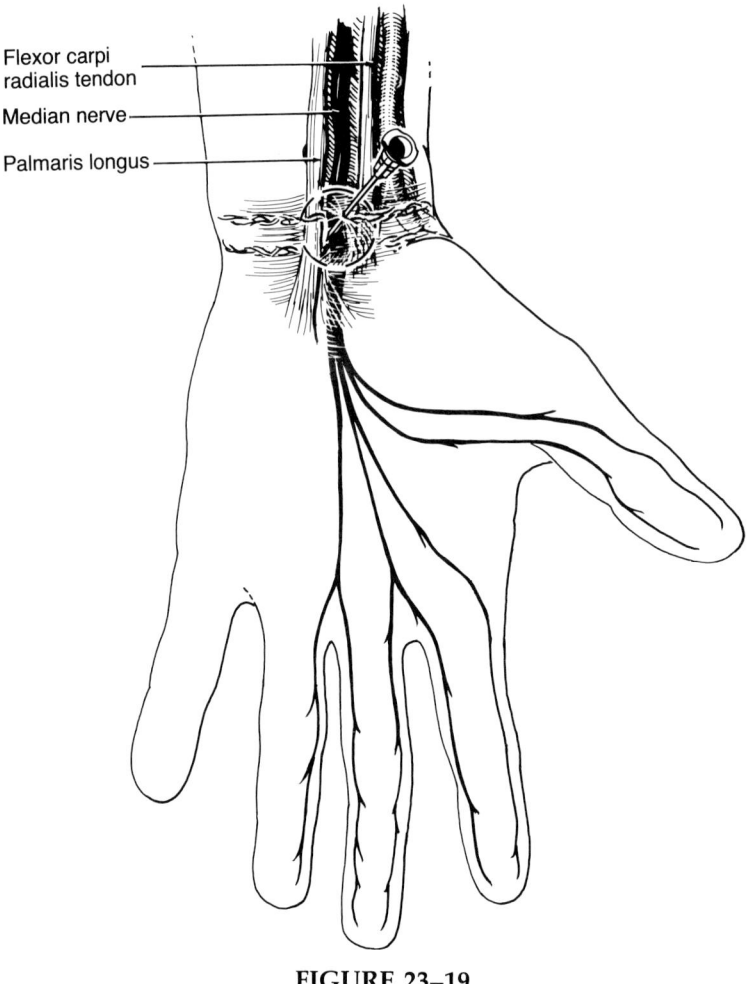

FIGURE 23-19

Paresthesias need not be sought before slowly injecting 5 ml of anesthetic. Rapid injection of local anesthetic will reliably produce a "pressure paresthesia" much like that often obtained during either supraclavicular block or caudal anesthesia.

If a paresthesia is obtained during needle insertion (usually felt in the index or long finger), the initial injection should be less than 1 ml. Be certain that the paresthesia is not intensified by injection of local anesthetic, a sign of possible intraneural injection. If the paresthesia recurs during injection, the needle should be withdrawn 1 to 2 mm and a repeat test dose performed before injecting the full 5 ml of anesthetic.

ULNAR NERVE BLOCK

Position the patient supine on the operating room table with the operative wrist's palmar surface uppermost. Cleanse the skin of the wrist and hand with antiseptic solution.

Palpate the styloid process of the ulna and the pisiform bone. Just medial to the styloid process lie (in sequence) the tendon of the flexor carpi ulnaris, the ulnar nerve, and the ulnar artery.

Create a skin wheal of local anesthetic between the pulse of the ulnar artery and the flexor carpi ulnaris tendon, between the level of the ulnar styloid and the pisiform bone. This is usually in line with the proximal wrist crease (Fig. 23–20).

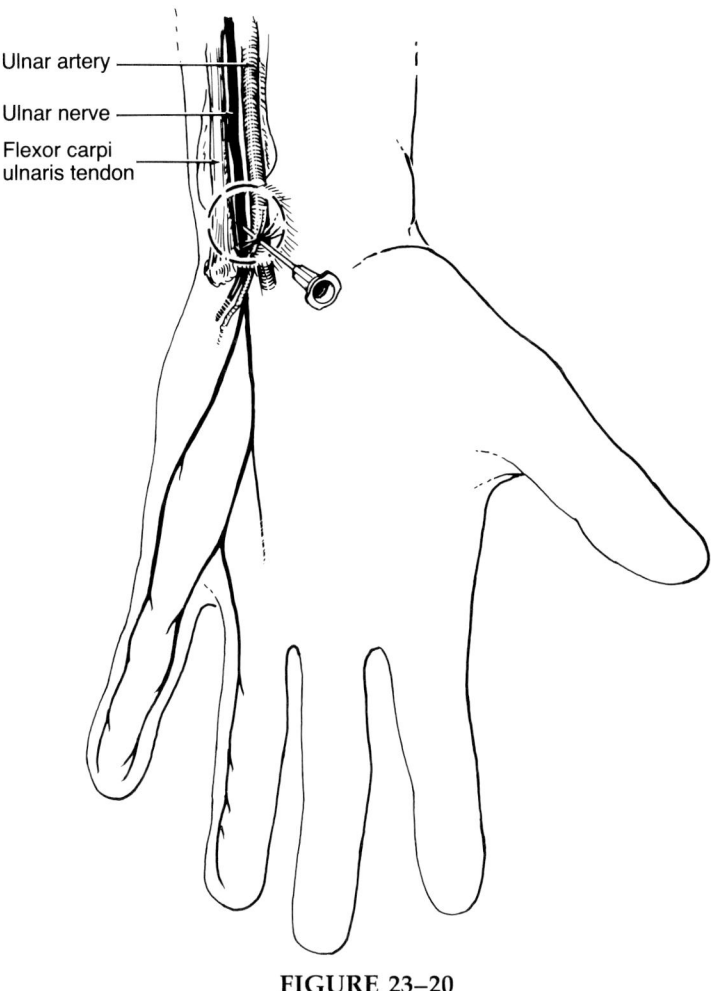

FIGURE 23–20

Advance a 22-gauge needle through the skin wheal, medial to the pulse of the ulnar artery and radial to the tendon of flexor carpi ulnaris. A "pop" may be felt as the needle passes through the superficial transverse carpal ligament. The ulnar nerve is relatively superficial to the median nerve and to the deep transverse carpal ligament.

If the artery is entered, the needle should be redirected in a slightly more medial direction. A paresthesia need not be obtained.

Aspiration should be carefully done before injecting local anesthetic owing to the close proximity of the ulnar artery. Moreover, if a paresthesia is obtained (to the little finger and/or ulnar side of the ring finger) the initial injection should be less than 1 ml to be certain that the needle tip is not located within the nerve. Five milliliters of local anesthetic should be slowly injected.

The dorsal branch of the ulnar nerve may emerge from the main trunk of the ulnar nerve proximal to the point of local anesthetic injection. Sometimes this dorsal branch must be anesthetized separately for complete anesthesia of the dorsal hand surface. In such cases, 2 ml of local anesthetic must be injected intradermally starting above the styloid process and continuing on around to the midpoint of the dorsal surface of the wrist.

RADIAL NERVE BLOCK

Position the patient supine on the operating room table. The arm should be abducted, the forearm extended, and the hand and wrist partially supinated. Cleanse the skin of the hand, wrist, and lower forearm with antiseptic solution (Fig. 23–21).

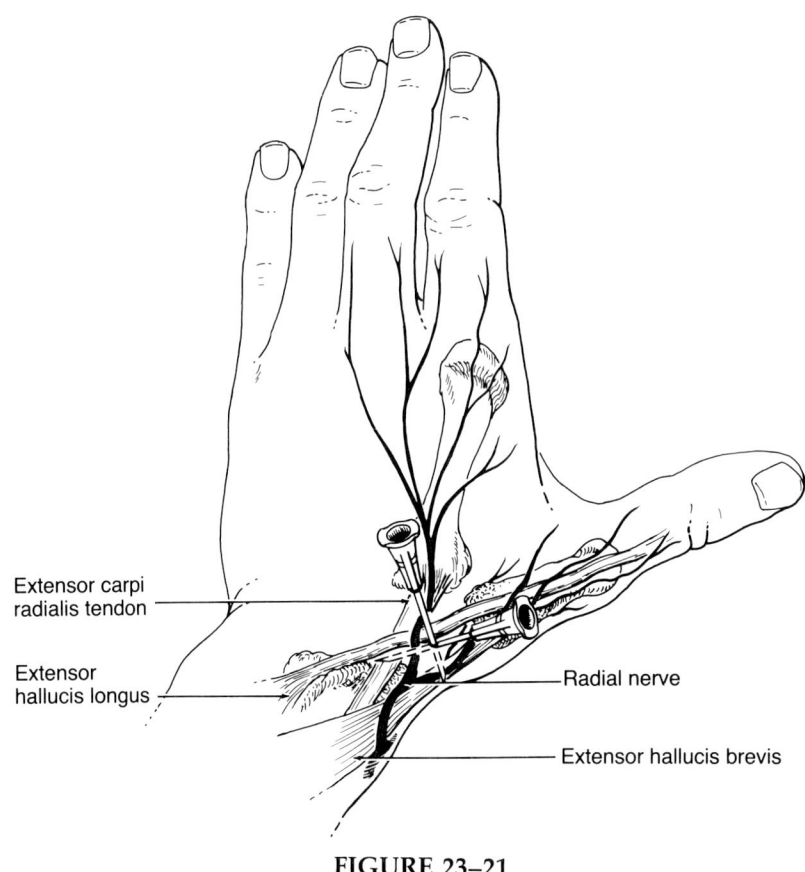

FIGURE 23–21

Local anesthetic is injected on the lateral aspect of the wrist, intradermally and subcutaneously, starting with the "anatomic snuffbox," 0.5 ml distal to the styloid process of the radius, and continuing over the dorsal surface of the hand up to the skin overlying the extensor carpi radialis and over the palmar surface of the hand to the skin overlying the radial pulse. Five milliliters of dilute local anesthetic (half the concentration used for median, ulnar, or brachial plexus block) is appropriate.

References

BRACHIAL PLEXUS BLOCK

Adriani J: Labat's Regional Anesthesia, pp 254–286. St. Louis, Warren H. Green, 1985
Eriksson E: Brachial plexus block—axillary approach. In Eriksson E (ed): Illustrated Handbook in Local Anaesthesia, ed 2, pp 82–84. London, Edward Arnold, 1979
Eriksson E: Brachial plexus block—supraclavicular approach. In Eriksson E (ed): Illustrated Handbook in Local Anaesthesia, ed 2, pp 79–81. London, Edward Arnold, 1979
Hughes TJ, Desgrand DA: Upper limb blocks. In Wildsmith JAW, Armitage EN (eds): Principles and Practice of Regional Anesthesia, pp 138–154. Edinburgh, Churchill Livingstone, 1987
Moore DC: Regional Block, pp 221–274. Springfield, IL, Charles C Thomas, 1965
Scott DB: Techniques of Regional Anesthesia, pp 90–115. Norwalk, CT, Appleton & Lange, 1989

Southworth JL, Hingson RA: Pitkin's Conduction Anesthesia, pp 448–471. Philadelphia, JB Lippincott, 1946

Thompson GE, Rorie DK: Functional anatomy of the brachial plexus sheaths. Anesthesiology 59:117–122, 1983

Winnie AP: Plexus Anesthesia. Philadelphia, WB Saunders, 1983

MUSCULOCUTANEOUS NERVE BLOCK

deJong RH: Modified axillary block: With block of the lateral antebrachial cutaneous (terminal musculocutaneous) nerve. Anesthesiology 26:615–618, 1965

Löfström B: Nerve block at the elbow. In Eriksson E (ed): Illustrated Handbook in Local Anaesthesia, ed 2, pp 86–89. London, Edward Arnold, 1979

NERVE BLOCKS AT THE WRIST

Hughes TJ, Desgrand D: Upper limb blocks. In Wildsmith JAW, Armitage EN (eds): Principles and Practice of Regional Anaesthesia, pp 138–154. Edinburgh, Churchill Livingstone, 1987

Löfström B: Nerve block at the wrist. In Eriksson E (ed): Illustrated Handbook in Local Anaesthesia, ed 2, pp 90–92. London, Edward Arnold, 1979

Moore DC: Regional Block, ed 4, pp 257–274. Springfield, IL, Charles C Thomas, 1965

24

Lower Extremity Nerve Blocks

Sciatic and Femoral Nerve Blocks

Blocks of the sciatic and femoral nerves provide satisfactory anesthesia for all lower extremity surgical procedures below the knee. Leg surgery at or proximal to the knee joint can also be accomplished with sciatic and femoral nerve blocks, provided that local anesthesia of the obturator and lateral femoral cutaneous nerves is also included. Operations on the leg in which a pneumatic tourniquet will be applied to the thigh also benefit from block of the obturator and lateral femoral cutaneous nerves, regardless of the site of the surgery.

LOCAL ANESTHETICS

Although every local anesthetic probably has been used for lower extremity nerve blocks, I recommend mepivacaine and bupivacaine. In outpatient surgery or whenever prolonged postoperative pain relief is unnecessary, I use mepivacaine 1.5%. For operations in which the surgery may last longer than 3 hours, or whenever postoperative pain relief is desired, I use bupivacaine 0.5%. I routinely add epinephrine 1:400,000 to plain solutions of mepivacaine or bupivacaine prior to injecting them for lower extremity blocks.

EQUIPMENT NEEDED

Sterile gloves
Antiseptic solution
20-ml syringe
Local anesthetic of choice
Epinephrine
Tuberculin syringe (to measure epinephrine)
25-gauge needle
3-inch or 4-inch "B-bevel" needle
Usual monitoring devices
Resuscitation drugs and equipment

SCIATIC NERVE BLOCK

The sciatic nerve, the largest in the body, has its origin in the lumbosacral plexus. Approximately 2 cm in width, the sciatic nerve emerges through the greater sciatic notch, courses behind the gluteus maximus muscle, and then enters the dorsal thigh. The nerve can be blocked at several locations. However, I believe it is most conveniently anesthetized where it emerges from the greater sciatic foramen.

Preparation and Positioning

Insert an intravenous cannula in the patient (if one is not already present). Attach the electrocardiographic leads, the blood pressure cuff, and the pulse oximeter probe for monitoring during the procedure. Position the patient with the operative leg uppermost and flexed at the knee. Palpate and mark (with a surgical marking pen) the position of the greater trochanter and the ipsilateral posterior-superior iliac spine. Connect the two points with a line. At the midpoint of the line, draw a perpendicular line in a caudal direction.

Injection of Anesthetic

Cleanse the skin of the buttock with antiseptic solution. The sciatic nerve lies beneath the perpendicular line, about 4 cm from its intersection with the trochanter–posterior-superior iliac spine line. Inject local anesthetic in the skin overlying the sciatic nerve. Insert a 3-inch "B-bevel" needle through the skin wheal perpendicular to the skin, and advance it until either the iliac bone is encountered or a paresthesia to the foot is elicited (Fig. 24–1). If bone is encountered, carefully note its depth beneath the skin (the sciatic nerve is no deeper than the iliac bone) and reinsert the needle in a fanwise fashion until a paresthesia is obtained. When a paresthesia is obtained, aspirate (to rule out intravascular placement of the needle) and then inject a test dose of 1 ml of local anesthetic. If the paresthesia is not intensified, inject the remaining 19 ml of local anesthetic.

If a paresthesia is elicited during injection of the 1-ml test dose, the needle should be withdrawn approximately 1 mm and a repeat test dose performed before injecting the remaining 18 ml.

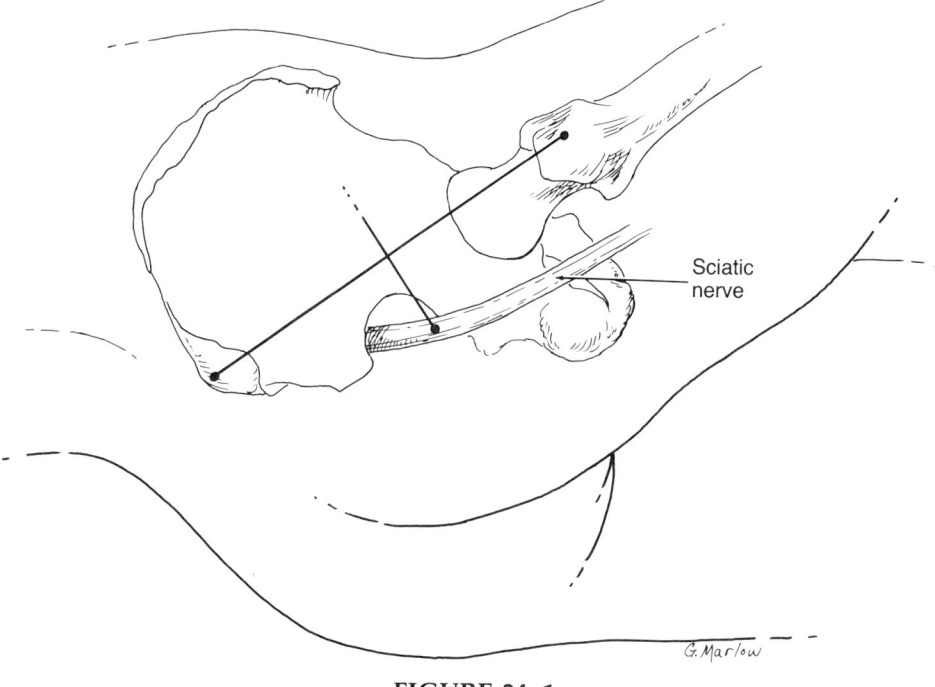

FIGURE 24–1

FEMORAL NERVE BLOCK

The femoral nerve, formed by branches of the lumbar plexus, passes into the upper leg beneath the inguinal ligament where it lies lateral to the femoral artery. Distal to the inguinal ligament, the femoral nerve branches into anterior and posterior trunks. The anterior group innervates the skin of the anterior surface of the thigh and the sartorius muscle; the posterior group innervates the quadriceps muscle in the thigh and the knee joint (including its medial ligament) and terminates in the saphenous nerve, which supplies sensory innervation to the skin on the medial side of the calf and foot.

Preparation and Positioning

Insert an intravenous cannula in the patient (if one is not already present). Attach the electrocardiographic leads, the blood pressure cuff, and the pulse oximeter probe for monitoring during the procedure. Identify the anterior-superior iliac spine, pubic tubercle, and inguinal ligament. Cleanse the skin of the anterior thigh and lower abdomen with antiseptic solution.

Injection of Anesthetic

Inject local anesthetic in the skin immediately lateral to the pulse of the femoral artery, 1 to 2 cm distal to the inguinal ligament. Insert a 3-inch or 4-inch 22-gauge needle through the skin wheal lateral to the vessel. The goal is to place the needle close to the artery without puncturing it. When the needle is properly inserted, it will pulsate, but blood will not be obtained. Attach a syringe to the needle and aspirate through the needle to ensure that neither the femoral artery nor vein has been entered (Fig. 24–2). Inject a total of 20 ml of local anesthetic in a fanwise fashion from the subcutaneous tissue to a depth of about 3 cm beneath the skin

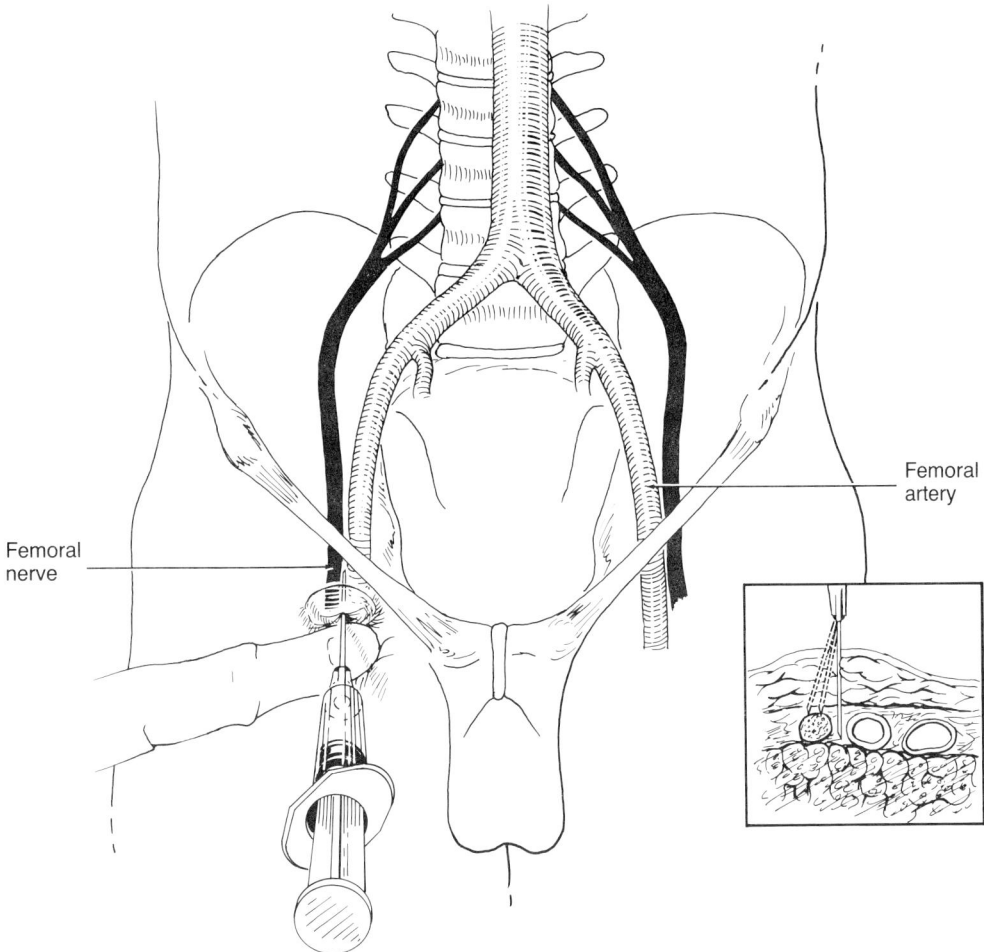

FIGURE 24–2

surface. Start the injections adjacent to the femoral artery and "fan" out 3 to 4 cm lateral to the femoral artery. Paresthesias are not necessary. Carefully check with aspiration before each injection to be certain that the needle does not lie within a blood vessel. If a paresthesia is obtained, inject 10 to 20 ml of local anesthetic at that point after aspiration and an initial 1-ml test dose to rule out intravascular and intraneural needle placement.

Block of the Lateral Cutaneous Nerve of the Thigh

The lateral cutaneous nerve of the thigh arises from the lumbar plexus, courses along the inner surface of the iliac muscle, and passes deep to the inguinal ligament about 1 cm medial to the anterior-superior iliac spine. The nerve emerges on the lateral side of the thigh where it is covered by the fascia lata. Entrapment of this nerve leads to the syndrome known as meralgia paraesthetica.

TECHNIQUE

Prepare the patient as described for femoral nerve block. Identify the anterior-superior iliac spine and the inguinal ligament. Inject local anesthetic in the skin 2 cm medial and inferior to the anterior-superior iliac spine at this point (Fig. 24–3). Next, inject 10 ml of local anesthetic fanwise above and below the fascia lata. The location of the fascia lata can be determined by the characteristic "pop" as the needle goes through it.

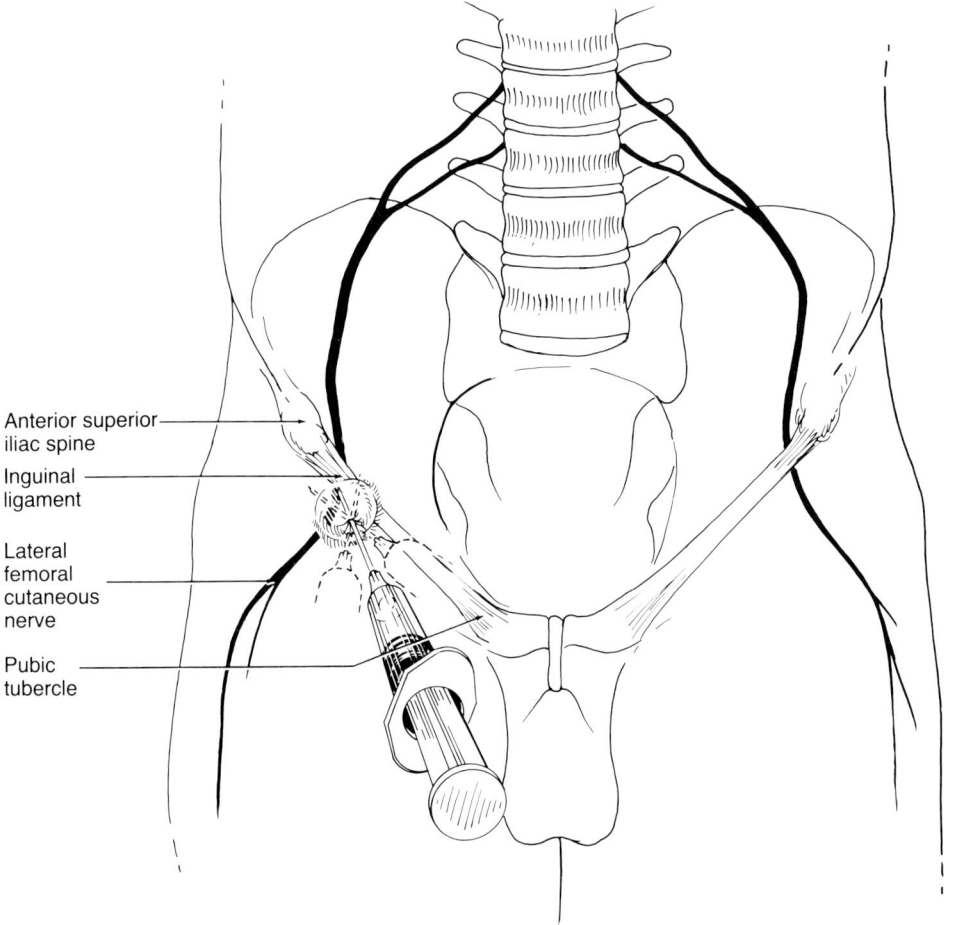

FIGURE 24–3

Obturator Nerve Block

The obturator nerve, a branch of the lumbar plexus, is often the "rate-limiting" step for accomplishing nerve block anesthesia for open surgical procedures on the knee joint. The nerve is blocked in the obturator canal where the nerve lies adjacent to the obturator artery and vein. The obturator nerve innervates a small area of skin on the medial side of the knee and lower thigh and provides motor innervation of the hip adductor muscles. The combination of sciatic and femoral nerve block is thus insufficient for open knee surgery in the absence of block of the obturator nerve.

TECHNIQUE

Position and prepare the patient as described for femoral nerve block. Identify the inguinal ligament, the anterior-superior iliac spine, and the pubic tubercle. Inject local anesthetic in the skin approximately 1 cm inferior and lateral to the pubic tubercle. Advance a 22-gauge 3-inch or 4-inch needle through the skin wheal until it contacts the pubic bone (Fig. 24–4). Reposition the needle slightly laterally and cranially until the tip passes over the bone and into the obturator canal. Carefully aspirate before injecting a total of about 15 ml of local anesthetic as the needle is slowly withdrawn from within the obturator canal.

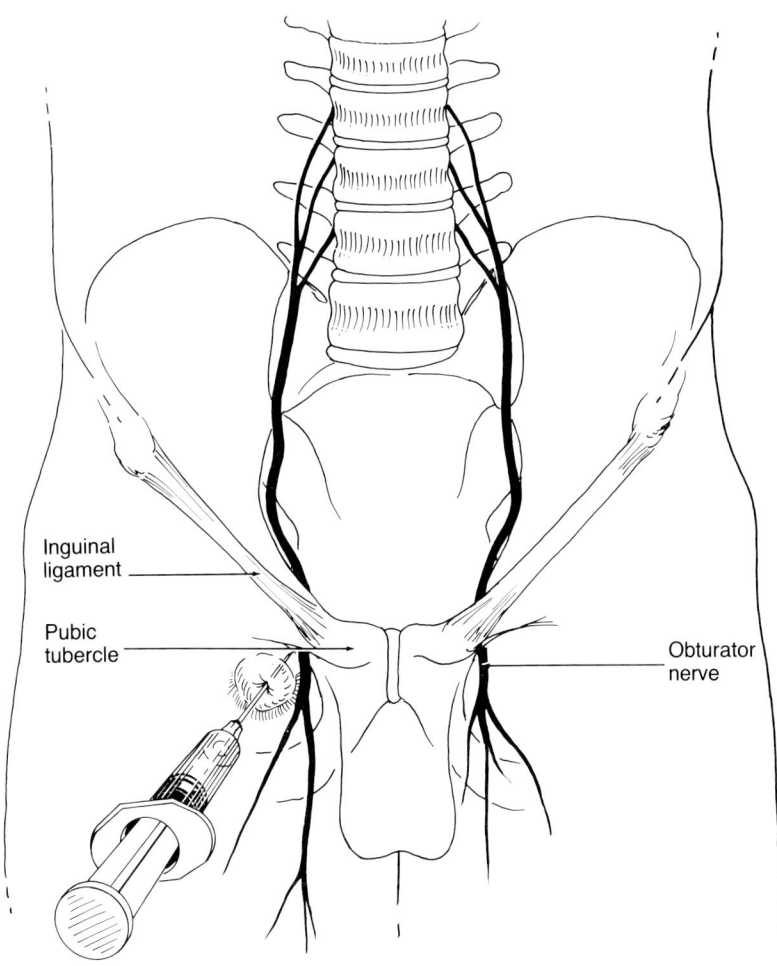

FIGURE 24–4

Knee Block

Regional anesthesia can be provided for diagnostic arthroscopy of the knee using the combination of sciatic, femoral, lateral femoral cutaneous, and obturator nerve blocks; spinal anesthesia; epidural anesthesia; caudal anesthesia; or through a combination of local infiltration and intra-articular local anesthetic that I refer to as "knee block." When knee block anesthesia is used, both the surgeon and the anesthetist must understand that supplemental anesthesia (either general anesthesia or a more extensive form of regional anesthesia) will be necessary if either an open operative procedure or a pneumatic thigh tourniquet is required.

To perform the block, I inject 30 ml of bupivacaine 0.5% with 1:200,000 epinephrine in the knee joint and 15 ml of lidocaine 1% in the skin around the knee. Epinephrine should always be added to the intra-articular local anesthetic solution to avoid the near-toxic levels of bupivacaine that might otherwise result.

EQUIPMENT NEEDED

Sterile gloves
Antiseptic solution
Lidocaine 1% 15 ml
Bupivacaine 0.5% 30 ml
Epinephrine
Tuberculin syringe (to measure epinephrine)
2 30-ml syringes
25-gauge needle
22-gauge 2-inch (or longer) needle
Usual monitoring devices
Resuscitation drugs and equipment

PREPARATION AND POSITIONING

Insert an intravenous cannula in the patient (if one is not already present). Position the patient supine on the operating room table. Attach the electrocardiographic leads, blood pressure cuff, and pulse oximeter probe for monitoring during the procedure. Cleanse the skin of the knee with antiseptic solution.

INJECTING THE ANESTHETIC

Inject 5 ml of lidocaine 1% at each of the superolateral, inferolateral, and inferomedial margins of the patella (starting 1 cm from the patella in each case) for a total dose of 15 to 20 ml (Fig. 24–5). These skin wheals provide cutaneous anesthesia for the intra-articular local anesthetic injection and for the insertion of the arthroscope and for any necessary probes or grasping forceps.

Next, with the knee flexed to approximately 45°, advance a 2-inch or longer needle through the superolateral skin wheal into the knee joint. Entry into the knee joint can be confirmed by aspiration (which will sometimes yield bloody or straw-colored joint fluid or, more commonly, nothing at all), by a palpable "pop," or by ease of injection of the local anesthetic (Fig. 24–6).

Slowly inject (over about 3 minutes) the 30 ml of bupivacaine 0.5% with 1:200,000 epinephrine into the knee joint. Usually a bulge can be palpated in all four quadrants as the joint space expands uniformly. The anesthesia will intensify over 10 to 15 minutes.

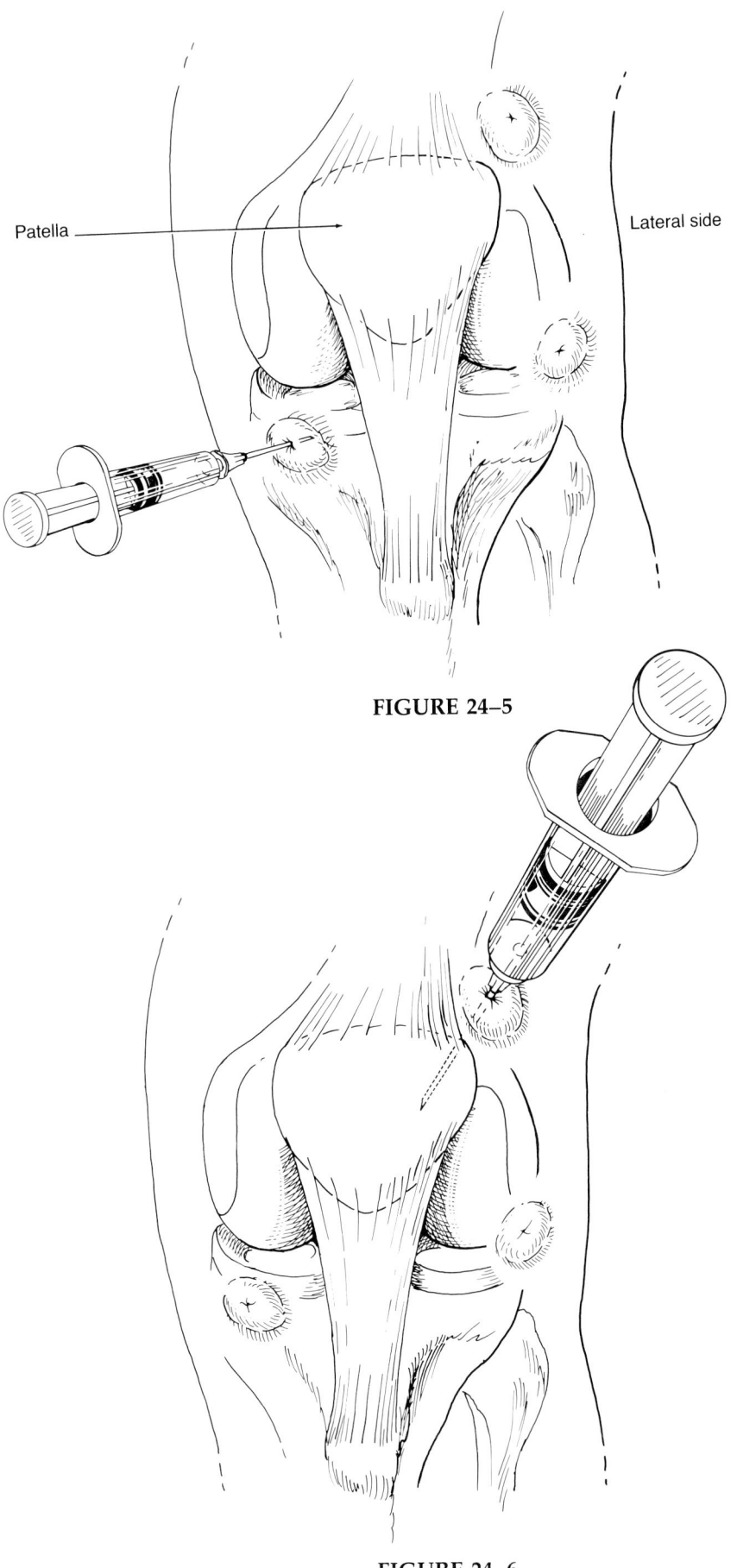

FIGURE 24–5

FIGURE 24–6

Ankle Block

Surgery of the toes and distal foot is well suited to regional anesthesia and, in particular, to ankle block anesthesia. "Ankle block" denotes the approximate location where the anesthetic is injected and does not mean that the technique is suitable for surgery on the ankle (Fig. 24–7). A *complete* ankle block involves injection and blockade of five peripheral nerves: superficial and deep peroneal, tibial, sural, and saphenous. Of these, the first four are branches of the sciatic nerve; only the saphenous nerve is a branch of the femoral nerve.

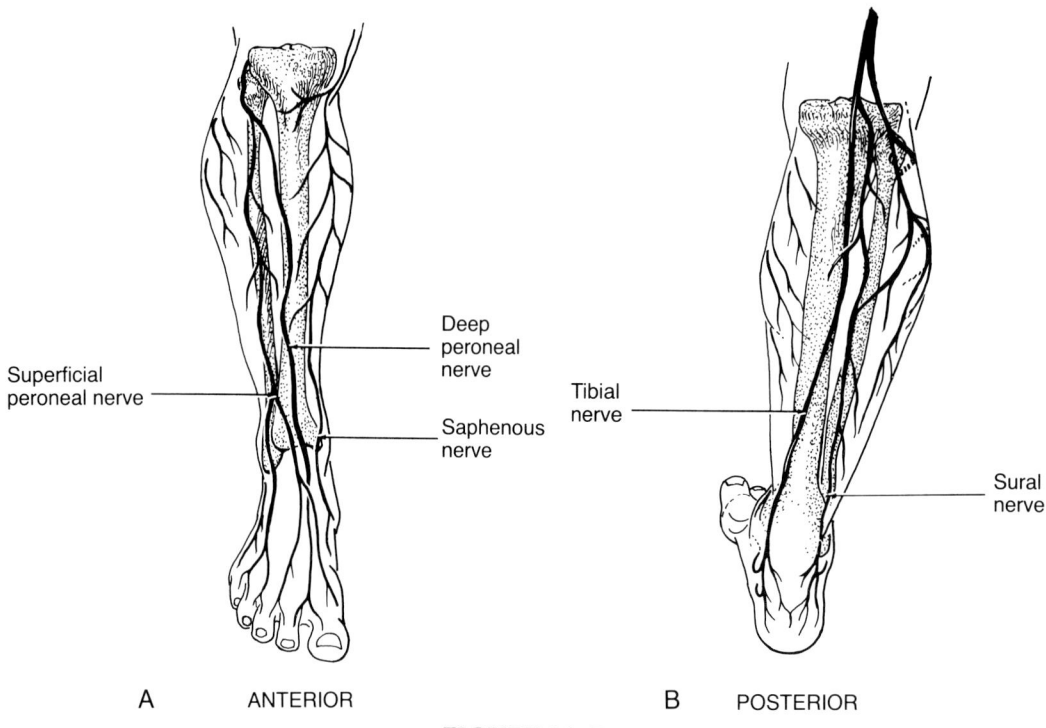

FIGURE 24–7

APPLICATIONS

For most indications the block need not include all five nerves. For example, if ankle block is selected for bunionectomy, anesthesia of superficial and deep peroneal, posterior tibial, and saphenous nerves, but not the sural nerve, needs to be obtained. Conversely, if surgery is planned to correct an isolated deformity of the little toe, anesthesia of superficial peroneal, sural, and tibial nerves will be required.

Ankle block anesthesia will certainly not be sufficient to provide anesthesia for inflation of a thigh tourniquet. However, my experience has been that most patients will tolerate exsanguination and ischemia from an Esmarch bandage wrapped around the lower leg for the brief duration required for most toe surgery.

The onset of the anesthesia should be carefully monitored so that any required supplementation can be given in a timely fashion. For example, if the planned surgery is limited to the great toe (and anesthesia is incomplete), supplementation can take the form either of reinjection of the sural, saphenous, and peroneal nerves or of digital nerve block of the great toe.

LOCAL ANESTHESIA

I use bupivacaine 0.5% with 1:400,000 epinephrine to block the sural, deep peroneal, and tibial nerves and bupivacaine 0.25% with 1:400,000 epinephrine for subcutaneous and cutaneous infiltration to block saphenous and superficial peroneal nerves.

EQUIPMENT NEEDED

Sterile gloves
Antiseptic solution
Local anesthetic
Epinephrine
Tuberculin syringe (to measure epinephrine)
10-ml syringe
25-gauge and 22-gauge needles
Resuscitation drugs and equipment
Rolled blanket or towel

PREPARATION AND POSITIONING

Insert an intravenous cannula if one is not already present. After positioning the patient supine on the operating room table, cleanse the ankle and foot with antiseptic solution.

DEEP PERONEAL NERVE BLOCK

Identify the dorsalis pedis artery and the tendons of the extensor hallucis longus and tibialis anterior muscles on the dorsal surface of the foot (Fig. 24–8). The deep peroneal nerve lies deep to the tendon of extensor hallucis longus, at approximately the same depth beneath the skin as the dorsalis pedis artery.

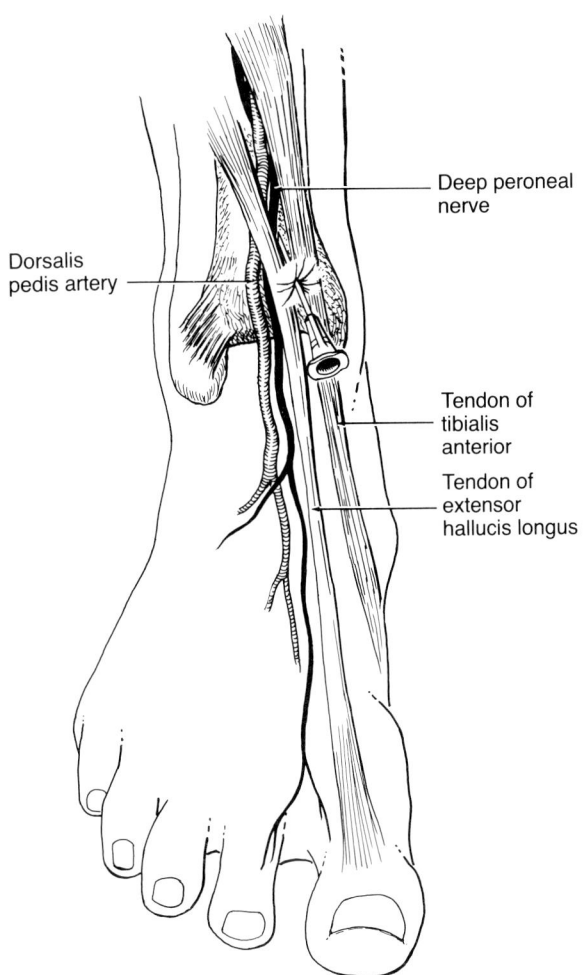

FIGURE 24–8

Inject local anesthetic in the skin between the tendons at the level of the malleoli, then advance the needle alongside and beneath the extensor hallucis longus tendon, seeking a paresthesia if possible, to the great or second toe. In the absence of a paresthesia, advance the needle until bone is contacted and then inject 5 ml of local anesthetic in a fanwise fashion while withdrawing the needle.

TIBIAL NERVE BLOCK

Place a rolled towel beneath the patient's lower leg to elevate the foot and ankle. The tibial nerve is located on the medial side of the foot posterolateral to the posterior tibial artery, posterior to the medial malleolus and medial and anterior to the Achilles tendon (Fig. 24–9). After raising a skin wheal with local anesthetic, insert the needle posterior (and usually lateral) to the posterior tibial artery (or, if the pulse is not palpable, medial and anterior to the Achilles tendon), and advance it toward the posterior border of the medial malleolus until a paresthesia is obtained (rarely) or the tibia is encountered. Inject 5 to 10 ml of anesthetic at the site of the paresthesia or, in its absence, fanwise while withdrawing the needle.

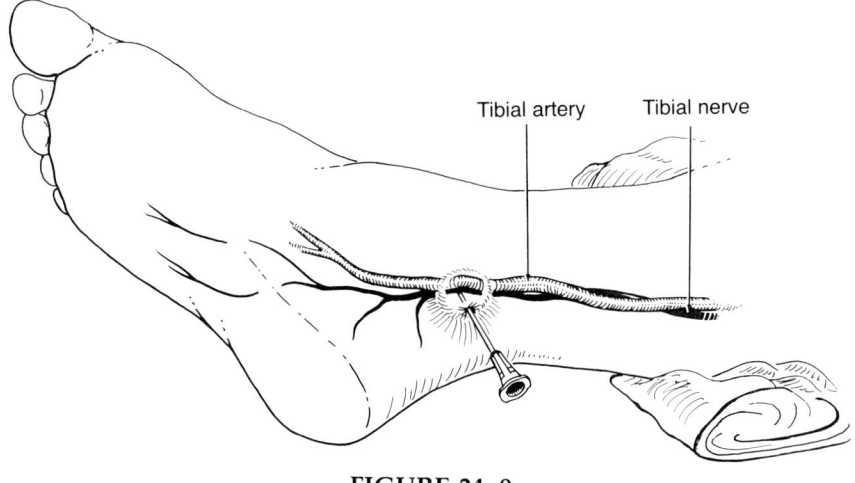

FIGURE 24–9

SURAL NERVE BLOCK

Place a rolled towel beneath the patient's lower leg to elevate the foot and ankle. Create a skin wheal of local anesthetic on the lateral side of the foot between the lateral malleolus and the Achilles tendon (Fig. 24–10). Inject 3 to 5 ml of local

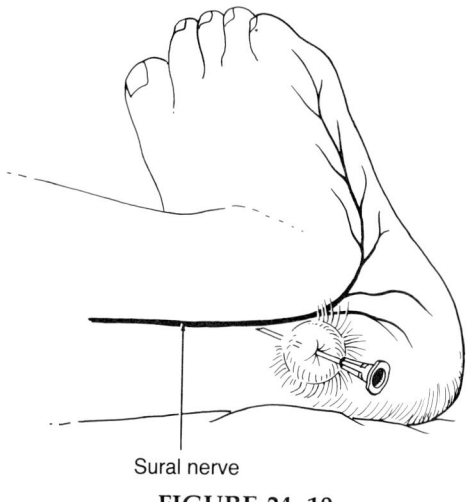

FIGURE 24–10

anesthetic (fanwise) in the subcutaneous tissue between the malleolus and tendon. A paresthesia is usually not obtained.

SUPERFICIAL PERONEAL AND SAPHENOUS NERVE BLOCKS

The superficial peroneal and saphenous nerves, although they may be blocked individually, are more conveniently anesthetized by injecting a "ring" of local anesthetic in the cutaneous and subcutaneous tissue (Fig. 24–11).

Starting at the upper and medial border of the medial malleolus (the long saphenous vein will usually be apparent here), inject 10 ml of local anesthetic while advancing the needle subcutaneously to the medial border of the lateral malleolus. Usually this can be accomplished with two needle insertions. If sural nerve block has not been performed, the injection can proceed circumferentially and the sural block can be eliminated. I favor blocking the sural nerve separately.

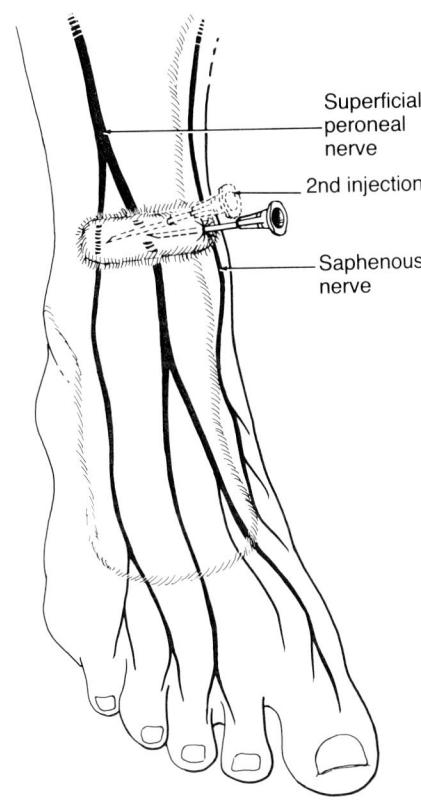

FIGURE 24–11

References

LOWER EXTREMITY NERVE BLOCKS PROXIMAL TO THE KNEE JOINT

Adriani G: Labat's Regional Anesthesia, pp 370–375. St. Louis, Warren H. Green, 1985
Löfström B, Englesson S: Nerve block in the region of the hip joint. In Eriksson E (ed): Illustrated Handbook in Local Anaesthesia, ed 2, pp 101–110. London, Edward Arnold, 1979
Macrae WA: Lower limb blocks. In Wildsmith JAW, Armitage EN (eds): Principles and Practice of Regional Anaesthesia, pp 155–163. New York, Churchill Livingstone, 1987
Moore DC: Regional Block, ed 4, pp 275–293. Springfield, IL, Charles C Thomas, 1965
Scott DB: Techniques of Regional Anaesthesia, pp 116–127. Norwalk, CT, Appleton & Lange, 1989
Southworth JL, Hingson RA: Pitkin's Conduction Anesthesia, pp 615–619. Philadelphia, JB Lippincott, 1946

KNEE BLOCK

Butterworth JF IV, Carnes RC III, Samuel MP, Janeway D, Poehling GG: Effect of adrenaline on plasma concentrations of bupivacaine following intra–articular injection of bupivacaine for knee arthroscopy. Br J Anaesth 65:537–539, 1990

Eriksson E: Local anaesthesia for arthroscopy. In Eriksson E (ed): Illustrated Handbook in Local Anaesthesia, ed 2, pp 149–150. London, Edward Arnold, 1979

Halperin N, Axer R, Hirschberg E, Agasi M: Arthroscopy of the knee under local anesthesia and controlled pressure irrigation. Clin Orthop Rel Res 134:176–179, 1976

Pevey JK: Outpatient arthroscopy of the knee under local anesthesia. Am J Sports Med 6:122–127, 1978

ANKLE BLOCK

Adriani J: Labat's Regional Anesthesia, pp 380–384. St. Louis, Warren H. Green, 1985

Löfström B: Nerve block at the ankle. In Eriksson E (ed): Illustrated Handbook in Local Anaesthesia, ed 2, pp 112–115. London, Edward Arnold, 1979

Macrae WA: Lower limb block. In Wildsmith JAW, Armitage EN (eds): Principles and Practice of Regional Anaesthesia, pp 155–167. Edinburgh, Churchill Livingstone, 1987

Southworth JL, Hingson RA: Pitkin's Conduction Anesthesia, pp 641–646. Philadelphia, JB Lippincott, 1946

25

Spinal Anesthesia

Spinal anesthesia, first described by August Bier in 1899, is a useful regional technique applicable to most surgical procedures below the umbilicus. In the past, spinal anesthesia was used during upper abdominal, thoracic, and even head and neck surgical procedures. However, with the widespread application of "balanced" general anesthetic techniques with neuromuscular paralysis and controlled ventilation, most clinicians do not favor the use of spinal anesthesia alone for such cases. Combinations of regional (commonly epidural, not spinal) and general anesthesia continue to be popular for abdominal and thoracic surgery.

In brief, spinal anesthesia consists of performing a lumbar puncture (usually with a 22-gauge or smaller needle), followed by the injection of a local anesthetic solution into the cerebrospinal fluid. Depending on the patient's position (i.e., sitting, supine, lateral decubitus, Trendelenburg) and on the baricity of the anesthetic solution (i.e., the ratio of its specific gravity to that of cerebrospinal fluid), the upper extent of spinal anesthesia may range from sacral to cervical dermatomes.

Indications

The relative indications for spinal anesthesia include lower abdominal, perineal, and lower extremity surgery; desire to avoid instrumentation of the airway (e.g., recent food ingestion, airway polyps); desire to avoid cardiovascular depression associated with general anesthetics; and patient reluctance to lose consciousness (e.g., parturients).

Choices

The basic choices the anesthetist makes during spinal anesthesia include (1) *needle size* (smaller needles produce fewer post–lumbar puncture headaches but are more difficult to use), (2) *local anesthetic* (the identity of which influences the onset, duration, and "quality" of anesthesia), (3) *baricity* of the anesthetic solution (one can use hyperbaric, isobaric, or hypobaric solutions that influence the extent and duration of the anesthesia), (4) *site* of lumbar puncture (which has a minimal influence on the extent of anesthesia), and (5) patient *positioning* after local anesthetic injection (which influences the extent of anesthesia produced by hypobaric and hyperbaric solutions). Finally, the anesthetist may choose to perform either a "single shot" or a "continuous" spinal anesthetic. In the latter technique a cannula is inserted through the spinal needle so that repeated local anesthetic injections can be made as needed.

In general, the smallest possible spinal needle should be used to reduce the incidence of post–lumbar puncture headache. In patients younger than age 40, 25-gauge or smaller needles should be used, if possible. Patients with spinal abnormalities (e.g., scoliosis, severe osteoarthritis) may require the use of larger (usually 22-gauge) spinal needles for successful lumbar puncture. In patients older than age 60, the incidence of post–lumbar puncture headache is so low that a 22-gauge needle may be used routinely without fear of an excessive incidence of headache.

LOCAL ANESTHETICS

In the United States, the most commonly used spinal anesthetics are hyperbaric solutions of lidocaine, bupivacaine, or tetracaine. The first two are premixed by the manufacturer with dextrose (which makes them hyperbaric); tetracaine must be mixed with dextrose by the anesthetist (usually with an equal volume of 10% dextrose) to make it hyperbaric. Hyperbaric lidocaine is suitable for surgery lasting 1 hour or less (unless a continuous catheter technique is employed). Either bupivacaine or tetracaine may be used for longer procedures (up to 2½ to 3 hours); however, I prefer bupivacaine. Anesthesia for surgery lasting longer than 3 hours is best accomplished with a single injection of hyperbaric tetracaine to which 200 μg of epinephrine has been added (epinephrine increases the duration of both sensory and motor block, and the extent of motor block achieved) or with a continuous spinal technique. Epinephrine has a limited influence on the duration of hyperbaric lidocaine or hyperbaric bupivacaine.

DOSES OF LOCAL ANESTHETICS

Increasing the dose of hyperbaric tetracaine solutions has less influence on the extent ("level") of anesthesia than on the duration and "quality" (a measure of the incidence of satisfactory anesthesia) of the block. Thus, in a given patient, hyperbaric solutions of tetracaine block comparable numbers of spinal segments regardless of whether 10 or 15 mg is used. Lower doses of hyperbaric anesthetic solution are more often associated with pain during surgery than higher doses of hyperbaric anesthetic solutions.

In general, 75 to 100 mg of lidocaine, 12 to 15 mg of bupivacaine, or 10 to 15 mg of tetracaine will achieve solid, mid-thoracic dermatomal levels (T3–T6) of anesthesia in adult patients who are turned supine immediately following hyperbaric injection of anesthetic solution. Many clinicians reduce the dose of spinal anesthetic solution for pregnant patients; however, I use 12.5 to 15 mg of bupivacaine (depending on whether the injection is made with the patient sitting (15 mg) or in the lateral decubitus position (12.5 mg)) and have not noted excessively high levels of anesthesia during cesarean delivery.

BARICITY OF LOCAL ANESTHETIC SOLUTIONS

Although hyperbaric solutions are most often used (particularly when upper thoracic dermatomal levels of anesthesia are needed), both isobaric and hypobaric solutions also have an important place in anesthesia. Local anesthetic solutions intended for epidural injection (as well as spinal tetracaine solution as it comes from the manufacturer, or niphanoid tetracaine crystals mixed with saline or cerebrospinal fluid) are very nearly isobaric with cerebrospinal fluid. The advantage of isobaric solutions is that patient positioning has *no* influence on the extent of anesthesia. The onset of anesthesia with isobaric solution is gradual and of longer duration than that produced by an equal dose of hyperbaric solution. However, the upper extent of anesthesia is more unpredictable. Isobaric lidocaine (3 to 4 ml of the 2% epidural solution) is appropriate for perineal and lower extremity surgery of 2 hours' duration or less. A similar volume of isobaric 0.5% bupivacaine may be used for perineal and lower extremity operations anticipated to require 3 hours or less of anesthesia. Addition of epinephrine to isobaric solutions has a limited influence on the duration or quality of anesthesia. When a tourniquet will be used during lower extremity surgery, I recommend the use of a hyperbaric technique to obtain mid-thoracic dermatomal levels of sensory anesthesia. Tourniquet (ischemic) pain may not be inhibited by spinal anesthetic levels as high as the T10 dermatome.

Finally, hypobaric solutions may be used in selected instances. In the past, I have injected 3 to 4 ml of hypobaric tetracaine (10 mg tetracaine mixed with 5 ml of sterile, preservative-free water) with the patient positioned in Buie's ("jackknife") position for anorectal procedures (hemorrhoidectomy, pilonidal cyst excision, proctoscopy). More recently, I have used isobaric (epidural) solutions of lidocaine or bupivacaine for this purpose. Hypobaric solutions are useful for patients with hip fractures because the injured hip can be positioned in the operative (superior) position during and after the lumbar puncture. If a hyperbaric solution were used, the injured (operative) side would receive less anesthetic and be less likely to achieve full anesthesia unless the patient were turned supine after the injection. In this situation, I have found isobaric epidural bupivacaine 0.5% solutions to be more convenient than either hypobaric or hyperbaric techniques.

Patient positioning influences the distribution of the anesthesia after injection of either hypobaric or hyperbaric anesthetic solutions. When using hyperbaric solutions, one may inject the local anesthetic with the patient sitting and leave the patient in this position for 5 minutes to achieve a so-called saddle block. As the term implies, the goal is to anesthetize only those areas that would make contact with a saddle if the patient were to be seated on a horse. The saddle block is useful for many perineal procedures (e.g., application of forceps for delivery, cervical cerclage, removal of condylomata).

It is also possible to perform the lumbar puncture and inject hyperbaric anesthetic solutions with the patient sitting and then rapidly shift the patient to a supine position and achieve the mid-thoracic dermatomal levels of anesthesia. I often use this technique in parturients who require cesarean delivery. Hyperbaric spinal anesthetic solutions may be injected with the operative site in an inferior position (e.g., in the left lateral decubitus position when a left total knee replacement is the procedure) to achieve the so-called one-legged spinal. Usually, these are not completely unilateral blocks (depending on the anesthetic selected and the amount of time the patient is left with the operative site in an inferior position).

Paresthesias

If a paresthesia is obtained during insertion of the spinal needle, its location should be clearly identified. Brief paresthesias to the legs or feet coincidental with passage of the needle tip through the dura are usually inconsequential. Paresthesias not accompanied by the appearance of cerebrospinal fluid at the hub of the needle usually indicate that the tip of the needle has wandered away from the midline of the interspace. Paresthesias that persist, or that recur or intensify during injection of local anesthetic, suggest that the needle tip is located within a nerve and demand that injection of local anesthetic be discontinued immediately. Reposition the needle before resuming injection of local anesthetic.

Midline paresthesias (felt in the buttocks or rectum) are worrisome and suggest that the spinal needle may be in contact with the spinal cord itself. In these cases, the needle should be removed and replaced in a more caudad interspace.

Hypotension During Spinal Anesthesia

During any spinal anesthetic, the anesthetist should be prepared to administer a vasopressor if the patient's blood pressure should fall below a predetermined level. I nearly always treat decreases in systolic pressure to 90 mm Hg or decreases in mean arterial pressure of 20% or more. Hypotension during spinal anesthesia is caused by thoracolumbar sympathetic block induced by the local anesthetic. Inhibition of sympathetic neural outflow reduces the tone of arterial resistance vessels and increases venous pooling of blood. If high levels of sympathetic blockade are achieved (T1–T4), block of the sympathetic cardioaccelerator fibers (which are believed to emerge with the uppermost thoracic nerve roots) may lead to bradycardia. The extent of sympathetic blockade may greatly exceed the extent of sensory anesthesia measured by pinprick. Thus, hypotension requiring correction may occur even with low dermatomal levels of sensory anesthesia.

The techniques that most physiologically correct the hypotension induced by spinal anesthesia per se will reverse both the drop in resistance (by α-adrenergic stimulation) and the venous pooling (with a β-adrenergic agonist and/or fluid administration). I recommend either intravenous fluid administration (10 ml/kg) and infusion of the selective α-agonist phenylephrine (typical infusion rates are 30 to 100 μg/min); bolus administration of the mixed α- and β-adrenergic agonist ephedrine (typical doses are 5 to 10 mg); or careful infusion of the mixed α- and β-adrenergic agonist epinephrine (typical infusion rates are 2 to 6 μg/min). There are data that suggest that ephedrine may be preferable to phenylephrine or epinephrine for correction of hypotension in parturients.

Sedation

Many patients tolerate regional anesthesia better if they are given incremental doses of sedative medication during the anesthesia and surgery. I recommend midazolam (administered incrementally in 0.015-mg/kg doses up to 0.15 mg/kg). Small incremental doses of fentanyl (1 to 2 μg/kg) may also be used. A potentially disastrous cause of hypotension during spinal anesthesia is hypoventilation due to oversedation. For this reason, pulse oximetry should be used during spinal as well as general anesthetics.

Post–Lumbar Puncture Headache

The anesthetist should visit all patients postoperatively and question them regarding symptoms of post–lumbar puncture headache. Such symptoms include positional headache (worse when the patient sits or stands upright than when the patient lies supine), photophobia, and nausea. Post–lumbar puncture headaches are more common in younger, female, and (especially) pregnant patients. The use of larger spinal needles (i.e., 22-gauge or larger) also carries a greater risk of headache. If the headache seems clearly a post–lumbar puncture headache (and not musculoskeletal or vascular), and if the headache persists for 2 days or more, the patient should be offered an epidural blood patch. The patch is accomplished by performing an epidural puncture (with a standard epidural needle) at the same interspace at which the initial dural puncture was accomplished. Five-milliliter increments of the patient's venous blood, collected aseptically by an assistant at the time of epidural puncture, are injected through the epidural needle. A sterile intravenous extension tube connecting the assistant's syringe to the hub of the epidural needle helps preserve complete sterility. The blood is injected until the patient feels a sensation of "fullness" in the back or down the sides of the legs. Usually this will require 10 to 20 ml of blood. After application of the blood patch, the headache usually disappears almost immediately.

Contraindications

Spinal anesthesia should never be performed if the patient refuses the procedure. Other absolute contraindications to spinal anesthesia include intracranial hypertension from mass lesions (tumors or hematomas), in which loss of lumbar cerebrospinal fluid could lead to brain herniation, and infection (either localized to the site of lumbar puncture or septicemia), in which lumbar puncture might lead to epidural or meningeal seeding of bacteria. I do not recommend lumbar puncture to patients with coagulation disorders or those with undiagnosed, progressive neurologic deficits. However, I will perform spinal anesthetics in patients who will undergo anticoagulant therapy after the lumbar puncture.

Technique

EQUIPMENT NEEDED

Sterile gloves
Antiseptic solution
Spinal anesthesia kit (containing spinal needle, syringes, needles, local anesthetics, skin preparation sponge)
Vasopressor
Mayo stand or table
Sitting stool
Drugs and equipment for general anesthesia
Usual monitoring devices
Resuscitation drugs and equipment

PREPARATION AND POSITIONING

An intravenous infusion should be started. Attach the electrocardiographic leads, the pulse oximeter probe, and the blood pressure cuff. Administer intravenous crystalloid solution to the patient (5–10 ml/kg) to blunt the effects of the spinal anesthesia–induced sympathetic block. Dehydrated patients or patients with cardiac failure may require greater or lesser volumes of intravenous fluid.

Position the patient either in a lateral decubitus position with the back curved out toward the operator or seated and leaning over a Mayo stand (Fig. 25–1). Patients frequently have difficulty understanding how best to position themselves during lumbar puncture, particularly in the lateral decubitus position. Such phrases as "arch your back toward me like an angry cat" or "push your back against my hand" can be helpful. Make sure that the patient's shoulders are perpendicular to the floor. Deviations from perpendicular may mislead the operator into inserting the spinal needle lateral to the midline. Adjust the operating room table to a comfortable height. I prefer to be seated while performing lumbar puncture.

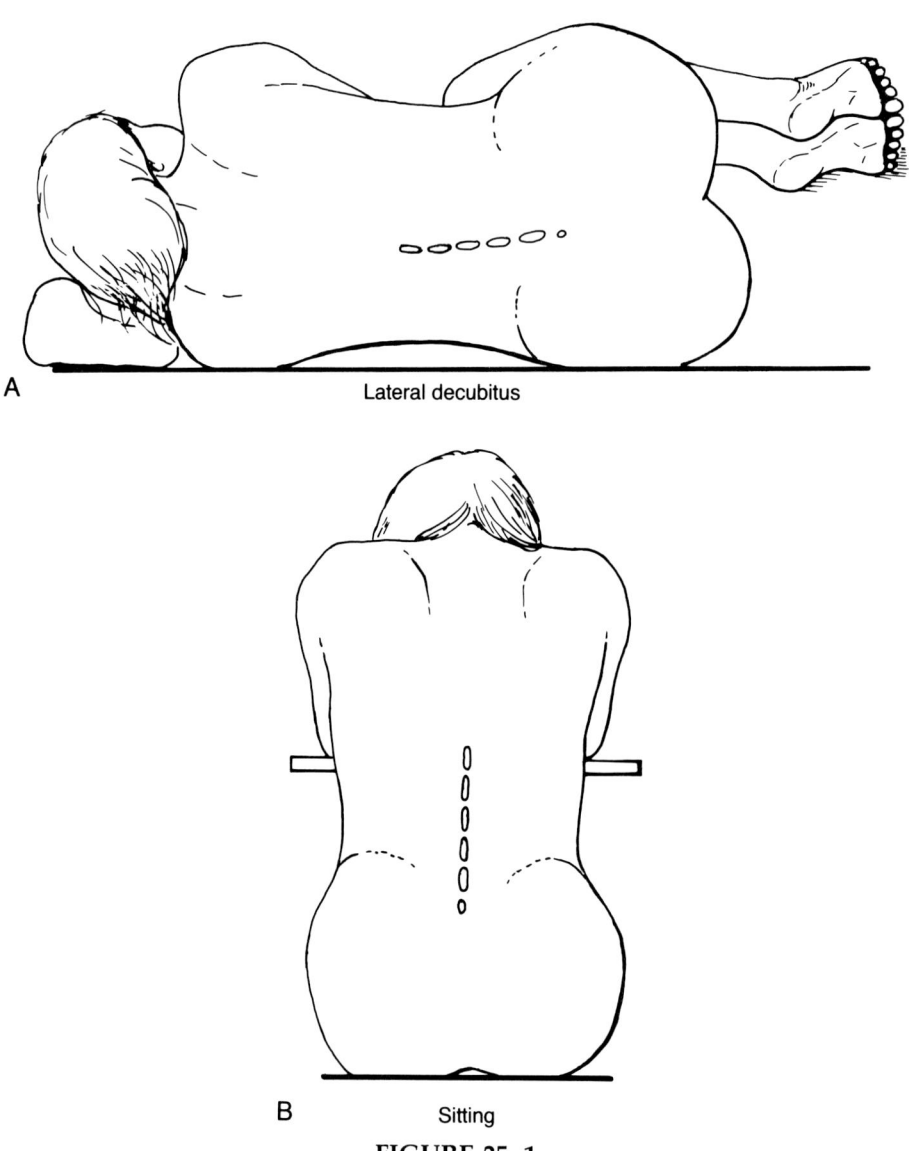

FIGURE 25–1

It is helpful to place a drape under the patient to prevent the wash solution from dampening the sheet on the operating room table. Cleanse the skin of the back with three applications of antiseptic solution. Antiseptic solution should be applied from uppermost flank down (Fig. 25–2). The solution will tend to drip downward; thus, strict adherence to an "expanding circumferential" skin preparation technique is pointless.

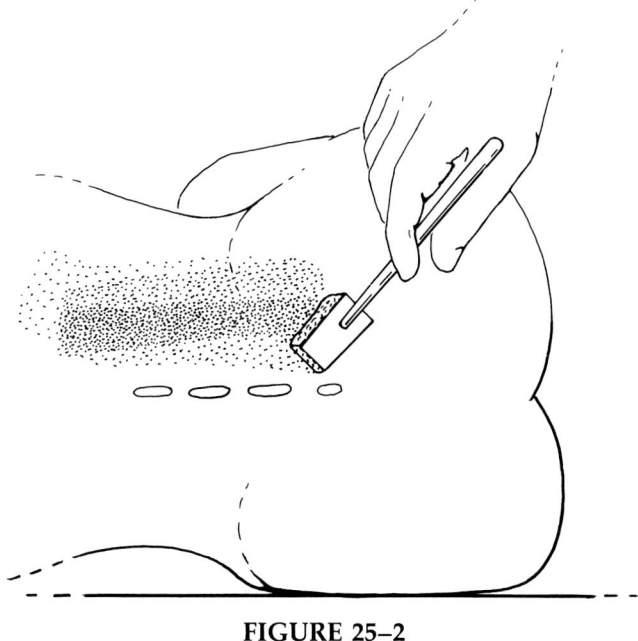

FIGURE 25–2

Place a fenestrated drape so that the site of intended lumbar puncture is clearly visible (Fig. 25–3). The drapes provided in spinal anesthesia kits usually incorporate adhesive strips to prevent them from sliding out of position. It is sometimes helpful to identify the intended site of puncture and other landmarks (e.g., spinous process, posterior-superior iliac spine) with a surgical marking pen before applying the antiseptic solution and drape.

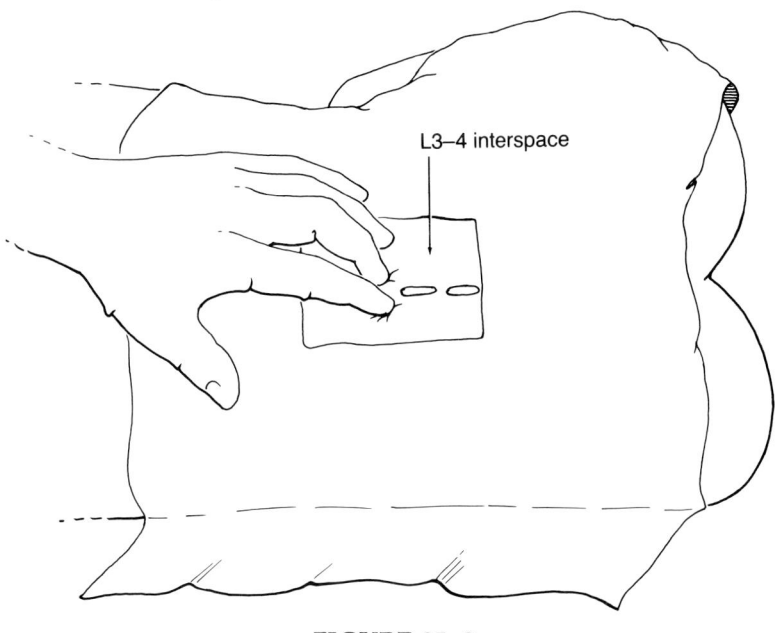

FIGURE 25–3

SELECTING AN INTERSPACE

The midpoint of an interspace is best identified by placing the index and middle fingers of the nondominant hand on either side of the interspace. I recommend keeping these fingers in place until the introducer or spinal needle has been placed

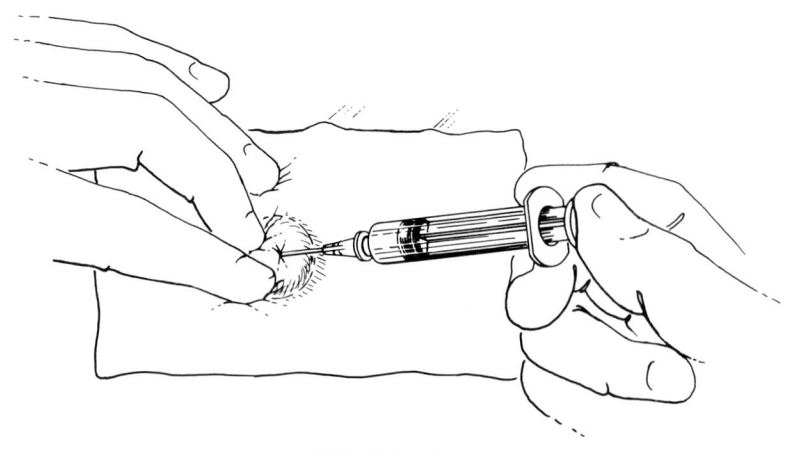

FIGURE 25–4

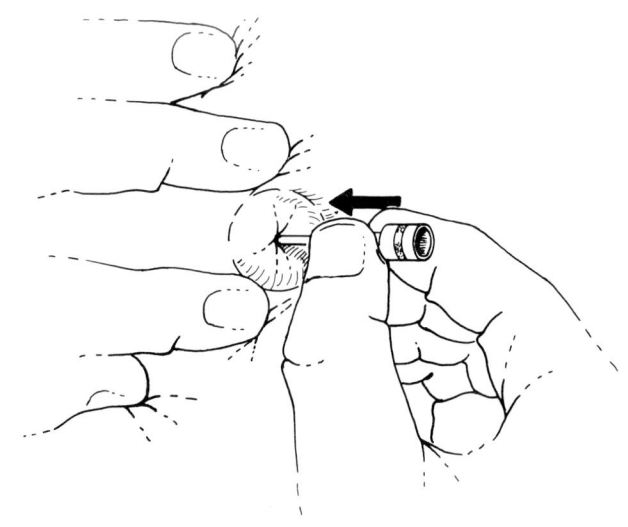

FIGURE 25–5

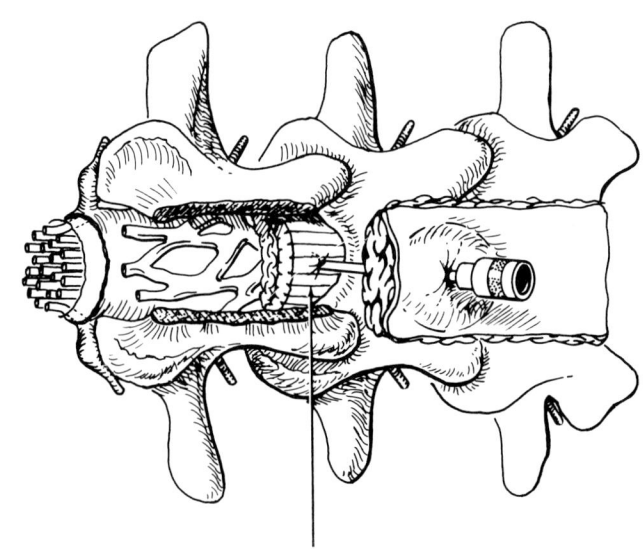

Ligamentum flavum

FIGURE 25–6

in the ligamentum flavum and recommend using the following interspaces (in order of preference): L2–3, L3–4, L4–5, L5–S1. The Tuffier line, which connects the posterior-superior iliac spines, normally crosses the L4–5 interspace. The conus medullaris of the spinal cord normally ends above the L2–3 interspace in adults; therefore, lumbar puncture through the interspaces cranial to the L2–3 interspace carry a much higher risk of cord impalement.

NEEDLE INSERTION

Inject local anesthetic (usually 1–2 ml of 1% lidocaine) into the skin and subcutaneous tissue at the site of the intended lumbar puncture (Fig. 25–4). When I use a 25-gauge or smaller spinal needle, I routinely use a 20-gauge introducer. Insert the introducer until resistance is encountered, indicating that its tip has encountered the ligamentum flavum (Fig. 25–5). Be careful not to advance the relatively large-bore introducer through the dura (Fig. 25–6).

Advance the spinal needle (through the introducer, if one has been used) in the midline in a slightly cephalad direction. With experience, the anesthetist can usually feel the needle traverse the ligamentum flavum and then the dura (Fig. 25–7). The beginner would be well advised to remove the stylet from time to time while advancing the spinal needle to ensure that he does not advance the needle all the way through the spinal canal and out the other side, perhaps into an intervertebral disk (Fig. 25–8).

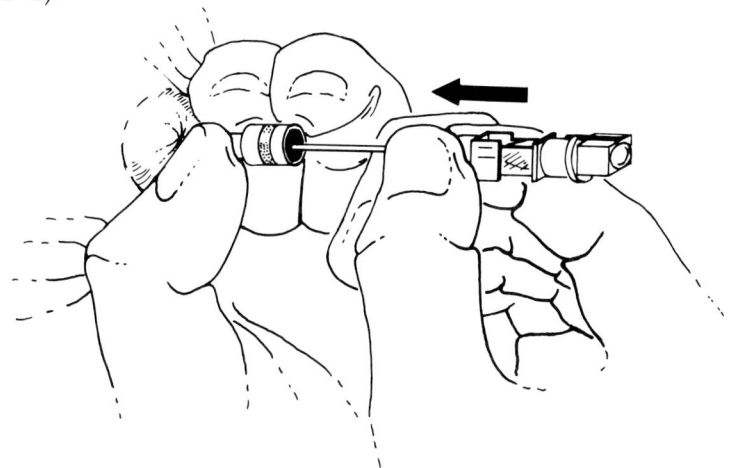

FIGURE 25–7

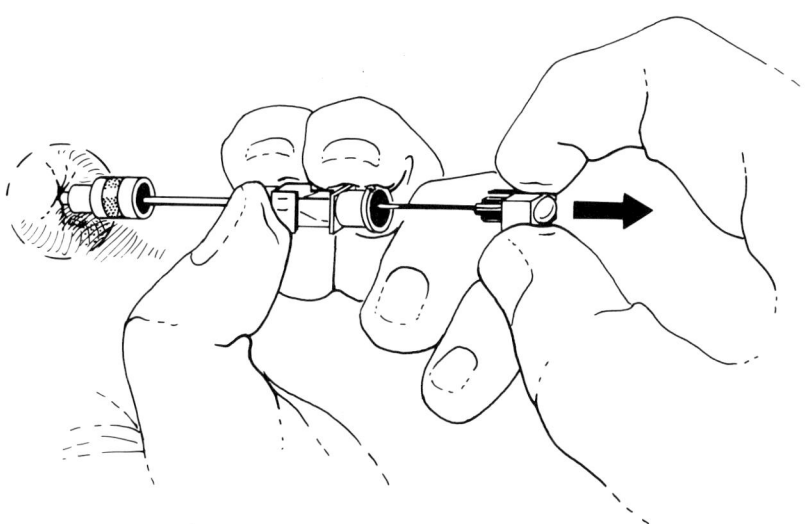

FIGURE 25–8

ASPIRATION OF CEREBROSPINAL FLUID AND INJECTION OF ANESTHETIC

Confirm that cerebrospinal fluid flows freely from the spinal needle before injecting any anesthetic solution. Cerebrospinal fluid flow through 22-gauge needles is relatively fast; unfortunately, 25-gauge, 26-gauge, and 27-gauge needles do not permit rapid flow of cerebrospinal fluid (Fig. 25–9). More impatient anesthetists may resort to aspiration with a syringe.

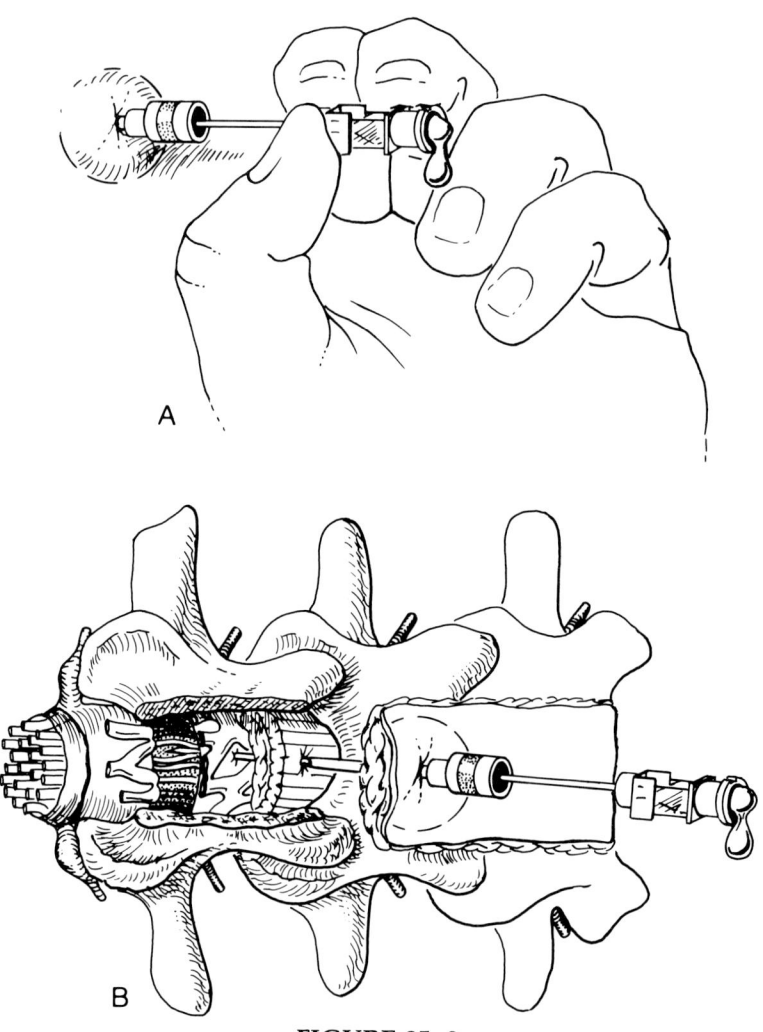

FIGURE 25–9

Aspiration of cerebrospinal fluid into a syringe containing local anesthetic solution produces birefringent swirls within the local anesthetic solution (Fig. 25–10). The local anesthetic should be injected slowly (over about 5 seconds) and care taken not to advance or withdraw the needle during injection of the anesthetic.

Following a difficult lumbar puncture, many anesthetists confirm that the needle tip has remained within the spinal theca during anesthetic injection by aspirating fluid from the spinal needle after completing the injection. The aspirate should be reinjected before the needle is removed. I usually omit this extra step.

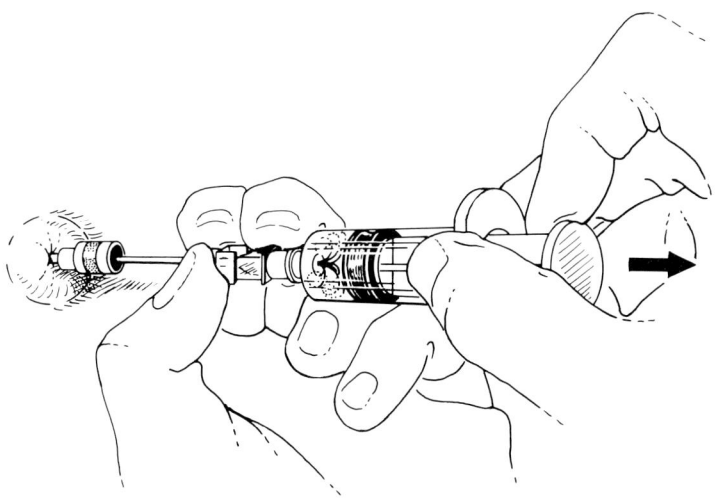

FIGURE 25–10

After injecting the anesthetic, withdraw the needle and return the patient to a supine position unless saddle block anesthesia is desired, in which case the patient should remain sitting for several minutes. Monitor the onset of anesthesia carefully so that the surgical incision can be made in a timely fashion. It is unnecessary to stab the patient repeatedly with a sharp needle to determine whether spinal anesthesia is present. Insensibility to cold (using an ice cube, a laryngoscope handle, or a wet alcohol swab) or light touch (using the operator's index finger) will reliably determine the approximate extent of spinal anesthesia. I recommend charting the upper limit (dermatome) of spinal anesthesia on both right and left sides at 5- to 10-minute intervals.

Charts of cutaneous sensory nerve distribution by spinal segments are provided in Figure 25–11.

CONTINUOUS SPINAL ANESTHESIA

Continuous spinal anesthesia is accomplished by inserting a fine cannula through the spinal needle (after placing the tip of the needle within the subarachnoid space) so that repeated injections of local anesthetic can be made as needed throughout the surgical procedure. Cannulae are available that will pass through spinal needles as small as 26 gauge. When using a continuous technique, I favor small incremental doses of hyperbaric lidocaine (25 mg) administered at 5-minute intervals to establish the block. The block may be maintained (when it starts to recede below the level achieved during the initial injections) with additional small doses of hyperbaric lidocaine or with small doses (e.g., 2.5 mg) of hyperbaric bupivacaine for those cases in which prolonged anesthesia will be required (>2 hr). Alternatively, isobaric lidocaine (2% epidural solution) or isobaric bupivacaine (0.5% epidural solution) given in 2-ml increments may be used to produce a slowly developing lower thoracic dermatomal level of spinal anesthesia.

DIFFICULT SPINAL PUNCTURE

In general, if a difficult lumbar puncture is anticipated (e.g., in a grossly obese patient, a patient with spinal anomalies, or a patient with a severe connective tissue disease), the patient should be placed in the sitting position before any attempt at lumbar puncture. The most common scenario leading to a difficult lumbar puncture is that the operator has mistakenly directed the needle tip away from the midline. In the sitting position (relative to the lateral decubitus position), sagging redundant skin is less likely to obscure the location of the midline. In rare instances, a paramedian approach (inserting the spinal needle about a finger's breadth lateral to the spinous process, and aiming it about 30° medial and craniad into the interspace) may be required for successful lumbar puncture.

References

Adriani J: Labat's Regional Anesthesia, ed 4, pp 385–443. St. Louis, Warren H. Green, 1985

Butterworth JF IV, Piccione W Jr, Berrizbeitia LD, Dance G, Shemin RJ, Cohn LH: Augmentation of venous return by adrenergic agonists during spinal anesthesia. Anesth Analg 65:612–616, 1986

Greene NM: Physiology of Spinal Anesthesia, ed 3. Baltimore, Williams & Wilkins, 1981

Lee JA, Atkinson RS: Sir Robert MacIntosh's Lumbar Puncture and Spinal Analgesia Intradural and Extradural. Edinburgh, Churchill Livingstone, 1978

Lemmon WT, Hager HG Jr: Continuous spinal anesthesia. In Southworth JL, Hingson RA (eds): Pitkin's Conduction Anesthesia, pp 827–837. Philadelphia, JB Lippincott, 1946

Palmer LA: Spinal anesthesia. In Southworth JL, Hingson RA (eds): Pitkin's Conduction Anesthesia, pp 726–826. Philadelphia, JB Lippincott, 1946

Rubin AP: Spinal anesthesia. In Wildsmith JAW, Armitage EN (eds): Principles and Practice of Regional Anaesthesia, pp 70–80. Edinburgh, Churchill Livingstone, 1987

Scott DB: Techniques of Regional Anaesthesia, pp 189–199. Norwalk, CT, Appleton & Lange, 1989

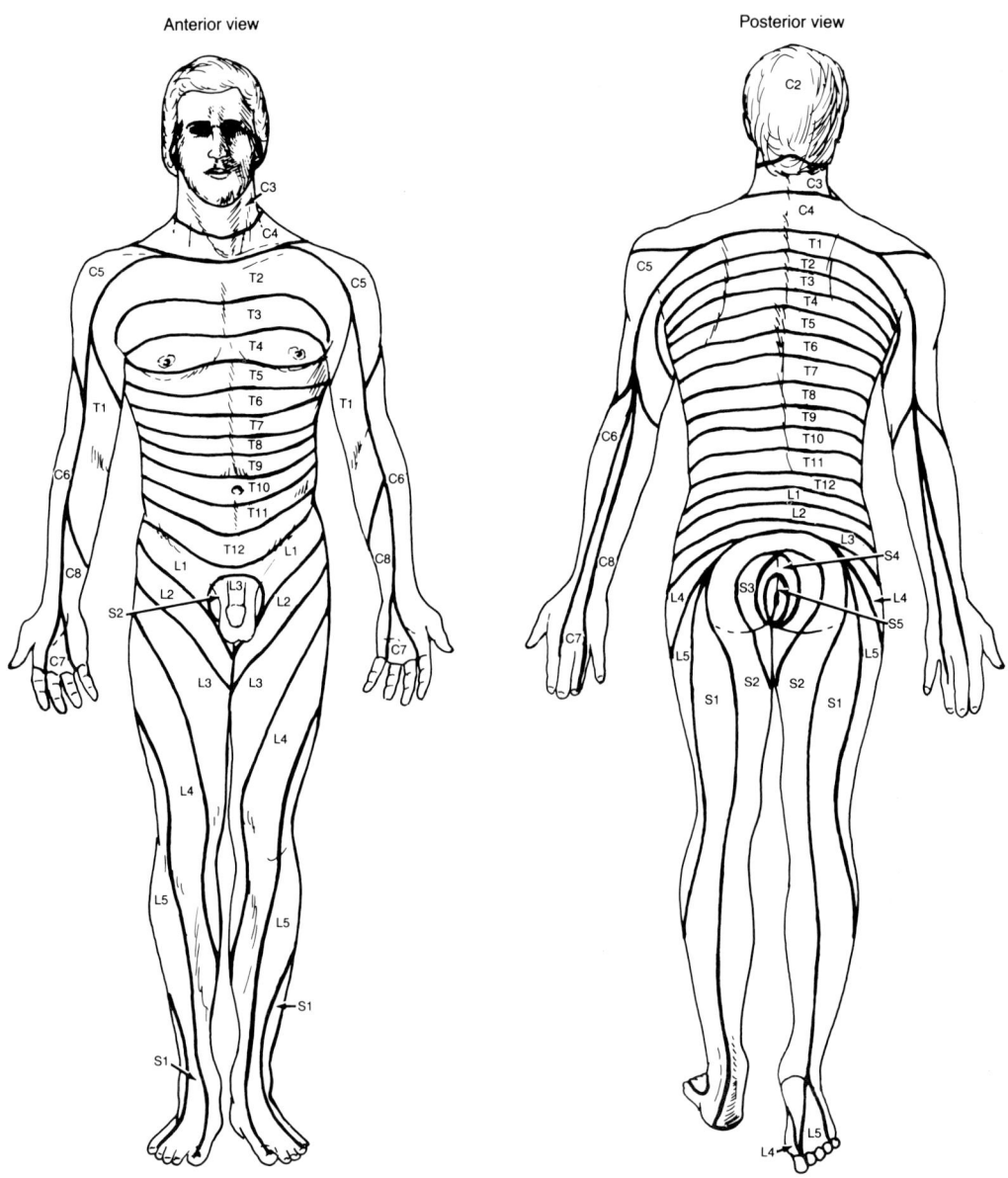

FIGURE 25–11. Dermatomal Chart.

26

Epidural Anesthesia

Continuous epidural anesthesia is ideally suited for lower abdominal, perineal, and lower extremity surgical cases of prolonged or unknown duration (e.g., vascular surgery in which embolectomies and additional bypass grafts are often unexpectedly required) or for pain relief in labor (in which the duration of the second stage of labor in a primiparous woman can range from 2 to 20 hours). An epidural catheter is also an ideal route through which postoperative pain relief can be provided, whether with narcotics, local anesthetics, or even α_2-adrenergic receptor agonists.

The approach to lumbar epidural puncture is similar to that for spinal anesthesia. The main differences between the two techniques include the depth of needle placement, the method by which correct needle placement is determined, the size and contour of the needles employed, and the volume of local anesthetic required. Epidural anesthesia has the advantage over spinal anesthesia (in the absence of an unintended dural puncture) of not being associated with headache. Epidural anesthesia has the disadvantages (relative to spinal anesthesia) of a longer onset time, less reliability (incomplete anesthesia is more common), less motor nerve block, and an increased risk of local anesthesia toxic side effects.

Epidural needles are usually 16 to 18 gauge in adults. Needles as small as 20 gauge have been used in pediatrics. The opening at the tip of nearly all epidural needles is directed toward the side. This feature is known as a "Huber" tip. The most commonly used epidural needle, the one described by Touhy, has this feature.

Identification of the Epidural Space

Entry into the epidural space is usually confirmed during epidural puncture by the use of one of two techniques: (1) "loss of resistance" or (2) the "hanging drop." I recommend the former but have used both. Both techniques rely on the low pressures (relative to atmospheric pressure) within the epidural space for their success. "Loss of resistance" is identified when the considerable resistance to attempted injection into the ligamentum flavum of either air or liquid is lost as the tip of the epidural needle passes through the ligamentum flavum into the epidural space. To use the "hanging drop" technique, the operator (after seating the needle tip in the ligamentum flavum) places a drop of liquid (usually local anesthetic or saline) at the external orifice of the epidural needle. When the needle exits the ligamentum flavum and enters the epidural space, the drop is (usually) aspirated into the needle. I believe that many trainees pay entirely too much attention to these two techniques for identifying the epidural space. Either technique should serve only to confirm what the anesthetist already believes regarding the location of the needle tip, based on what he feels as the needle is advanced. Thus, "loss of resistance" to attempted injection of air or saline by the dominant hand usually only confirms what the nondominant hand has already felt (a characteristic "grit" or "crunch" as the needle passes through the supraspinous and interspinous ligaments and "give" as the needle tip passes through the ligamentum flavum).

Site of Epidural Puncture

Some anesthetists select the site of epidural puncture based on the location of surgery (e.g., thoracic punctures for cases where the incision will be centered in thoracic dermatomes, lumbar insertions for surgeries on the lower extremities, or caudal epidural anesthesia for anorectal surgery). Although this approach has merit, it is also true that anesthesia can be provided for most abdominal and lower extremity surgery by injecting local anesthetics through a lumbar epidural catheter.

Although epidural puncture is most often accomplished in the lumbar region of the spine, cervical, thoracic, and caudal approaches to the epidural space all have their place. Cervical epidural anesthesia has limited value as a technique for providing anesthesia for surgery; rather, cervical epidural puncture is more commonly used for the diagnosis and treatment (with corticosteroids and local anesthetics) of chronic neck pain. Thoracic epidural anesthesia is well suited for providing sensory anesthesia and postoperative pain control during and after surgery of the upper abdomen and thoracic regions. Finally, the caudal (or sacral) approach to the epidural space may be used to provide surgical anesthesia for anorectal and lower abdominal and lower extremity surgery (if large doses of local anesthetic are used). Caudal analgesia with dilute bupivacaine (0.125%–0.25%) and/or morphine is commonly used in small children for postoperative pain relief. I believe that a discussion of cervical epidural anesthesia is beyond the scope of this book; however, the thoracic and caudal approaches will be described.

Lumbar Epidural Anesthesia

EQUIPMENT NEEDED

Sterile gloves
Antiseptic solution
Epidural kit (containing epidural needle, 5-ml glass syringe, 20-ml plastic syringe, 3-ml syringe for injection of local anesthesia, skin preparation sponges, local anesthetic for skin wheal, epidural catheter)
Local anesthetic of choice
Epinephrine
Tuberculin syringe (to measure epinephrine)
Vasopressor
Adhesive tape
Tincture of benzoin (optional)
Occlusive transparent dressing (especially if the catheter is to remain in place for postoperative analgesia) (optional)
Usual monitoring devices
Resuscitation drugs and equipment

PREPARATION AND POSITIONING

An intravenous infusion should be started. Attach the electrocardiographic leads, blood pressure cuff, and pulse oximeter probe for monitoring during the procedure. Position the patient either in the lateral decubitus position or in the sitting position so that the spinous processes are spread apart (Fig. 26–1). This can be accomplished in the lateral decubitus position by having the patient "bow" out his back, or in the sitting position by having the patient lean over a Mayo stand. I recommend asking the patient to arch his back "like an angry cat." Positioning for lumbar epidural anesthesia is identical to that for spinal anesthesia.

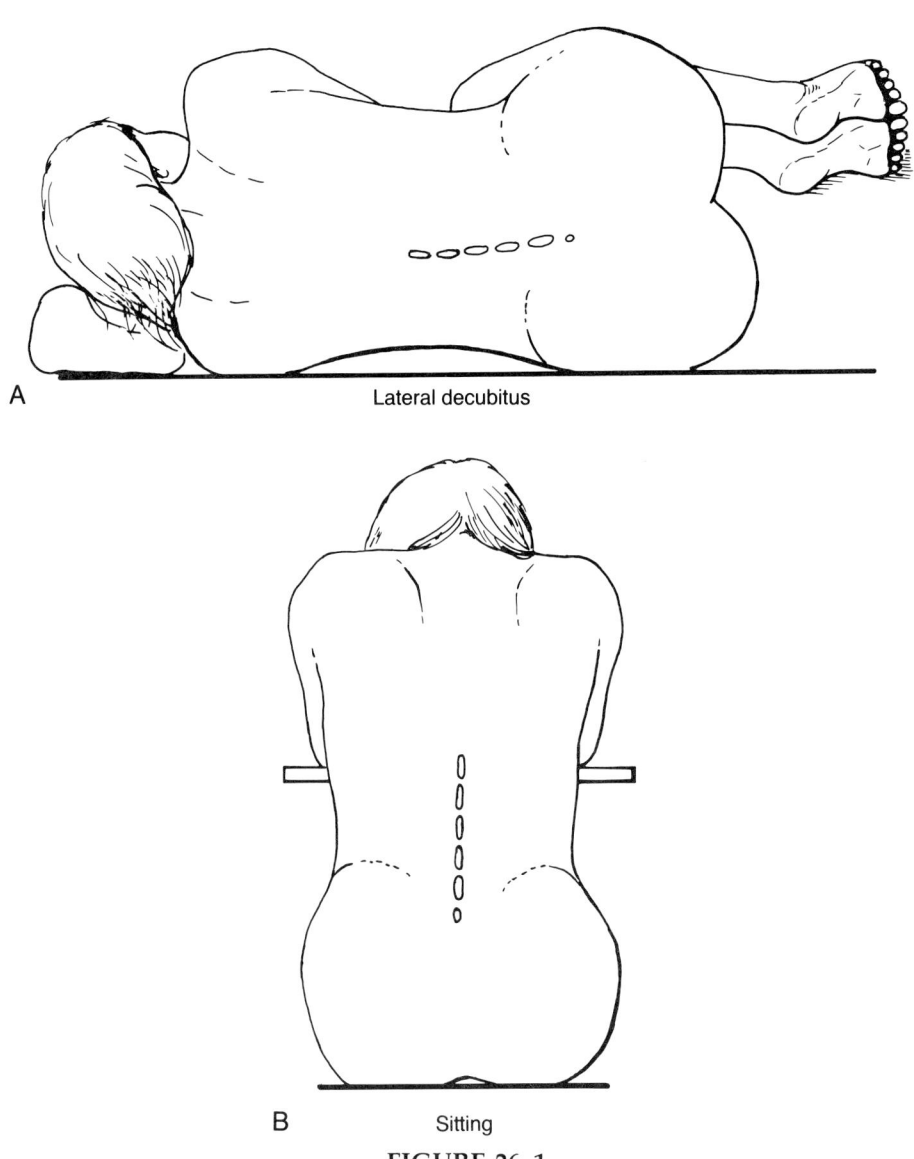

FIGURE 26–1

Cleanse the site of intended epidural puncture with antiseptic solution (Fig. 26–2). Wash the skin in a superior to inferior direction so that antiseptic solutions do not drip over already cleansed skin. In the lumbar region, I recommend the L2–3 and L3–4 interspaces. Identify the midpoint of the selected interspace by placing the index and middle finger of the nondominant hand on either side (Fig. 26–3). Inject local anesthetic (e.g., lidocaine 1%) in the skin overlying the interspace where epidural puncture will be attempted between the fingers and in the underlying tissues between the skin and the ligamentum flavum. The skin may be nicked with an 18-gauge needle to facilitate insertion of the epidural needle (Fig. 26–4).

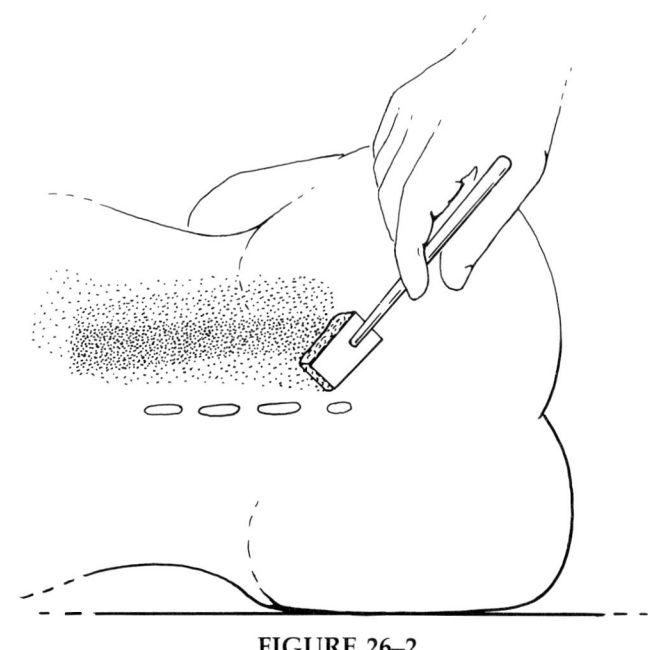

FIGURE 26–2

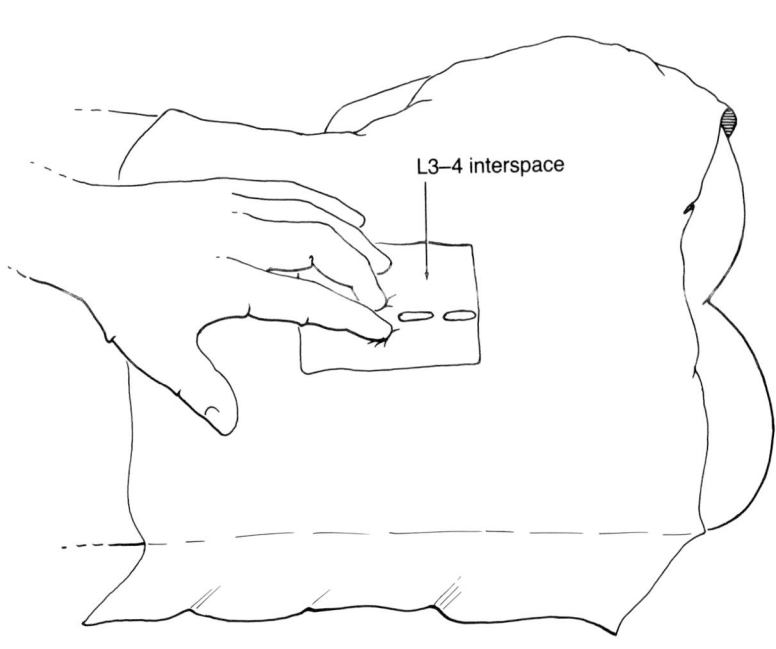

FIGURE 26–3

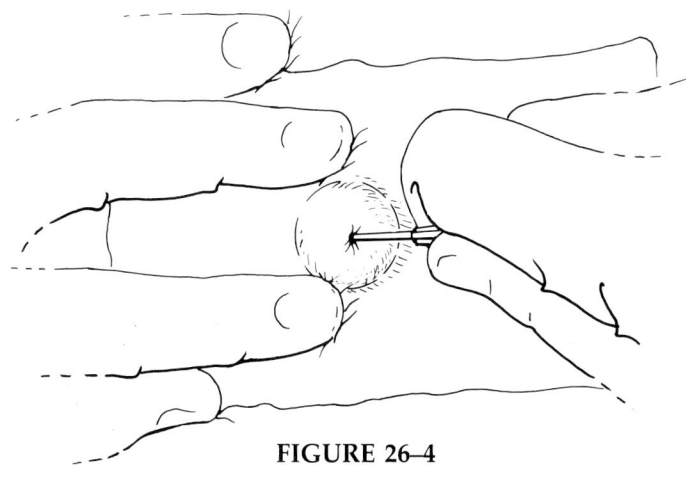

FIGURE 26–4

NEEDLE INSERTION

Insert the epidural needle (with the stylet in place) through the skin, supraspinous ligament, and interspinous ligament, into the ligamentum flavum (Fig. 26–5). With practice, the entry of the needle tip into the ligamentum flavum can usually be

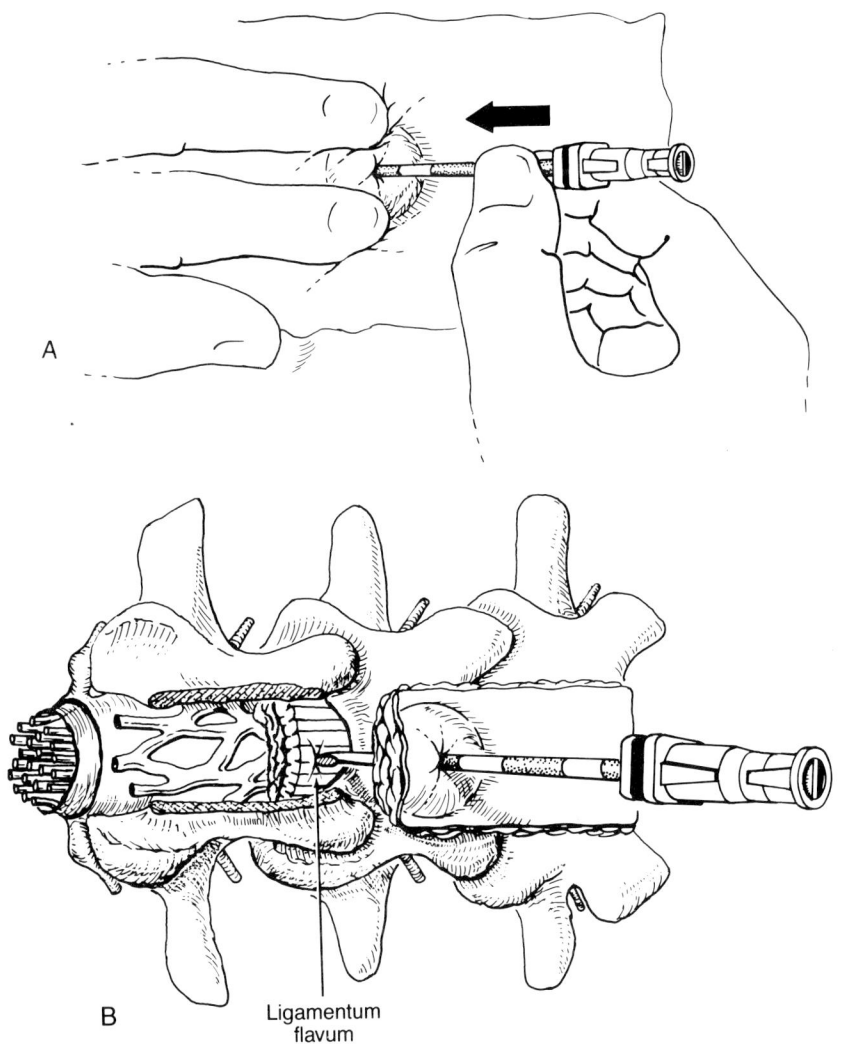

FIGURE 26–5

detected. When the operator releases an epidural needle inserted in the ligamentum flavum it will not sag (like an "arrow in the target"); conversely, if the needle is not yet in the ligament, the needle hub will sag when the needle is released.

Remove the stylet (Fig. 26–6). Dampen the plunger of the glass syringe, fill the syringe with either 0.9% saline or air (I favor air), and attach it securely to the epidural needle (Fig. 26–7).

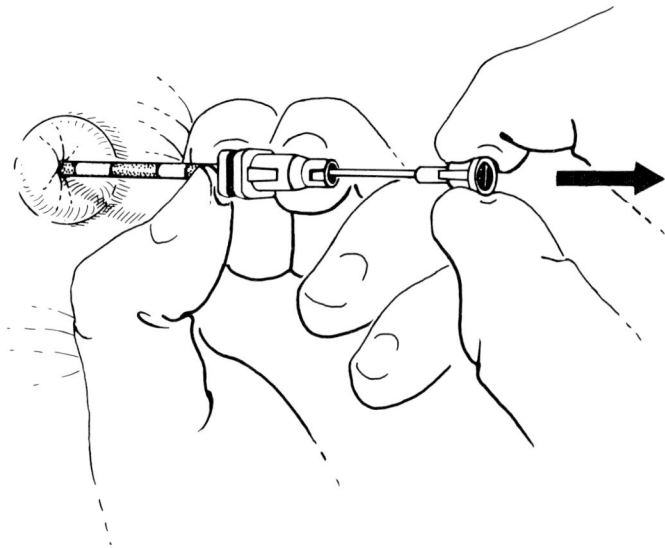

FIGURE 26–6

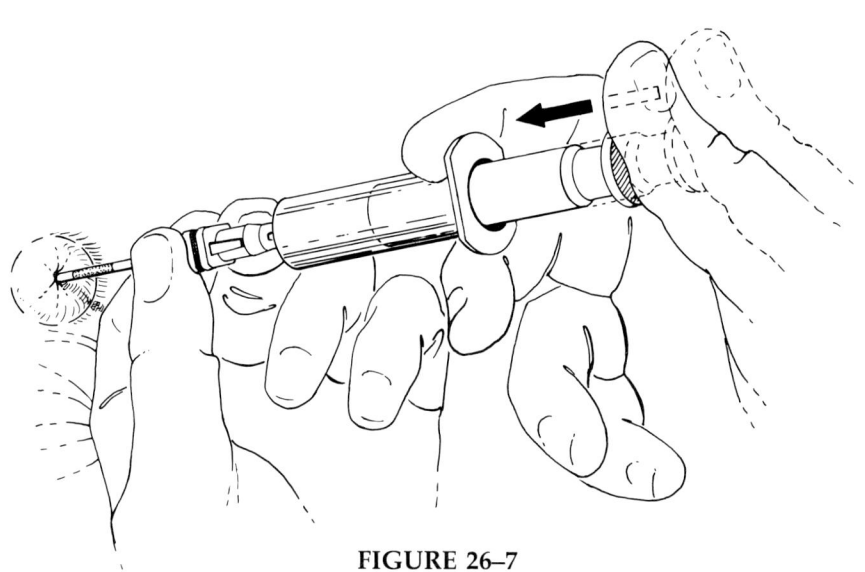

FIGURE 26–7

IDENTIFICATION OF EPIDURAL SPACE

With the dorsum of the nondominant hand securely against the patient's back, use the fingers of the nondominant hand to slowly advance the epidural needle through the ligamentum flavum. As the needle is advanced, the thumb of the dominant hand continuously "taps" on the plunger of the air-filled syringe (or continuously applies pressure on the plunger of the saline-filled syringe), confirming that resistance to injection (of air or saline) is present.

Advance the needle until "loss of resistance" is detected. While the tip of the needle remains in the ligamentum flavum, injection of air or saline will be difficult.

The instant that the needle tip emerges through the ligament, resistance to injection of air or saline drops to a minimum.

Sadly, injection of air or saline is also easily accomplished when the needle tip advances into the subarachnoid space. Thus, when loss of resistance is detected, the operator should remove the syringe, hoping *not* to see either a gush of cerebrospinal fluid or blood. If the former is obtained, the operator has the option of either performing spinal anesthesia or of removing the needle and attempting another epidural puncture at another interspace. A post–lumbar puncture headache is likely, as is the subsequent need for an epidural blood patch. If blood drips from the epidural needle (or can be aspirated through the syringe), the epidural needle tip lies within an epidural vein. The needle must be repositioned either in the same or another interspace.

Alternatively, the epidural space may be identified by placing a drop of saline or local anesthetic solution in the external opening of the epidural needle, after placing the needle in the ligamentum flavum (Fig. 26–8). When the needle tip passes through the ligament into the epidural space, the drop will usually be aspirated into the needle (Fig. 26–9).

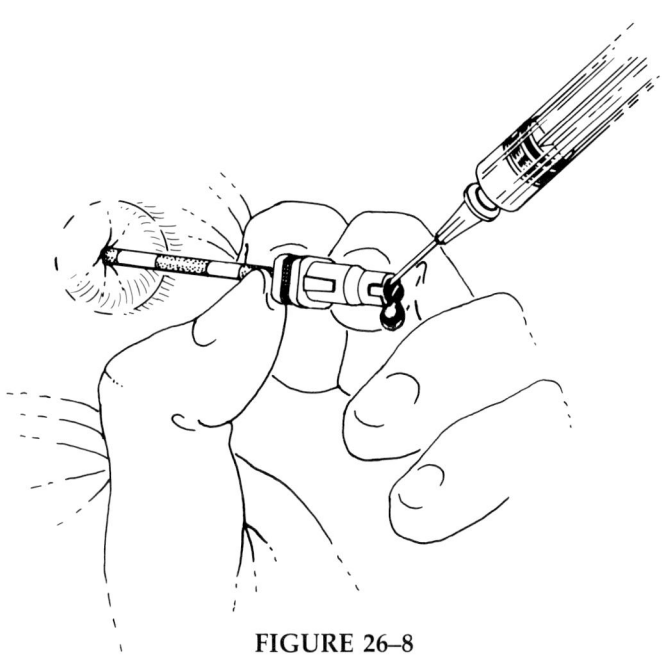

FIGURE 26–8

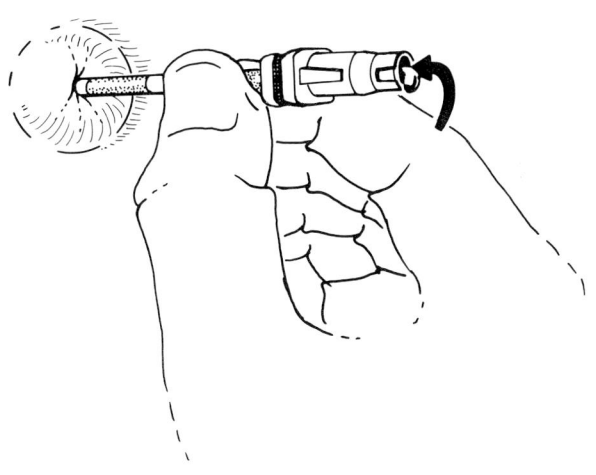

FIGURE 26–9

INSERTION OF EPIDURAL CATHETER

When the epidural needle seems appropriately sited within the epidural space, and neither blood nor cerebrospinal fluid can be aspirated, the anesthetist has the option of either injecting local anesthetic directly through the needle or of passing an epidural catheter through the needle, so that incremental injections of local anesthetic or narcotic can be made (Fig. 26–10). I nearly always pass an epidural catheter through the needle before injecting local anesthetic.

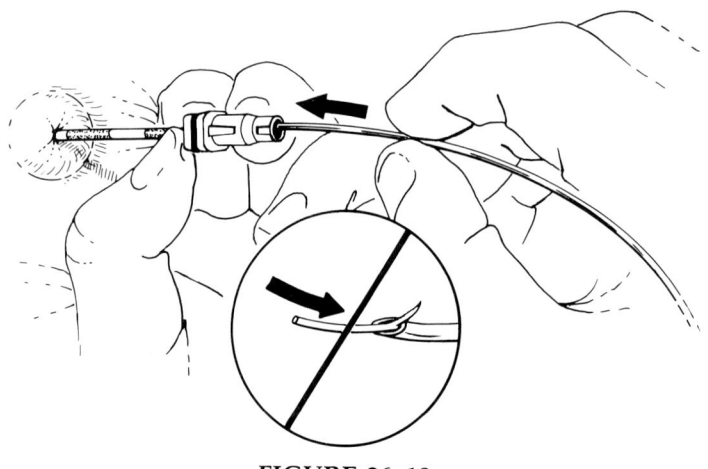

FIGURE 26–10

I customarily insert epidural catheters 2 to 3 cm beyond the tip of the epidural needle, with the bevel of the epidural needle directed cephalad (if possible) (Fig. 26–11). Unless the patient has large amounts of sagging, redundant skin threatening to drag out the epidural catheter with changes in position, or unless the catheter must be maintained in the epidural space for prolonged periods (days to weeks), I do not recommend inserting the catheter more than 3 cm beyond the tip of the epidural needle. The likelihood that a catheter will coil or pass out a nerve root sleeve seems to increase with the distance it is inserted into the epidural space.

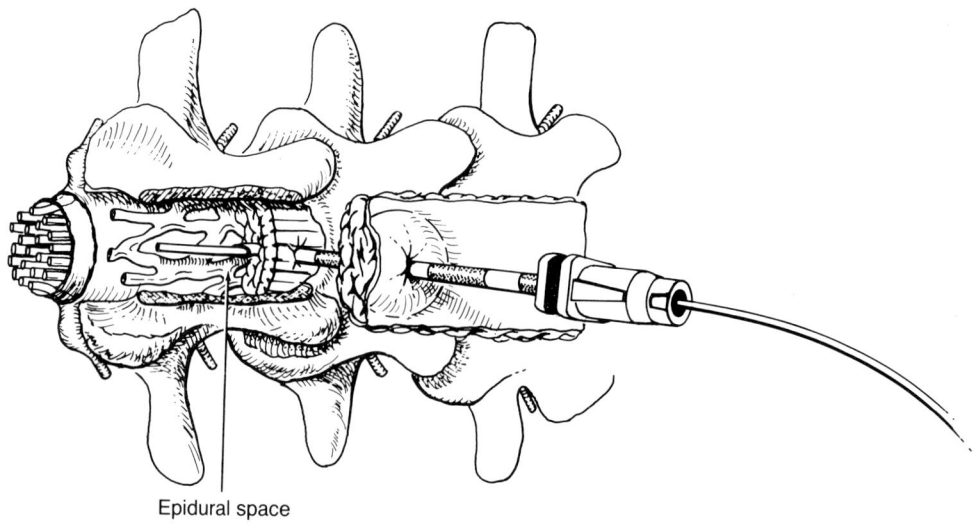

Epidural space

FIGURE 26–11

Sometimes the catheter will not pass through the needle tip in a cephalad direction. In such cases, I withdraw the catheter completely, turn the needle caudad, and attempt to pass the catheter. *If the catheter has already passed beyond the tip of the needle, the catheter should never be withdrawn through the needle, since the tip of the catheter might be sheared off and left behind in the epidural space. Alternatively, a "barb" may be formed on the catheter, making subsequent withdrawal of the catheter painful and nearly impossible (see Fig. 26–10).* If the catheter has passed beyond the needle tip and must be withdrawn, then *both needle and catheter must be withdrawn at the same time.*

When I am unable to pass the catheter with the needle bevel aimed in either a cranial or caudad direction, I sometimes find success by advancing the epidural needle an additional millimeter. Alternatively, I withdraw the epidural needle and replace it within the epidural space (either at the same or another interspace).

REMOVAL OF NEEDLE

After passing the catheter into the epidural space, withdraw the epidural needle while holding the epidural catheter in a constant position (Fig. 26–12). I recommend noting the distance (from the skin surface) of the outermost mark on the epidural catheter (I usually measure the marks against a finger or a syringe) before and after the needle is removed.

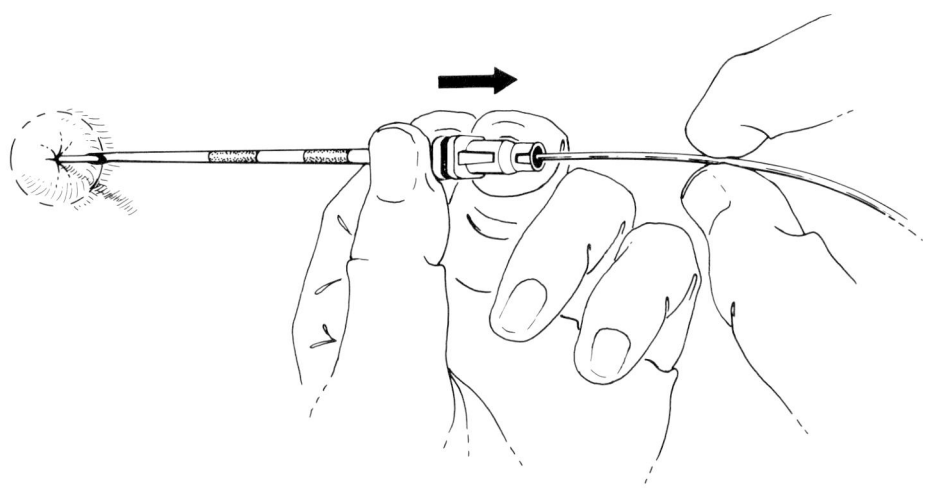

FIGURE 26–12

The catheter will often be pushed farther into the epidural space as the needle is removed. If so, the withdrawn catheter should be back to its initial position no more than 3 cm within the epidural space (Fig. 26–13).

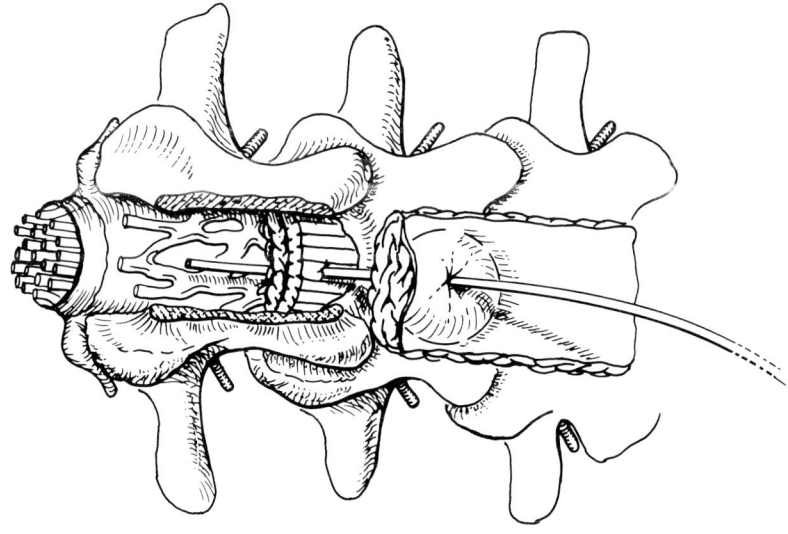

FIGURE 26–13

SECURING OF CATHETER

Tape the epidural catheter securely to the patient's back in such a way that it will not tend to kink. When the catheter will be used for postoperative pain relief, I apply tincture of benzoin to the skin and use three narrow SteriStrips to hold the catheter in place (Fig. 26–14). Place a small folded gauze pad under the catheter as it exits the skin to prevent the catheter from kinking at that point. Finally, secure the catheter to the skin of the back with 2-inch adhesive tape or with a narrow strip of SteriDrape (an adhesive, transparent material).

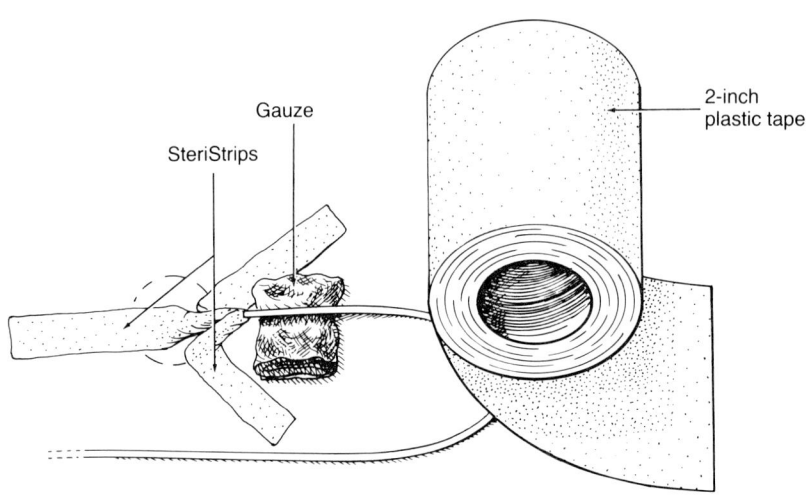

FIGURE 26–14

SPINAL TEST DOSE

All epidural catheters must be tested to be certain that they are not located beneath the dura or within an epidural vein. The fastest and most effective test for accidental intradural placement is to inject 50 to 75 mg of hyperbaric lidocaine (spinal anesthesia solution) through the epidural catheter (Fig. 26–15). If the catheter is subarachnoid, spinal anesthesia will become apparent within 2 to 3 minutes. However, for convenience, I normally use 3 ml of the epidural local anesthetic solution as the subarachnoid test dose. Onset of spinal anesthesia after injection of isobaric epidural anesthetic is more gradual; however, signs of spinal anesthesia will be perceived within 5 minutes.

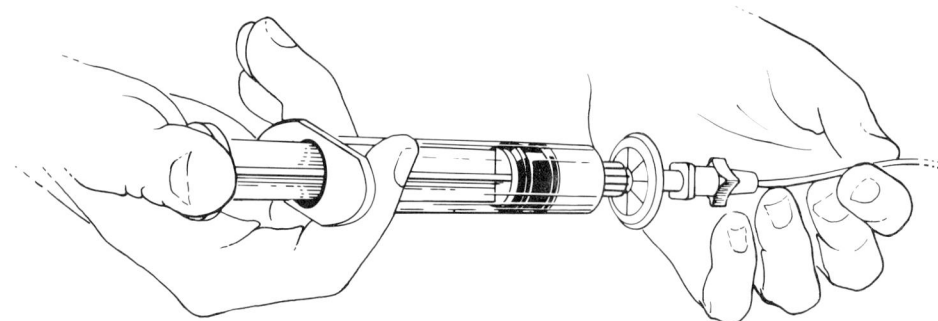

FIGURE 26–15

INTRAVENOUS TEST DOSE

If the "subarachnoid" test dose contains epinephrine and is injected intravenously, it will often produce hypertension and tachycardia, obviating the need for an "intravenous" test dose. If there is no response to the "subarachnoid" test dose, the best test for accidental intravenous catheter placement (in the nonobstetric population) is to inject a 5-ml bolus of epinephrine-containing (1:200,000 epinephrine) local anesthetic solution through the catheter. Blood pressure and heart rate should be monitored for the next 2 to 3 minutes. Twenty-five micrograms of epinephrine (in the "intravenous" test dose) injected intravenously will produce tachycardia and hypertension reliably, except in patients on β-adrenergic blockers, in whom it will produce hypertension and reflex *bradycardia* or no change in heart rate at all.

When local anesthetic solution is injected intravenously (i.e., through an epidural vein) the patient will usually also report symptoms of local anesthetic toxicity such as dizziness, tinnitus, an "ominous" feeling, circumoral numbness, and a metallic taste in the mouth. In pregnant patients presenting for relief of pain during labor, epinephrine is often omitted from test doses because (in animal studies) epinephrine tends to reduce uterine blood flow. When testing catheters inserted for labor analgesia, I recommend using first 3 ml (spinal test dose) and then an additional 5 ml of the non-epinephrine-containing local anesthetic solution (usually 2-chloroprocaine or bupivacaine). Signs of intravenous catheter placement in pregnant patients will consist of symptoms of intravenous local anesthetic injection or often simply the lack of satisfactory analgesia.

LOCAL ANESTHETIC DOSING

If the catheter appears to be located neither within the subarachnoid space nor within an epidural vein, there is a high likelihood that it is within the epidural space. The patient may be safely "dosed" with the local anesthetic of choice. I recommend that no more than 5 ml of anesthetic be injected at a time and that the operator pause for 1 minute between injections so that signs of intravenous local anesthetic toxicity will not go undetected. This is particularly important when using bupivacaine or etidocaine, for both of which the ratio between the doses that produce central nervous system and cardiovascular toxicity is nearly 1:1.

Lumbar epidural anesthesia requires fairly large volumes of local anesthetic relative to those required for spinal anesthesia. For analgesia during labor, my usual (total) dose is 10 to 12 ml of 2% 2-chloroprocaine or 0.25% bupivacaine to initiate the block. For lower extremity surgery, I usually give 15 ml of anesthetic (usually 2% lidocaine [or mepivacaine] with 1:200,000 epinephrine or 0.5% bupivacaine with 1:200,000 epinephrine). For abdominal surgery, I usually give no less than 20 ml of anesthetic with a lumbar catheter. Lower volumes are needed for abdominal surgery if a thoracic epidural catheter is used.

ONSET OF EPIDURAL ANESTHESIA

Epidural anesthesia requires at least 20 minutes to completely "set up" after injection, regardless of the local anesthetic employed. The local anesthetics of fastest onset, etidocaine and 2-chloroprocaine, are only a few minutes faster than the slowest (bupivacaine). As the anesthesia develops, always check to make sure that *bilateral* signs of anesthesia are present. I begin to worry whenever there seems to be some large disparity in the level or quality of anesthesia on the left and right sides of the patient. Refer to Figure 25–11 for charts of cutaneous sensory distribution by spinal segments.

Addition of epinephrine to epidural local anesthetic solutions increases the intensity of the motor block, delays local anesthetic absorption (and thus reduces the likelihood of toxic local anesthetic levels being achieved), prolongs the duration of some local anesthetics, and aids in the detection of intravenous placement of epidural catheters.

Hypotension

Hypotension is less of a problem with epidural anesthesia than with spinal anesthesia; nonetheless, vasopressors (I favor bolus doses of ephedrine or infusion of either phenylephrine or epinephrine) and intravenous fluid administration are often needed to maintain blood pressure during epidural anesthesia. The data are contradictory as to whether hypotension is greater when epinephrine-containing local anesthetic solutions are used than when "plain" local anesthetics are administered. The data are clear that cardiac output is better maintained when epinephrine is added to local anesthetic solutions injected for epidural anesthesia than when plain solutions are used. Differences between "plain" and epinephrine-containing local anesthetics likely result from selective β-adrenergic stimulation by sustained low concentrations of epinephrine, as a consequence of slow absorption of epinephrine from the epidural space.

Although the relevant data are now contradictory, most clinicians use intravenous fluid and ephedrine to correct hypotension during epidural anesthesia in parturients, owing to concern that phenylephrine and epinephrine (unlike ephedrine) may reduce uterine blood flow.

"Dysfunctional" Epidural Catheters

When an epidural catheter "doesn't work," I always suspect that its tip is located within a vein, particularly when epidural analgesia during labor is being attempted. I do not recommend prolonged attempts at partial withdrawal of the catheter, retesting, retaping, and so forth when the catheter is dysfunctional. I favor pulling the catheter out and starting over.

Thoracic Epidural Anesthesia

I do not recommend that anyone attempt a thoracic epidural puncture until he has *successfully* performed numerous lumbar epidural anesthesias. The first few visits to the epidural space qualify only as "social" visits. Before attempting thoracic epidural puncture, the anesthetist should find detection of loss of resistance a routine.

Generally, less local anesthetic solution will be required for epidural anesthesia when it is injected near the midpoint of the nerve roots to be blocked. Thus, for a subcostal cholecystectomy incision, an epidural catheter placed in the mid-thoracic region will more efficiently distribute local anesthetic solution than a lumbar epidural catheter. Whereas 20 to 30 ml of local anesthetic would be required to achieve somatic anesthesia for an upper abdominal incision if the local anesthetic were injected through a lumbar epidural catheter, only 10 to 15 ml will suffice if it were administered through a mid-thoracic epidural catheter.

I commonly infuse (7 to 15 ml/hr) dilute bupivacaine (0.075%) and morphine (0.005%) through the thoracic epidural catheters to provide postoperative analgesia after thoracic and abdominal vascular surgery. I have also used thoracic epidural anesthesia alone for mammary augmentations in awake outpatients.

TECHNIQUE

Unlike lumbar and caudal epidural anesthesia, the easiest approach to thoracic epidural puncture is paramedian, unless the fourth thoracic interspace (or higher) is selected, in which case the midline approach is preferable. After positioning and skin preparation as for lumbar epidural anesthesia, the anesthetist places the index finger of his nondominant hand alongside the spinous process below the interspace in which he intends to inject the anesthetic.

Inject lidocaine 1% in the skin lateral to the index finger's tip. Continue injecting local anesthetic down through all tissue layers (advancing the needle at a 90° angle to the skin) until the lamina of the next lower vertebra is encountered (Fig. 26–16). Carefully note the depth at which the lamina is encountered.

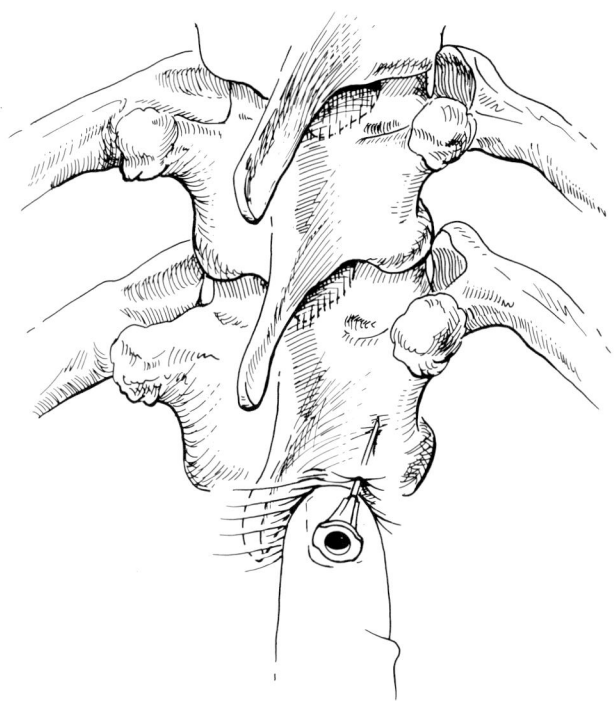

FIGURE 26–16

Advance the epidural needle (with stylet in place) in the same path as the exploring needle, so that the previously anesthetized lamina will be gently touched.

Redirect the epidural needle roughly 30° medially, and incline it cephalad roughly 30° (Fig. 26–17). Then advance the needle up and over the lamina into the ligamentum flavum (Fig. 26–18).

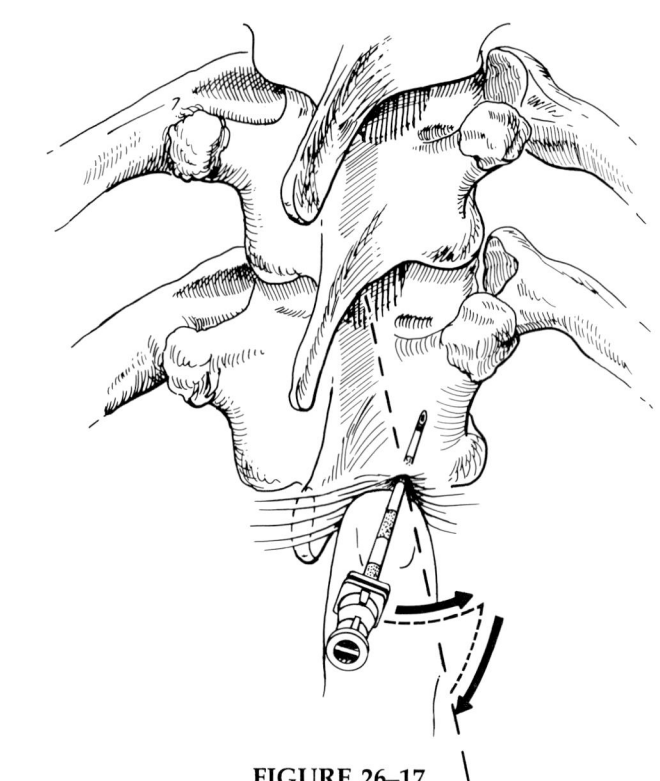

FIGURE 26–17

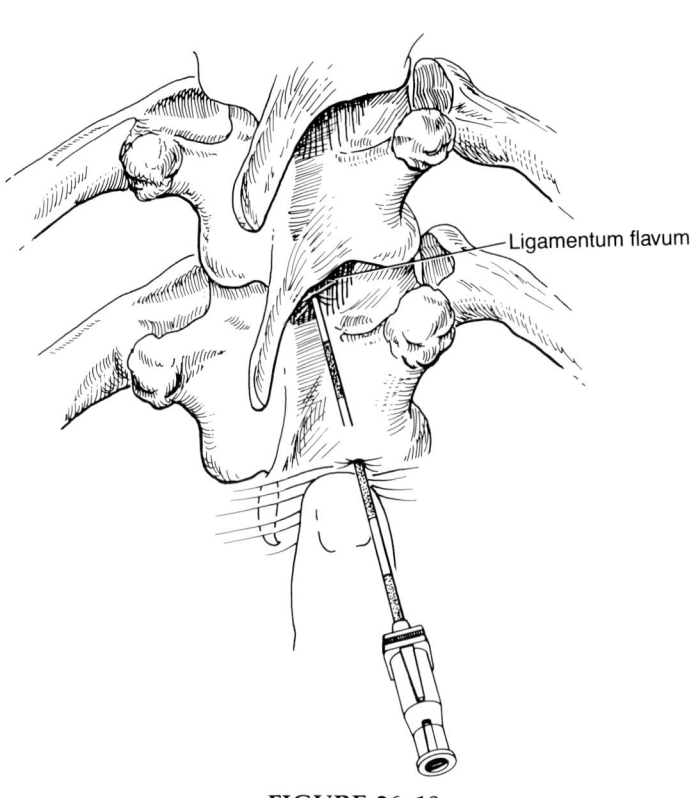

FIGURE 26–18

Fill the previously wetted glass syringe with air or saline and attach it to the epidural needle. Slowly advance the needle into the epidural space and confirm its proper location by loss of resistance to injection of air or saline.

Pass the catheter through the needle, remove the needle, and tape and test the catheter as described for lumbar epidural anesthesia.

Caudal Anesthesia

Caudal anesthesia is appropriate for anorectal and perineal procedures and for some superficial lower abdominal procedures. In children it is especially useful for providing postoperative pain relief using dilute bupivacaine and/or morphine.

Caudal anesthesia is in essence a sacral approach to the epidural space. As in other epidural techniques, the extent of caudal anesthesia depends on the volume of local anesthetic injected. I recommend 20 ml of solution (either 2% lidocaine with 1:200,000 epinephrine or 0.5% bupivacaine with 1:200,000 epinephrine) as a standard dose in adults to reliably anesthetize all sacral and lower lumbar segments. To achieve anesthesia up to and including the lower thoracic dermatomes, much higher doses (more than 30 ml) will be required.

As is true for other epidural techniques, the operator must be certain that the needle tip is located within the caudal epidural space and not within either subarachnoid space or within a blood vessel before local anesthetic is injected.

EQUIPMENT NEEDED

Sterile gloves
Antiseptic solution
Vasopressor
Local anesthetic of choice
Epinephrine
Tuberculin syringe (to measure epinephrine)
22-gauge spinal needle or 18-gauge 2-inch intravenous cannula
Usual monitoring devices
Resuscitation drugs and equipment

PREPARATION AND POSITIONING

Start an intravenous infusion and attach the electrocardiographic leads, blood pressure cuff, and pulse oximeter probe. Position the patient in either the lateral decubitus position or in the prone jack-knife position (Buie's position). I prefer the latter in adults, since this will usually be the position in which surgery is to be accomplished. Cleanse the area of the lower back superior to the gluteal cleft with antiseptic solution.

ANATOMY OF ANESTHETIC SITE

Identify the sacral hiatus by palpating the two posterior-superior iliac spines laterally and the sacral spines medially. Trace the sacral spines caudad, until an indentation is palpated in the midline. The two sacral cornua are on either lateral side of this indentation.

NEEDLE INSERTION

Inject cutaneous anesthesia with 1% lidocaine in the skin over the sacral hiatus (Fig. 26–19). Advance a 22-gauge spinal needle perpendicularly through the skin, subcutaneous tissue, and the sacrococcygeal ligament, contacting bone on the anterior side of the sacrococcygeal ligament (Fig. 26–20).

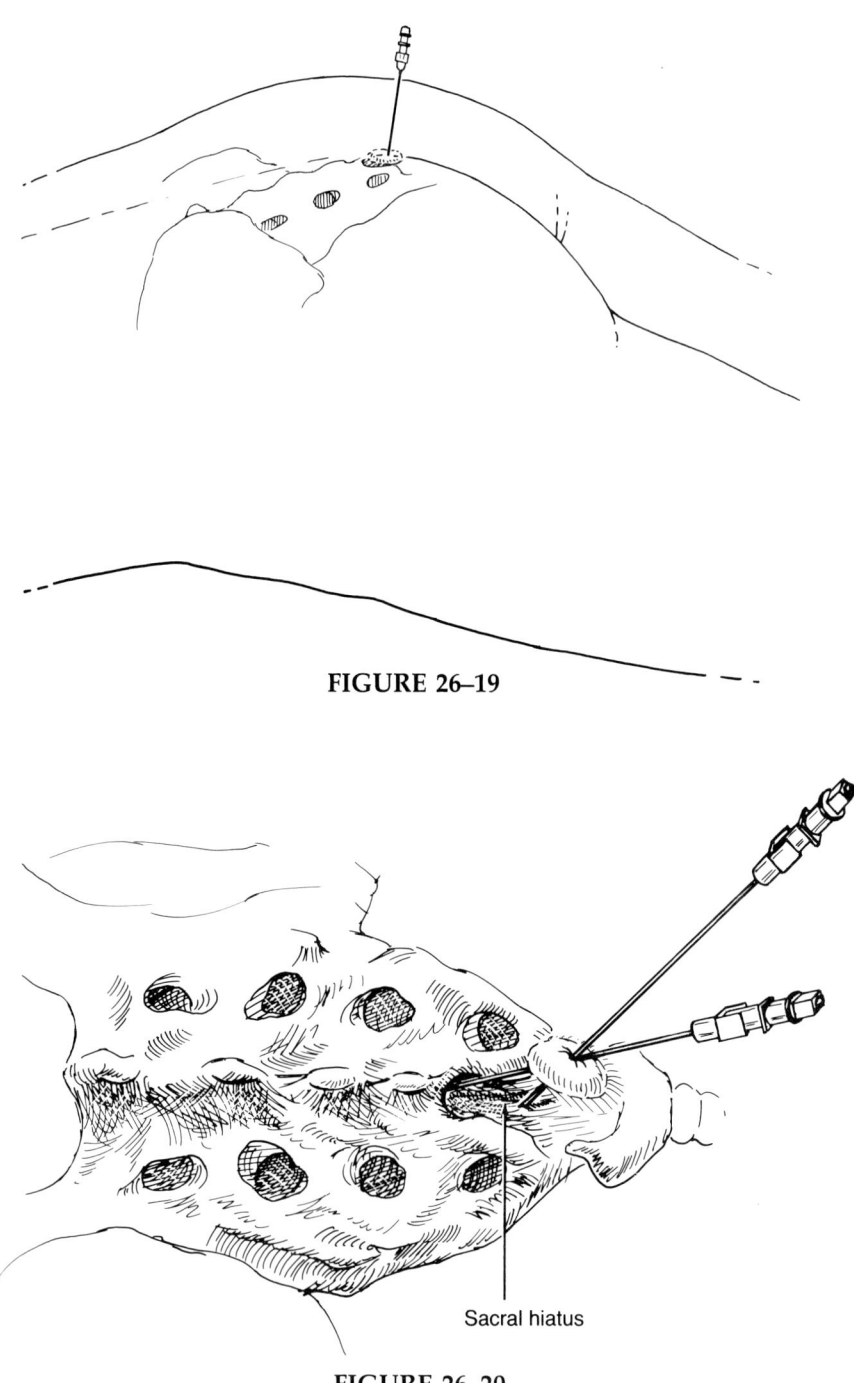

FIGURE 26–19

Sacral hiatus

FIGURE 26–20

Next, partially withdraw the needle and redirect it in a craniad direction for a distance of 2 to 3 cm. Advance the needle within the sacral spinal canal. Sometimes the operator will feel a "pop" or "give" as the needle is advanced within the canal, indicating passage into the caudal epidural space. Do not pass the needle under the periosteum of the bone on either side of the canal or excessively craniad (the lowermost extent of the dura is normally within 1 cm of the line connecting the posterior-superior iliac spines).

Remove the stylet and attach a syringe to the needle. If blood can be aspirated, do not inject local anesthetic until the needle has been repositioned. If cerebrospinal fluid can be aspirated, I recommend abandoning the caudal anesthetic and proceeding with a spinal anesthetic because of the risk of total spinal anesthesia when the large volume of local anesthetic to caudal anesthesia is injected near a dural puncture site.

TEST DOSING

If neither blood nor cerebrospinal fluid can be aspirated, administer a test dose of local anesthetic following the same format as for lumbar epidural anesthesia. Palpate the skin overlying the sacral hiatus as the local anesthetic is injected. A palpable "bulge" after injection suggests that the local anesthetic has not been placed within the caudal epidural space.

CONTINUOUS CAUDAL ANESTHESIA

Continuous caudal anesthesia can be performed with an epidural needle and an epidural catheter; however, I prefer an 18-gauge intravenous cannula and an intravenous extension tubing. I redose continuous caudal anesthetics on a similar schedule to lumbar epidural anesthetics.

USE OF CAUDAL ANALGESIA IN CHILDREN

I use the caudal approach to the epidural space to provide perioperative analgesia to young children undergoing lower abdominal and perineal procedures under general anesthesia. I inject the caudal anesthetic after induction of general anesthesia, either before surgery begins or after surgery is completed. I perform caudal puncture with a 22-gauge 2-inch spinal needle and inject 1 ml/kg (but no more than 20 ml) of 0.25% bupivacaine (without epinephrine) or 0.125% bupivacaine with 1:200,000 epinephrine. Injection of either local anesthetic solution yields more than 6 hours of analgesia. I caution against the use of epinephrine with 0.25% bupivacaine because it leads to an unacceptably high incidence of motor block (delaying the discharge of outpatients).

References

Adriani J: Labat's Regional Anesthesia, pp 352–370, 444–466. St. Louis, Warren H. Green, 1985

Bonica JJ, Akamatsu TJ, Berges PU, Morikawa K, Kennedy WF: Circulatory effects of peridural block: Effects of epinephrine. Anesthesiology 34:514–522, 1971

Bromage PR: Epidural Analgesia. Philadelphia, WB Saunders, 1978

Covino BG, Scott DB: Handbook of Epidural Anaesthesia and Analgesia. Orlando, FL, Grune & Stratton, 1985

Englesson S: Lumbar epidural anaesthesia. In Eriksson E (ed): Illustrated Handbook in Local Anaesthesia, pp 125–132. London, Edward Arnold, 1979

Hingson RA, Southworth JL: Peridural block and continuous caudal analgesia. In Southworth JL, Hingson RA (eds): Pitkin's Conduction Anesthesia, pp 669–725. Philadelphia, JB Lippincott, 1946

Kerkkamp HEM, Gielen MJM: Hemodynamic monitoring in epidural blockade: Cardiovascular effects of 20 ml 0.5% bupivacaine with and without epinephrine. Reg Anaesth 15:137–141, 1990

Löfström B: Caudal anaesthesia. In Eriksson E (ed): Illustrated Handbook in Local Anaesthesia, pp 133–138. London, Edward Arnold, 1979

Moore DC, Batra MS: The components of an effective test dose prior to epidural block. Anesthesiology 55:693–696, 1981

27

Intercostal Nerve Blocks

Intercostal (or rib) blocks are useful for providing postoperative analgesia after upper abdominal and thoracic surgical procedures. Intercostal blocks are less suitable for intraoperative anesthesia for any but the most superficial abdominal surgery unless accompanied by celiac plexus blockade and/or by general anesthesia.

Intercostal blocks are easy to perform; however, absorption of the injected local anesthetic is extremely rapid. Indeed, the same amount of local anesthetic injected for intercostal blocks will consistently yield higher blood levels than when administered for brachial or epidural blocks. Finally, the blocks carry a finite but small risk of pneumothorax.

Technique

EQUIPMENT NEEDED

Sterile gloves
Antiseptic solution
10-ml syringe
25-gauge and 22-gauge needles
Surgical marking pen
Bupivacaine (0.25 or 0.5%) 3 ml/nerve
Epinephrine
Tuberculin syringe (to measure epinephrine)
Usual monitoring devices
Resuscitation drugs and equipment

PREPARATION AND POSITIONING

Insert an intravenous cannula in the patient (if one is not already present). Attach the electrocardiographic leads, blood pressure cuff, and pulse oximeter probe to the patient for monitoring during the block. Position the patient so that the intercostal spaces to be injected are easily palpated. I prefer to position the patient prone with the arms above the head. This moves the scapulae laterally and superiorly and makes the blocks easier to accomplish. Alternatively, the sitting or lateral decubitus positions are acceptable.

MARKING OF INTERCOSTAL SPACES

Palpate the ribs immediately superior and inferior to each intercostal nerve to be blocked about a hand's breadth from the midline of the back and mark their position on the patient's back with a standard surgical marking pen (Fig. 27–1). Because of overlap of the area innervated by intercostal nerves, at least one intercostal nerve above and below the site of pain should be anesthetized.

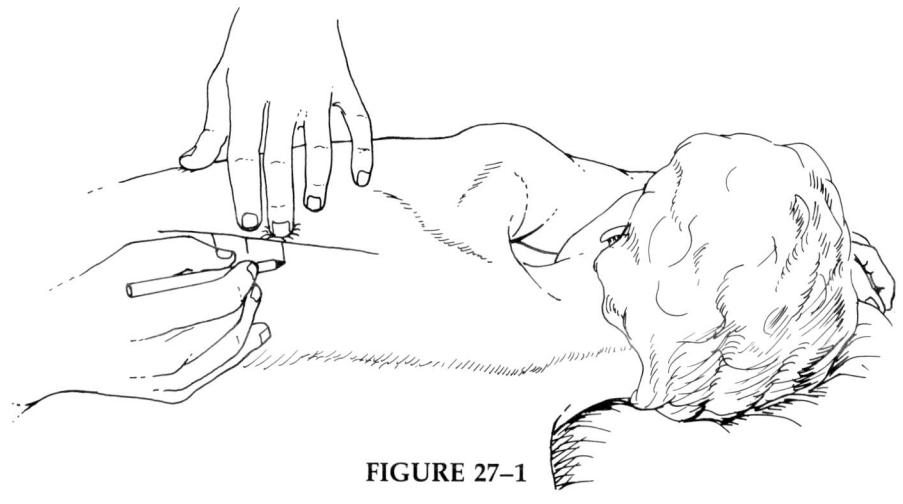

FIGURE 27–1

SKIN PREPARATION

Cleanse the skin overlying the previously marked sites of intended puncture with antiseptic solution. Inject a wheal of local anesthetic in the skin overlying each intercostal space.

NEEDLE INSERTION

Use the fingers of the nondominant hand to push the skin superiorly over the rib superior to the intercostal nerve to be blocked (Fig. 27–2). Advance a 22-gauge

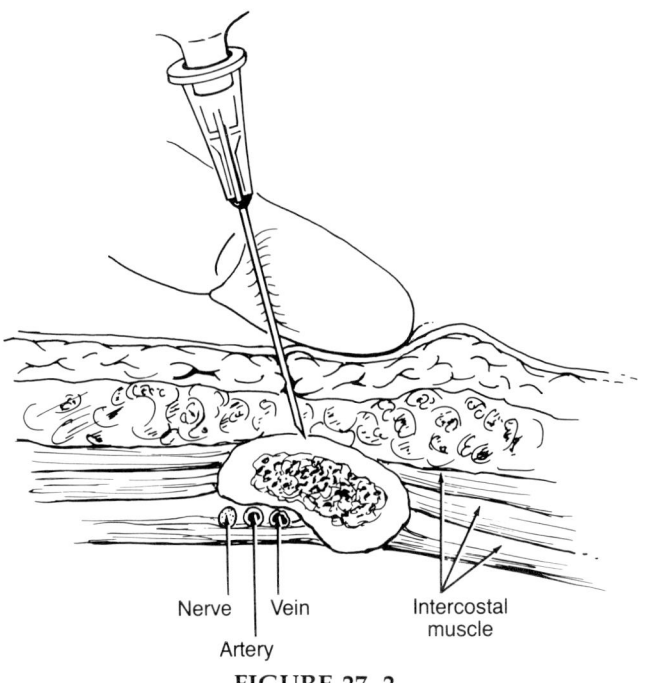

FIGURE 27–2

needle through the skin wheal at a slightly cranial angle to the skin until it touches the inferior part of the flat portion of the rib (Fig. 27–3). Carefully "walk" the needle inferiorly off the rib by allowing the overlying skin to gradually "creep" inferiorly (toward its normal location) while probing with the needle (Fig. 27–4). The neurovascular bundle lies about 0.5 cm deep (and slightly craniad) to the lower margin of the flat surface of the rib. While "walking" the needle off the rib, maintain the angle of entry of the needle slightly cranial. Under no circumstances should the needle be directed caudad. Before injecting the local anesthetic, check by aspirating through the needle to be sure that neither the intercostal vein nor artery has been entered. Three milliliters of local anesthetic containing 1:200,000 epinephrine should be sufficient for each intercostal nerve.

Subsequent intercostal nerves are blocked in a similar fashion.

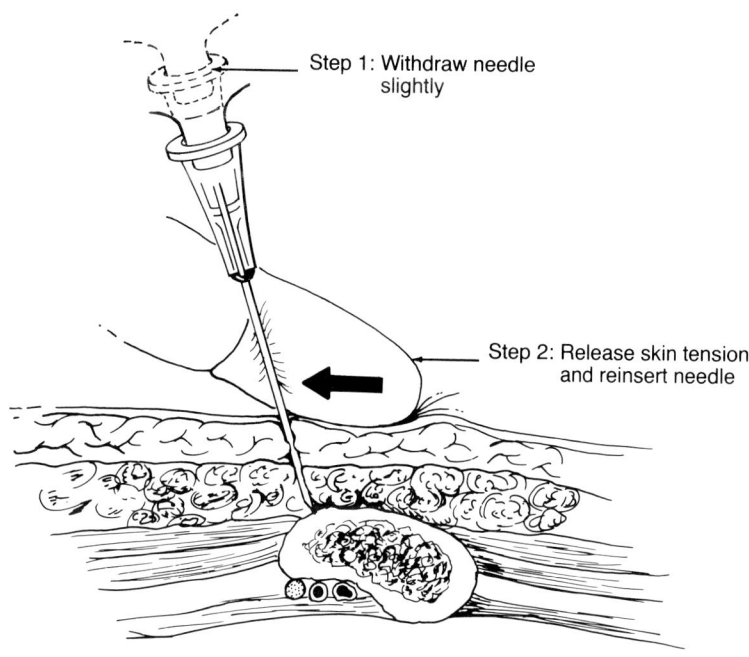

FIGURE 27–3

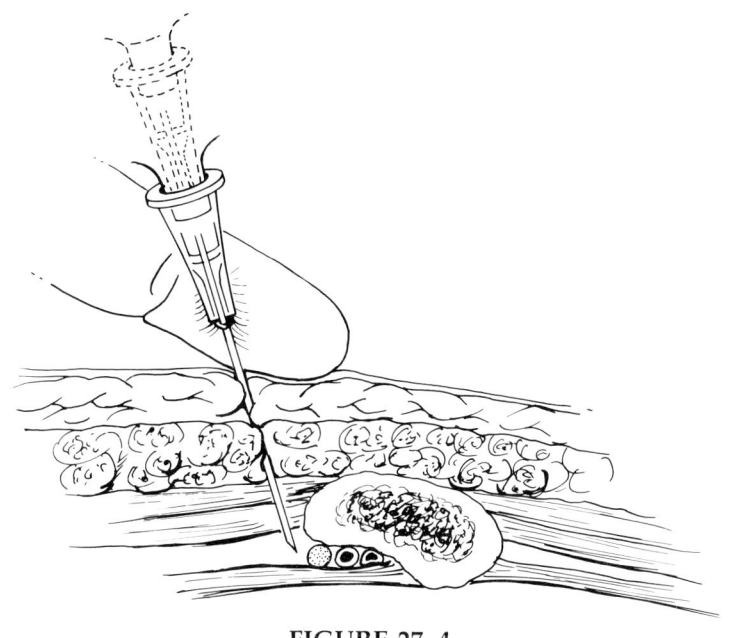

FIGURE 27–4

LOCAL ANESTHESIA

For postoperative analgesia, I recommend 0.25% bupivacaine with 1:200,000 epinephrine. For intraoperative anesthesia, I prefer 0.5% bupivacaine with 1:200,000 epinephrine.

References

Little DG: Regional anaesthesia of the trunk. In Wildsmith JAW, Armitage EN (eds): Principles and Practice of Regional Anaesthesia, pp 127–132. Edinburgh, Churchill Livingstone, 1987

Löfström B: Intercostal nerve block. In Eriksson E (ed): Illustrated Handbook in Local Anaesthesia, pp 93–95. London, Edward Arnold, 1979

Moore DC: Regional Block, pp 163–166. Springfield, IL, Charles C Thomas, 1965

Southworth JL, Hingson RA: Pitkin's Conduction Anesthesia, pp 472–516. Philadelphia, JB Lippincott, 1946

Tucker GT, Mather LE: Properties, absorption, and disposition of local anesthetic agents. In Cousins MJ, Bridenbaugh PO (eds): Neural Blockade in Clinical Anesthesia and Management of Pain, pp 47–110. Philadelphia, JB Lippincott, 1988

28

Cervical Plexus Block

Blocks of the cervical plexus are useful for providing regional anesthesia for operations on the neck. Deep cervical plexus blocks can be used for procedures as extensive as thyroidectomy. I use superficial cervical plexus blocks most commonly for patients undergoing carotid thromboendarterectomy or to provide analgesia during pulmonary artery cannulation by the internal jugular approach. By keeping the patient conscious during carotid surgery, he can serve as his own monitor of cerebral function when the carotid artery is cross-clamped. I usually do not perform deep cervical plexus blocks for carotid surgery. The risks of deep plexus block (accidental local anesthetic injection into vertebral or carotid arteries, epidural or subdural spaces, or phrenic nerve) seem unwarranted, given the safety and ease with which local anesthetic can be injected in the carotid sheath, should there be discomfort during deep dissection. I reserve deep cervical plexus blocks for extensive or invasive neck surgery in which general anesthesia is relatively contraindicated or for carotid thromboendarterectomy performed by surgeons unwilling to supplement patchy superficial blocks.

Technique of Superficial Cervical Plexus Block

EQUIPMENT NEEDED

Sterile gloves
Antiseptic solution
Local anesthetic of choice
Epinephrine
Tuberculin syringe (to measure epinephrine)
10-ml syringe
25-gauge and 22-gauge needles
Usual monitoring devices
Resuscitation drugs and equipment

PREPARATION AND POSITIONING

Start an intravenous infusion. Position the patient supine on the operating room table. Attach the electrocardiographic leads, blood pressure cuff, and pulse oximeter probe for monitoring during the procedure. Cleanse the skin of the neck and upper shoulder with antiseptic solution. Turn the patient's head to the side opposite that on which the cervical plexus block is to be performed. Identify the point of intersection between the external jugular vein and the inferior margin of the sternocleidomastoid muscle. Sometimes it will be necessary either to have the patient lift his head off the pillow to define the margins of the sternocleidomastoid muscle, or to have the patient perform a Valsalva maneuver to identify the course of the external jugular vein. When the external jugular vein cannot be identified, palpate and identify the transverse process of the third cervical vertebra by counting craniad from the Chassaignac tubercle (the most prominent transverse process, C6) toward the mastoid prominence.

INJECTION OF LOCAL ANESTHETIC

Inject 10 ml of 0.5% bupivacaine with 1:400,000 epinephrine in a fanwise fashion beneath the external jugular vein where it crosses the sternocleidomastoid muscle (or dorsad to the sternocleidomastoid muscle at the C3 level if the vein cannot be seen), and continue the injection along the inferior border of the sternocleidomastoid muscle 3 cm craniad and caudad to the initial injection (Fig. 28–1).

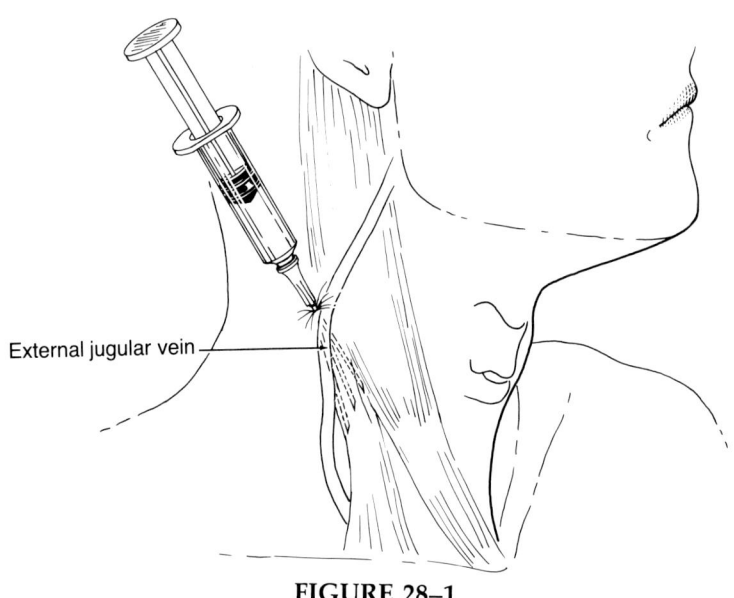

FIGURE 28–1

It may also be helpful to inject 5 ml of local anesthetic solution into the sternocleidomastoid muscle itself at approximately the same level as the first 10 ml of anesthetic injection, to relax the muscle and reduce discomfort from muscle spasms induced by self-retaining retractors. This injection may also further anesthetize the superficial cervical plexus as it travels through and around the muscle.

Test the extent of anesthesia so that any necessary supplementation can be provided in a timely fashion.

INTRAOPERATIVE ANALGESIA

Following a successful superficial cervical plexus block, patients usually will experience no discomfort until the carotid sheath is exposed. Innervation of the carotid fascial sheath is provided by the nerves of the deep cervical plexus and also from cranial nerves; therefore, superficial cervical plexus block will not reliably eliminate all pain perception at this depth of the incision. If the patient reports discomfort I request that the surgeon, after a negative aspiration (given the proximity of both the internal jugular vein and the carotid artery), inject 2 to 3 ml of local anesthetic into the carotid sheath itself. Often the surgeon will spray the carotid artery and the contents of the carotid sheath with local anesthetic for surface anesthesia of the vascular structures prior to making the incision into the carotid artery. Excess local anesthetic can be aspirated into the wall suction device.

Technique of Deep Cervical Plexus Block

PREPARATION AND POSITIONING

Position and prepare the patient on the operating room table as described for superficial cervical plexus block. Palpate the mastoid process and the Chassaignac tubercle (the transverse process of C6). Palpate the transverse process of C2 1 to 2 cm caudad to the mastoid prominence and in line with the Chassaignac tubercle. In the same way, palpate and mark the transverse processes of C3 and C4. Cleanse the skin of the neck with antiseptic solution.

INJECTION OF LOCAL ANESTHETIC

Inject local anesthetic into the skin overlying the C2, C3, and C4 transverse processes. Insert a 22-gauge 1½-inch needle through the uppermost skin wheal aiming the needle slightly caudad. Advance the needle until it touches the transverse process of C2 (Fig. 28–2). After contacting the transverse process, check by aspiration to be sure that the tip of the needle is not within a blood vessel (e.g., the vertebral artery). Inject a test dose of local anesthetic (less than 1 ml would be appropriate). If there is no response to the test dose, inject an additional 4 ml of bupivacaine 0.5% with 1:400,000 epinephrine. Withdraw the needle approximately 1 cm, check placement by aspiration, and then inject an additional 5 ml of local anesthetic.

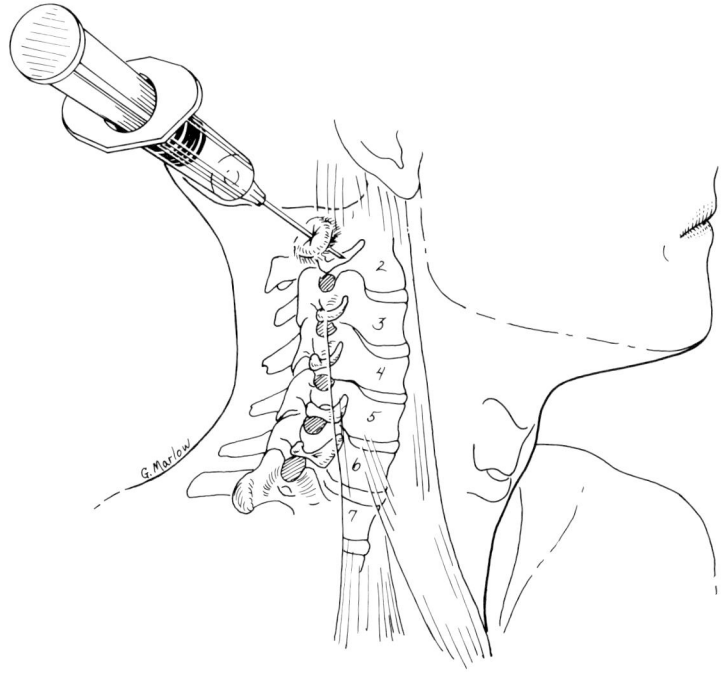

FIGURE 28–2

Repeat the local anesthetic injection at the transverse processes of C3 and C4. Paresthesias are usually not obtained. However, if a paresthesia should occur (felt in the back of the head or on the neck), this would indicate correct needle placement.

The onset of anesthesia from deep cervical plexus block should be carefully monitored so that supplementation, if required, can be administered in a timely fashion.

References

Adriani J: Labat's Regional Anesthesia, pp 236–251. St. Louis, Warren H. Green, 1985

Löfström B: Cervical nerve block. In Eriksson E (ed): Illustrated Handbook of Local Anaesthesia, pp 77–78. London, Edward Arnold, 1979

Moore DC: Regional Block, pp 112–122. Springfield, IL, Charles C Thomas, 1965

Neill RS: Head, neck and airway. In Wildsmith JAW, Armitage EN (eds): Principles and Practice of Regional Anaesthesia, pp 168–175. Edinburgh, Churchill Livingstone, 1987

Scott DB: Techniques of Regional Anaesthesia, pp 74–77. Norwalk, CT, Appleton & Lange, 1989

Southworth JL, Hingson RA: Pitkin's Conduction Anesthesia, pp 395–447. Philadelphia, JB Lippincott, 1946

Till JS, Toole JS, Howard VJ, Ford CS, Williams D: Declining morbidity and mortality of carotid endarterectomy: The Wake Forest University Medical Center Experience. Stroke 18:823–829, 1987

von Bahr V: Local anesthesia for thyroid surgery. In Eriksson E (ed): Illustrated Handbook in Local Anaesthesia, pp 43–45. London, Edward Arnold, 1979

29

Use of the Electrical Nerve Stimulator for Regional Anesthesia

In any regional anesthesia procedure in which paresthesias must be elicited for nerve location, use of an electrical nerve stimulator will obviate the need for the needle to contact the nerve directly. In brief, a needle is passed *near* the nerve, allowing brief pulses of electric current to depolarize the nerve, ultimately leading to a motor response. The nerve may be identified by the muscle(s) that respond to the electric pulses.

Electrophysiology

A nerve fires when a stimulating current (usually measured in milliamperes) exceeds its threshold. The amount of current required to stimulate a motor nerve is small both in absolute terms and in comparison to that required to elicit the sensation of pain in a sensory nerve. However, it is critical that the nerve be stimulated by current passed from the tip of the needle, near to the site of local anesthetic injection, rather than from along the length of the needle. Specially designed, insulated regional block needles are available (however, noninsulated block needles work nearly as well because the current density is highest at the needle tip).

Nerve stimulators used in regional anesthesia typically emit pulses of constant duration. For nerve location during regional anesthesia, I recommend using a stimulator that permits the current to be adjusted, and which provides a digital display of the milliamperes actually delivered to the nerve. The *negative* terminal of the stimulator should be connected to the block needle. The *positive* lead of the stimulator should be attached to an electrocardiograph skin patch electrode placed on nearby skin.

Technique

EQUIPMENT NEEDED (IN ADDITION TO USUAL BLOCK EQUIPMENT)

Insulated block needle
Adjustable nerve stimulator

Cable and alligator clips
Electrocardiographic patch electrode

PREPARATION AND POSITIONING

Position and prepare the patient for the specific nerve block procedure to be performed. Attach the skin (ground) electrode and needle electrode to the nerve stimulator.

NEEDLE INJECTION AND NERVE LOCATION

Insert the needle through the skin as appropriate for the block being attempted. With standard stimulators, adjust the intensity of the current to approximately 3 mA. The subject should barely feel each pulse of electricity (Fig. 29–1). These pulses (delivered at 1 Hz) should *not* be uncomfortable. Advance the needle until the motor response elicited in the nerve to be blocked is maximal. For example, during brachial plexus block, one should elicit a motor response in the fingers or wrist.

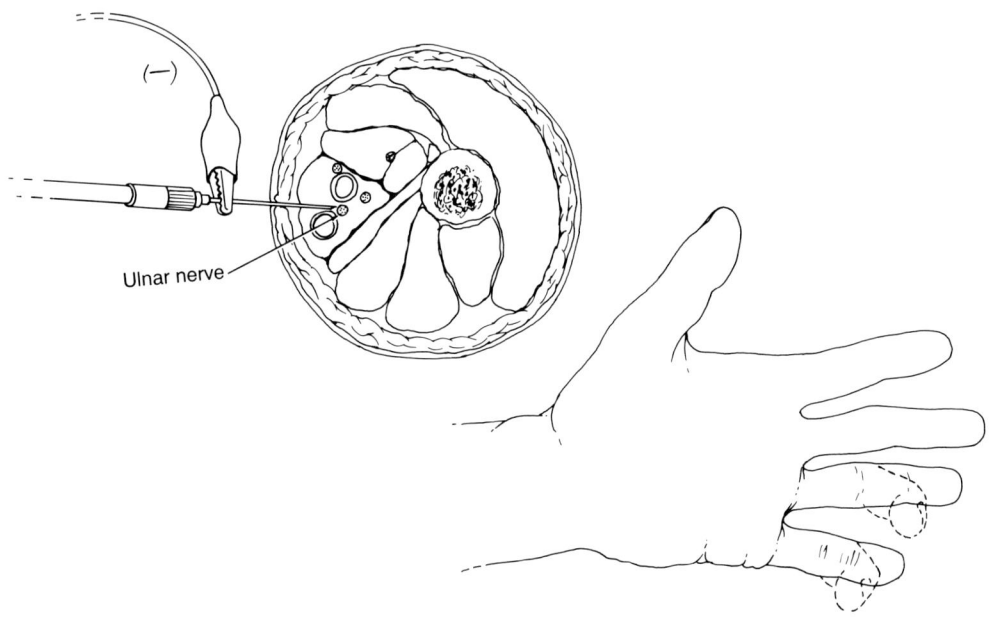

FIGURE 29–1

Carefully advance and/or withdraw the needle to identify the point of maximal motor response. Reduce the stimulus intensity to 1 mA. The motor response to electrical pulses should be maintained. Inject 2 ml of local anesthetic (after aspiration has confirmed that the needle tip is extravascular). If the needle is correctly placed, the motor response to electrical stimulation will be eliminated almost immediately. Next, inject the remainder of the local anesthetic after appropriate test dosing.

References

Carley LR, Raymond SA: Threshold measurement: Applications to excitable membranes of nerve and muscle. J Neurosci Methods 9:309–333, 1983

Charlton JE: The management of regional anaesthesia. In Wildsmith JAW, Armitage EN (eds): Principles and Practice of Regional Anaesthesia, pp 46–47. Edinburgh, Churchill Livingstone, 1987

Greenblatt GM, Denson JS: Needle nerve stimulator-locator: Nerve blocks with a new instrument for locating nerves. Anesth Analg 41:599–602, 1962

Koons RA: The use of the Block-Aid monitor and plastic intravenous cannulas for nerve blocks. Anesthesiology 31:290–291, 1969

IV

POSITIONING THE PATIENT ON THE OPERATING ROOM TABLE

30

Operation of the Surgical Table

The surgical table is designed to optimally position the patient for surgery. Tables are of two main varieties: (1) manually operated mechanical tables and (2) electrically operated motorized tables. Manually operated surgical tables have a handle on the left side that when rotated inclines the operating room table and patient. A crank under the head of the table controls the kidney rest. On the right side, a handle and clutch control flexing the table, raising and lowering the back and leg supports, and tilting the table to the left or right. A foot control raises and lowers the table height (Fig. 30–1). Movements of motorized tables are achieved by depressing the appro-

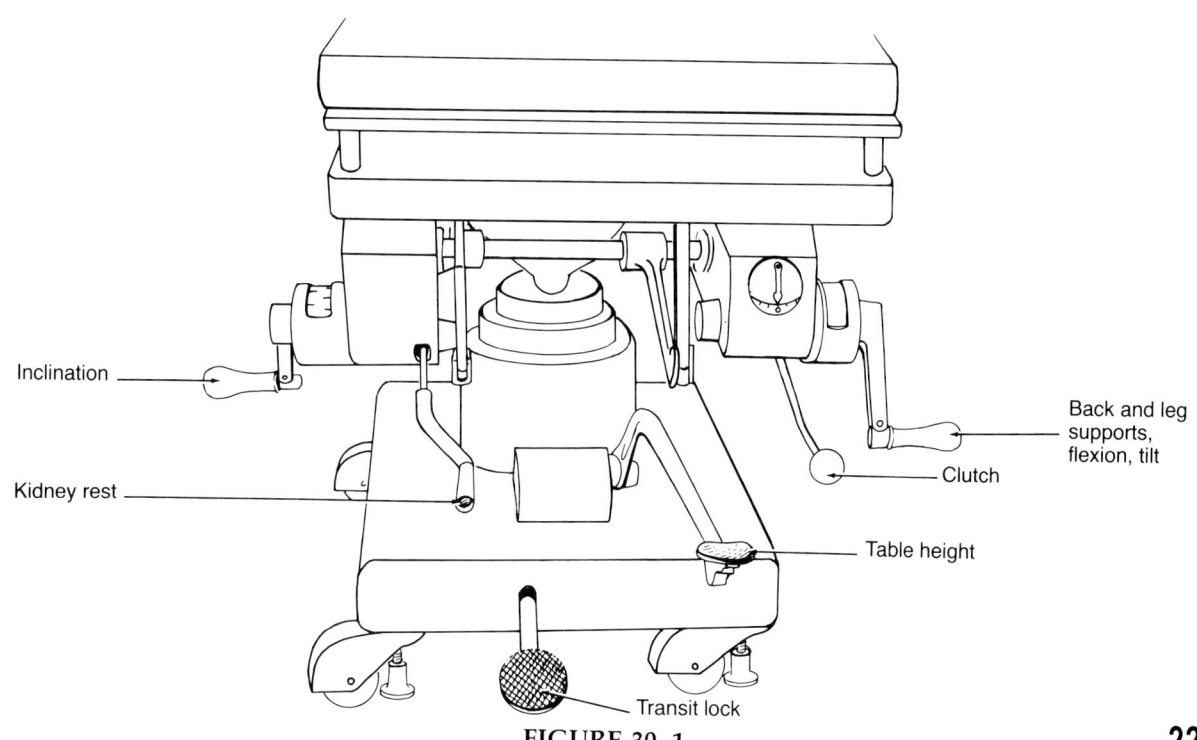

FIGURE 30–1

priate button (Fig. 30–2). In either case, the tables have an identical repertoire of permitted movements.

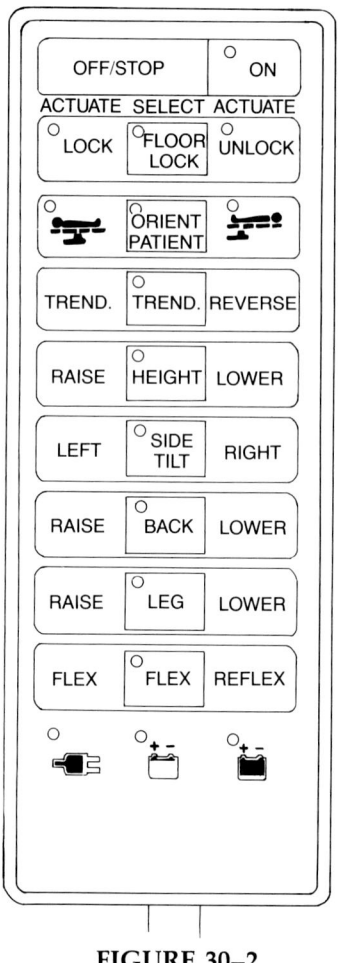

FIGURE 30–2

Movements of the Operating Room Table

TRENDELENBURG AND REVERSE-TRENDELENBURG POSITIONS

Trendelenburg, a 19th-century surgeon, positioned his patients head down to facilitate exposure of the pelvic viscera during urologic surgery. Although the position he described included both head-down tilt and knee flexion, in current vernacular "Trendelenburg" position denotes only a head-down tilt.

The patient is placed in the Trendelenburg position by rotating the left-hand control in a clockwise direction, or on electrical tables by depressing the appropriate button (Fig. 30–3). I often place patients in the Trendelenburg position to facilitate central venous cannulation or pelvic surgical exposure or to prevent air bubbles from embolizing to the cerebral circulation after aortic or mitral valve replacement.

Elevating the patient's head above the level of the heart into the so-called reverse-Trendelenburg position is accomplished by rotating the handle in a counterclockwise direction or by depressing the appropriate button. This position is rarely used since it may lead to severe hypotension from dependent venous pooling.

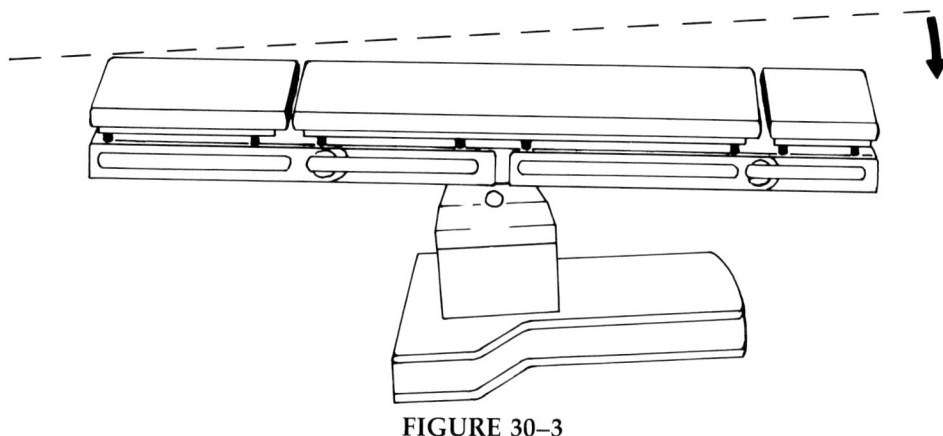

FIGURE 30–3

FLEXING THE TABLE

Operating room tables can be "flexed" so that the back and leg supports of the table may be either lowered or raised in concert (Fig. 30–4). Flexing the table facilitates closure of transverse abdominal incisions and forms a part of other surgical postures (e.g., the "sitting" position).

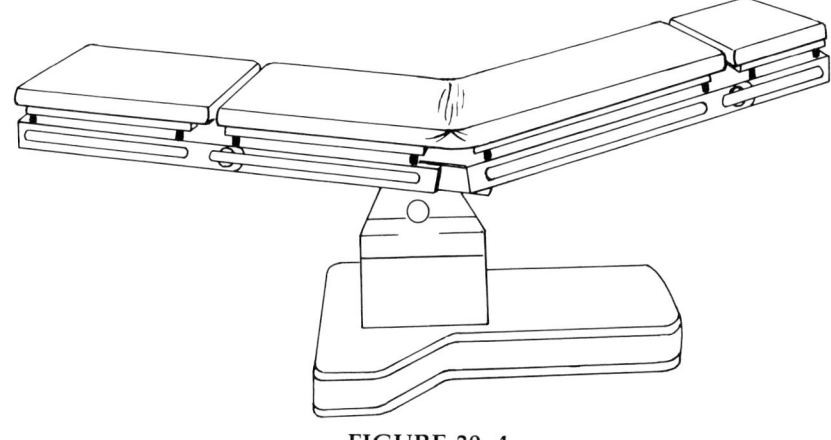

FIGURE 30–4

ADJUSTMENT OF BACK SUPPORT

The back support of the operating room table can be raised or lowered independently of the lower body section of the table (Fig. 30–5). To adjust the back section, shift the clutch control into the "back" position and crank the right-hand control either clockwise to raise the back section or counterclockwise to restore the back of the table to horizontal.

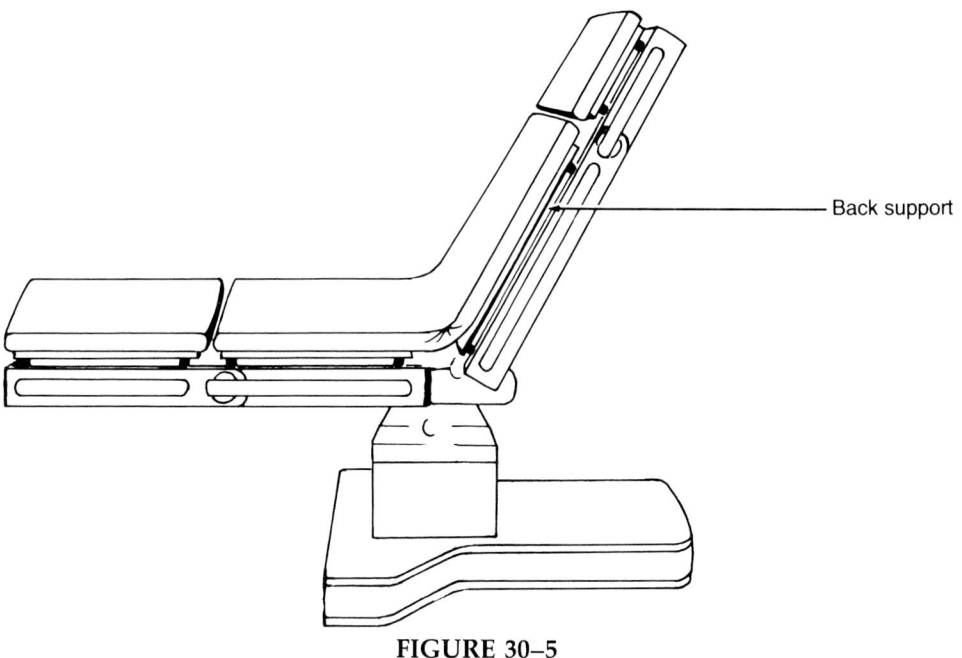

FIGURE 30–5

ADJUSTMENT OF FOOT SUPPORT

Lowering the foot support of the table permits the patient to assume the "meniscectomy position" with the legs flexed at the knees and permits the surgeon to have easy access to the patient in "lithotomy position" with both legs elevated in stirrups (Fig. 30–6). Whenever the foot support is adjusted it is important to determine that no part of the patient's body (e.g., a finger) is at risk of being crushed.

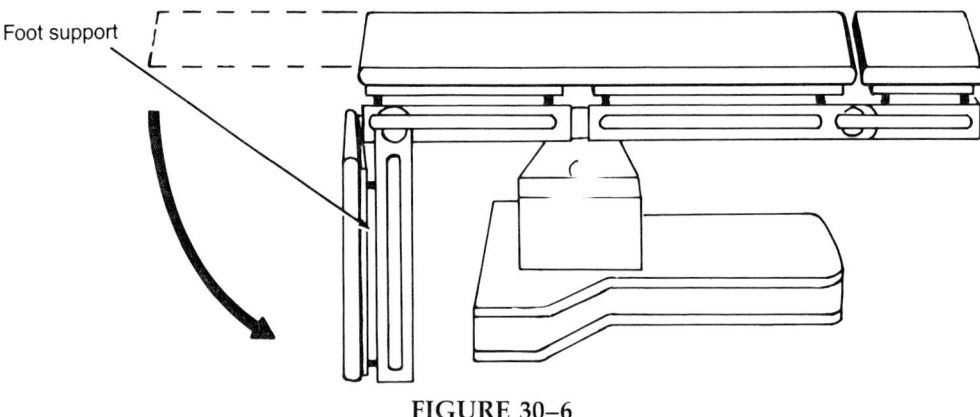

FIGURE 30–6

KIDNEY REST

In the past, the kidney rest was commonly raised during upper abdominal surgery to facilitate exposure of the biliary drainage system. The more frequent use of cholangiography (which requires that the kidney rest not be used so that the radiograph film cassette can be inserted beneath the patient) has virtually eliminated the use of the kidney rest during general surgery. At present, the kidney rest serves to facilitate exposure during kidney surgery in the flexed, lateral decubitus position (Fig. 30–7).

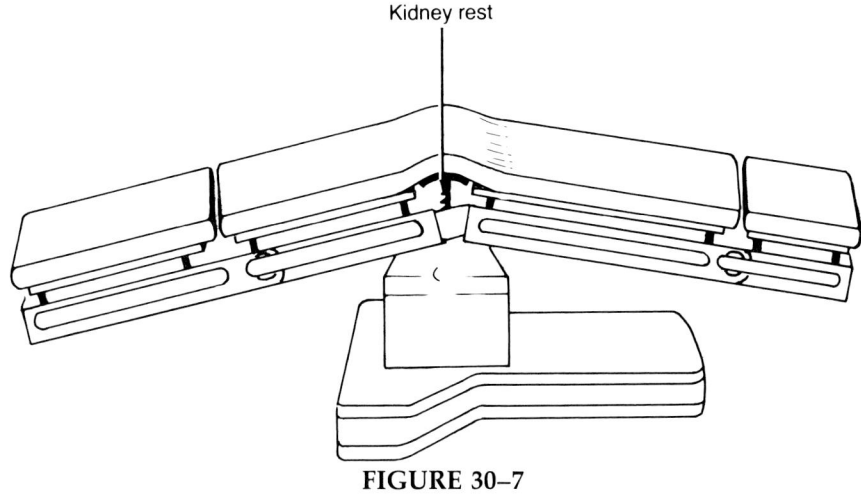

FIGURE 30–7

On both motorized and manual operating room tables, the kidney rest is raised with a small hand crank located under the surgical table, on the left side.

ARM SUPPORTS

Usually, at least one of the patient's arms will be abducted and supported on an arm rest during surgery in the supine position. To reduce the likelihood of injury to the brachial plexus, I prefer to abduct only one arm as much as 90%. I usually put additional padding between the arm and the cushioned arm rest, hoping to reduce the likelihood of ulnar nerve injury (Fig. 30–8).

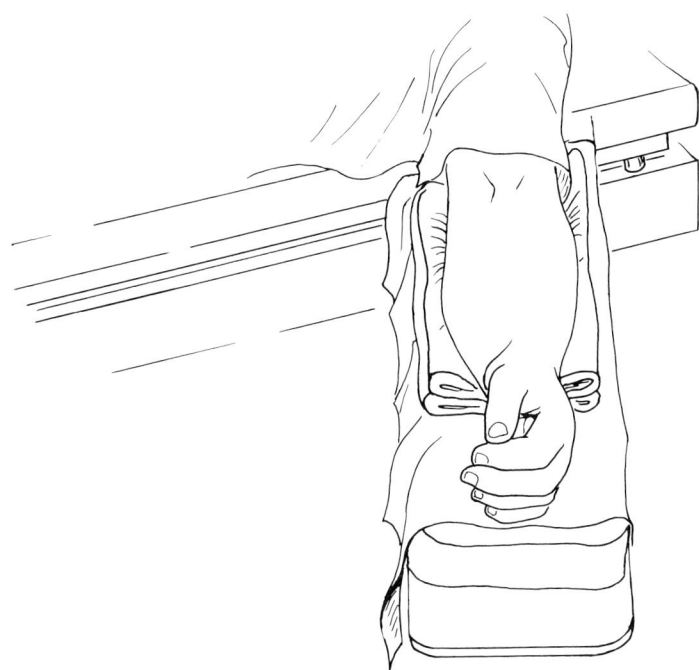

FIGURE 30–8

31

Patient Positions

Supine Position

Nearly all patients are anesthetized, and most undergo surgery in the supine position. Although no movement of the anesthetized patient is required to accomplish this position, there remain a few pitfalls in this most common of surgical postures. Unsedated patients (e.g., during regional anesthesia) who must remain supine and immobile quickly become restless and uncomfortable. Such patients will benefit from slight elevation of the back and foot supports, slight flexion, and a slight head-down tilt (Trendelenburg) to produce the "lawn chair" position (Fig. 31–1).

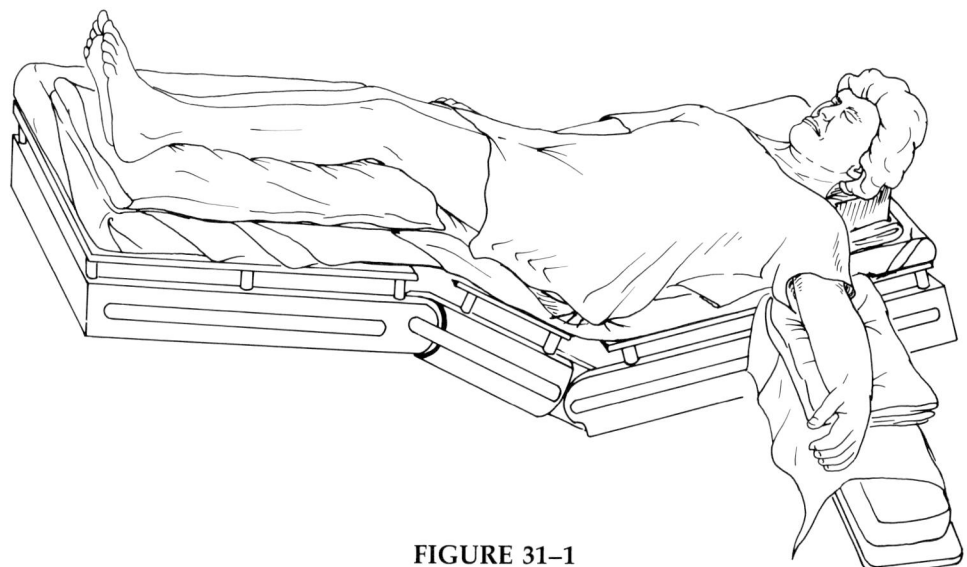

FIGURE 31–1

Anesthetized patients may develop cranial alopecia if their heads are allowed to rest on the unpadded mattress of the surgical table for prolonged periods. Foam head cradles effectively protect against this (probably ischemic) complication. I also routinely place a pillow behind the lower legs of patients who will remain supine during general anesthesia to improve venous drainage and reduce the strain on the lower back.

Pregnant women and patients with large intra-abdominal tumors may develop the supine hypotension syndrome from compression of the aorta and abdominal vena cava against the spine. I routinely place a "wedge" under the right side of all pregnant women to displace the gravid uterus off the great vessels (Fig. 31–2).

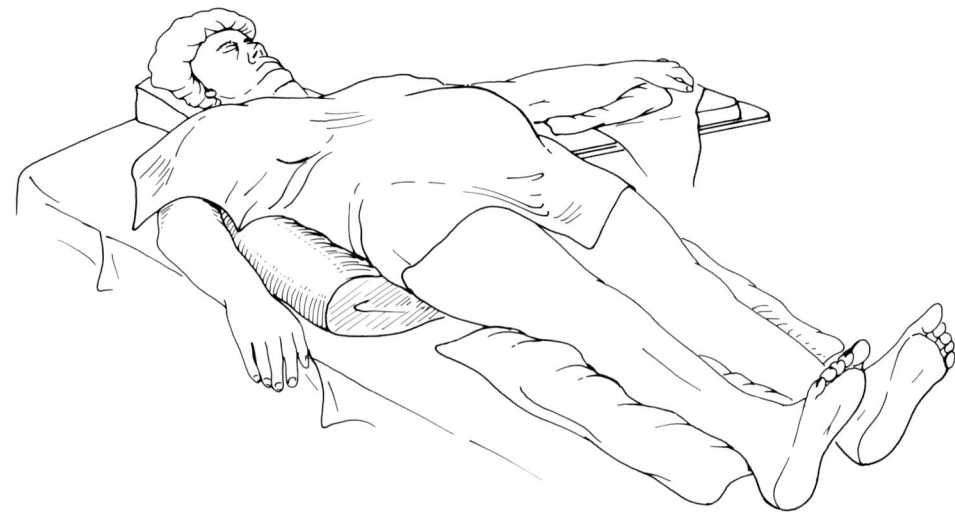

FIGURE 31–2

Lithotomy Position

The lithotomy position, a variation on the supine posture, is used during most perineal gynecologic procedures (e.g., vaginal hysterectomy) and many genitourinary procedures (e.g., cystoscopy). To achieve the lithotomy position, first attach the leg holders (or stirrups) on either side of the table. Flex both of the patient's legs together at the hip and knee (Fig. 31–3). Place both legs in the leg holders (or stirrups) at the same time. Determine that neither peroneal nerve is impinged on by the leg support. Lower the foot section of the table out of the way after ensuring that no body parts will be crushed (Fig. 31–4).

Returning to the supine position from the lithotomy position requires the same sequence of maneuvers in reverse order and in reverse direction.

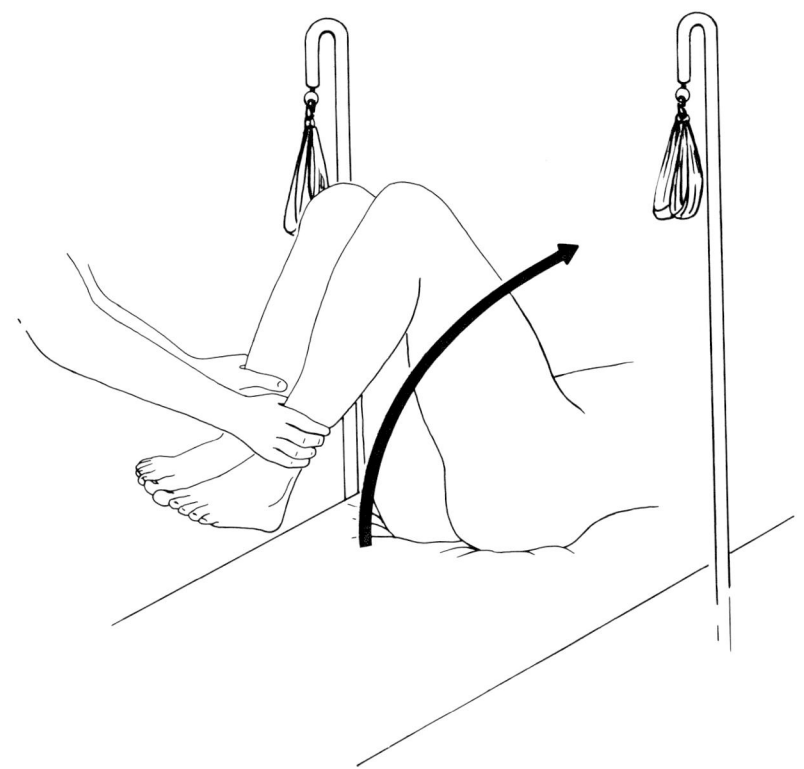

FIGURE 31–3

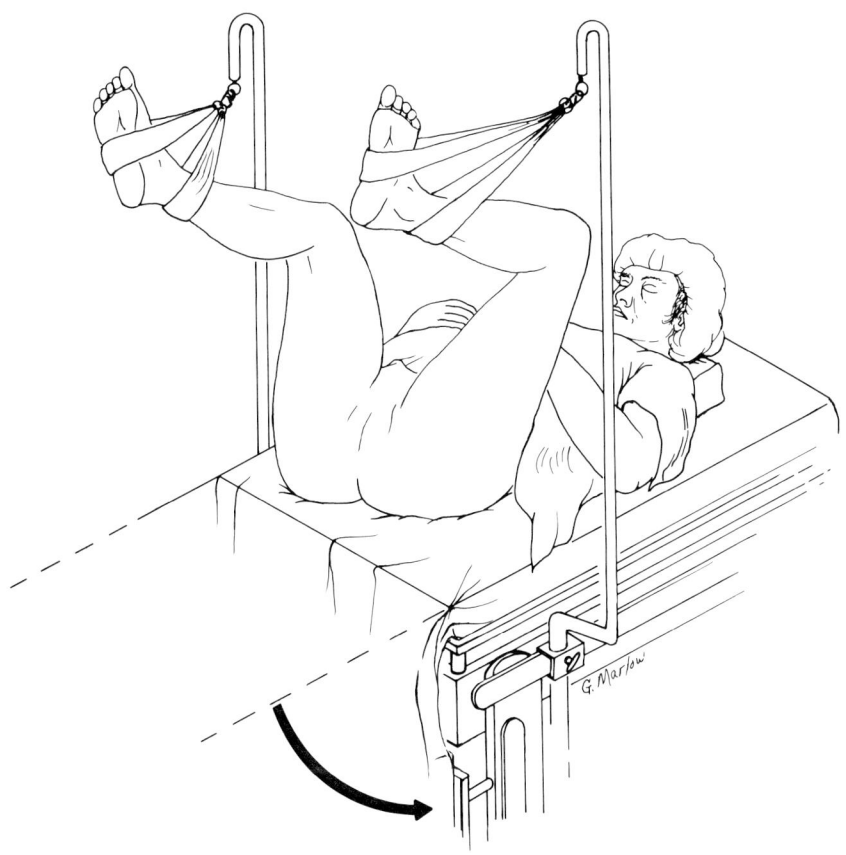

FIGURE 31–4

Lateral Decubitus Position

Patients often undergo pulmonary and renal surgery in the lateral decubitus position. Typically, patients are anesthetized while supine and then are moved to the lateral decubitus position after tracheal intubation. Since the patient must be physically lifted to accomplish the turn, make sure that a sufficient number of assistants are available. The anesthetist will be responsible for head and tracheal tube position and for the security of monitoring devices during the move. When the assistants are ready, the anesthetist should give a signal to start the turn. Usually, transition to the lateral decubitus position is accomplished in two steps: (1) *rotating* the patient onto the side and (2) *shifting* the patient's back toward the edge of the table (Fig. 31–5). Normally, a foam or rolled blanket axillary roll is put beneath the patient to prevent compression of the brachial plexus in the axilla.

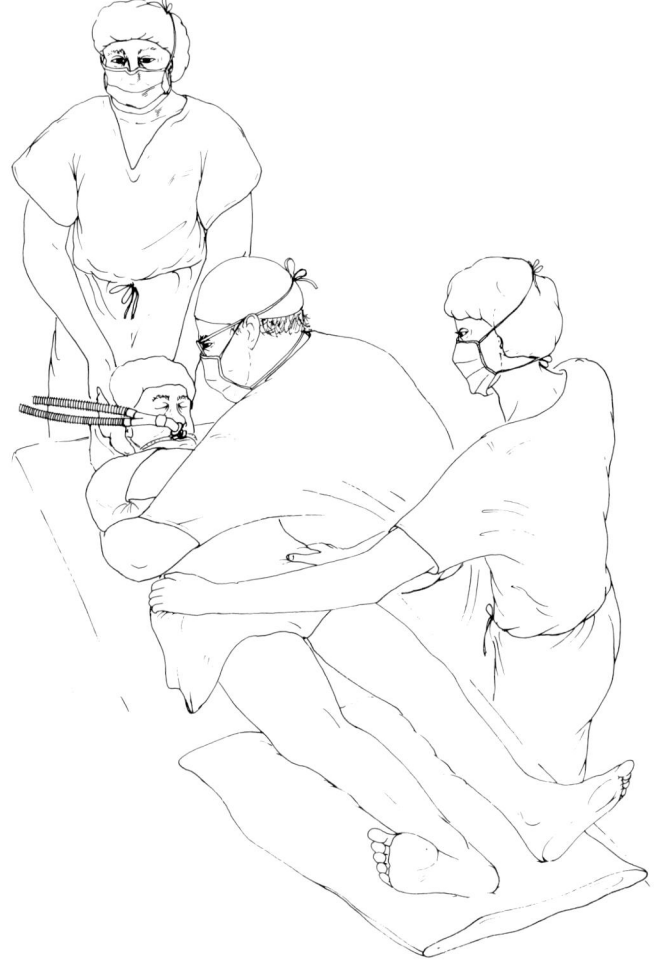

FIGURE 31–5

After the move is complete, recheck the tracheal tube position by auscultation, capnography, and pulse oximetry to be sure that it has not migrated into a mainstem bronchus or out of the trachea. Support and pad the patient's head to prevent excessive tension being placed on the connective tissue at the neck or on the ear. Flex the patient's legs at the hips and knees for stabilization. Place a pillow between the legs to prevent bony protuberances from abutting one another. Position the dependent arm on a padded arm rest. Tape four blankets together in a stack to support the upper arm on the dependent arm. Use wide (3-inch) adhesive tape to stabilize the bundle of blankets in place and the arm on top of the blankets (Fig. 31–6). Alternatively, support the upper arm on an adjustable arm rest. The latter must be adjusted so that it does not project into the axilla of the upper extremity. Usually, strips of wide (3-inch) adhesive tape are placed across the upper hip and shoulder and under the operating room table on either side to stabilize the patient in place during the surgery.

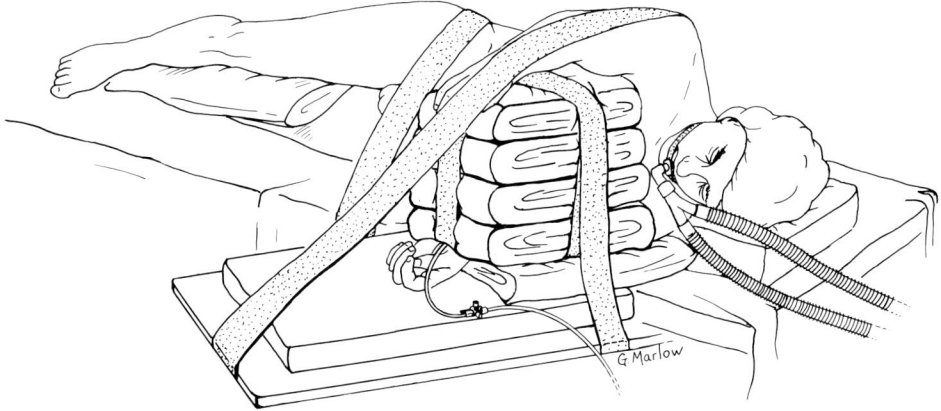

FIGURE 31–6

Prone Position

The prone position is used most often for operations on the lumbar, thoracic, and cervical spine. Patients who will be operated on in the prone position usually will be anesthetized on a stretcher and then carefully "rolled" onto the operating room table. The anesthetist will be responsible for the position of the head and neck during the move except when the spine is unstable. If the spine may be unstable (e.g., after injury), all movements of the patient's head and neck must be supervised by the neurosurgeon.

Always be sure that there are a sufficient number of assistants available before attempting to reposition a patient. The anesthetist should signal when the patient is to be "rolled" onto the arms of the assistants (Fig. 31–7). The arms remain at the

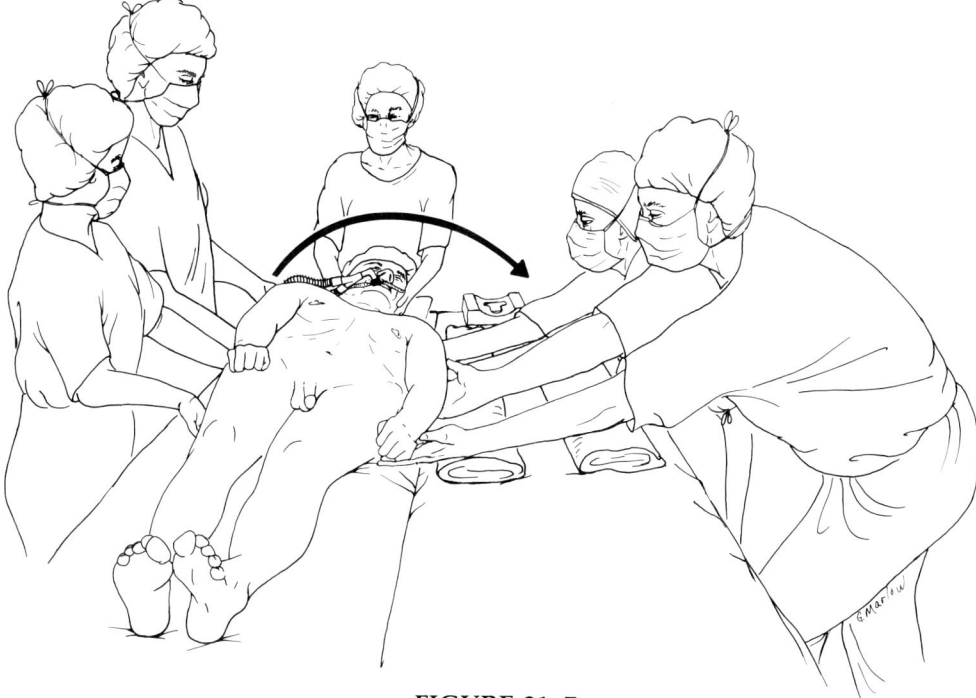

FIGURE 31–7

patient's sides while the turn is accomplished. The shoulders will usually be elevated off the operating room table by the chest rolls, permitting the arms to be positioned comfortably above the head on the arm rests. Pad both elbow areas to prevent ulnar nerve injury. The assistants then must lift the patient onto the chest rolls previously positioned on the operating room table. The chest rolls (I use taped, rolled blankets) should be positioned between the clavicles and the anterior-superior iliac spines on each side. When the chest rolls are correctly located they will not impede ventilation. The abdominal contents should sag downward between the chest rolls.

Place the head on a foam head cradle, a "horseshoe" headrest, or a pin fixation device (Fig. 31–8). The goal is to stabilize the head while avoiding undue pressure on the soft tissues of the face. Check that the eyes, nose, ears, and genitalia are not compressed. After completing the move, always recheck the position of the endotracheal tube with auscultation, capnography, and pulse oximetry to be certain that it has not migrated.

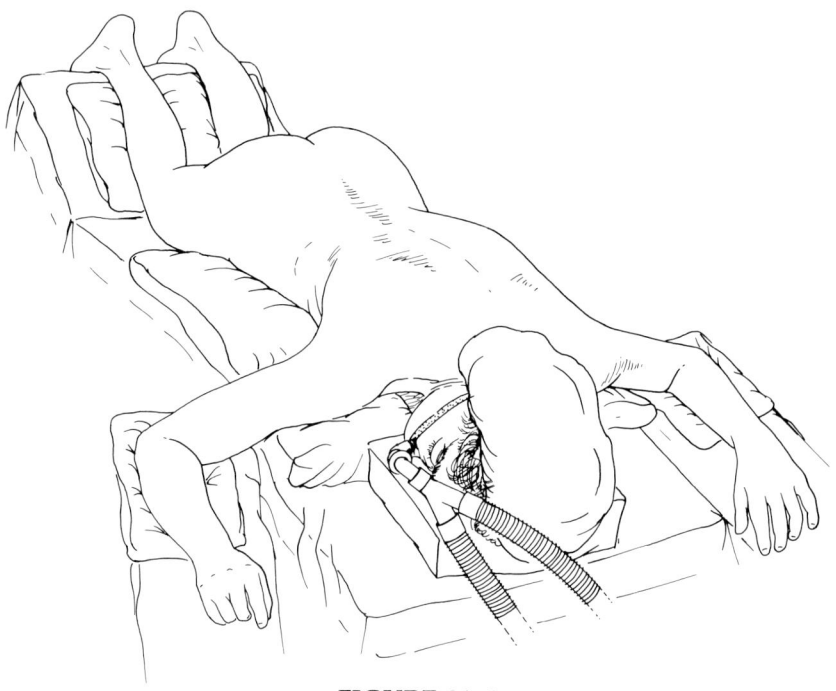

FIGURE 31–8

A variety of frames and devices have been developed to prevent increased intra-abdominal pressure during surgery conducted on prone patients. These devices may be substituted for the chest roll technique described previously. Batson's venous plexus permits free communication between the vena cava and the epidural veins. Proper positioning reduces the intra-abdominal pressure, thus reducing the pressure in the inferior vena cava and epidural veins and decreasing venous bleeding during spinal surgery.

Sitting Position

The sitting or "head elevated" position is commonly used in neurosurgery for operations in the posterior cranial fossa, cerebellopontine angles, and cervical spine. Advantages of the sitting position include unencumbered access to the patient for both the surgeon and the anesthetist. Blood drains by gravity from the wound. Ventilation is not impaired. The anatomic structures are presented in their natural position. Counterbalanced against these advantages of the sitting position is the increased incidence of venous air emboli during surgery.

The sitting position is accomplished through a coordinated series of movements. These changes in posture must be accomplished slowly. Too rapid changes can result in precipitous hypotension. Fully flex the surgical table (Fig. 31–9). Fully raise the back section of the surgical table (Fig. 31–10). Incline the table in Trendelenburg's

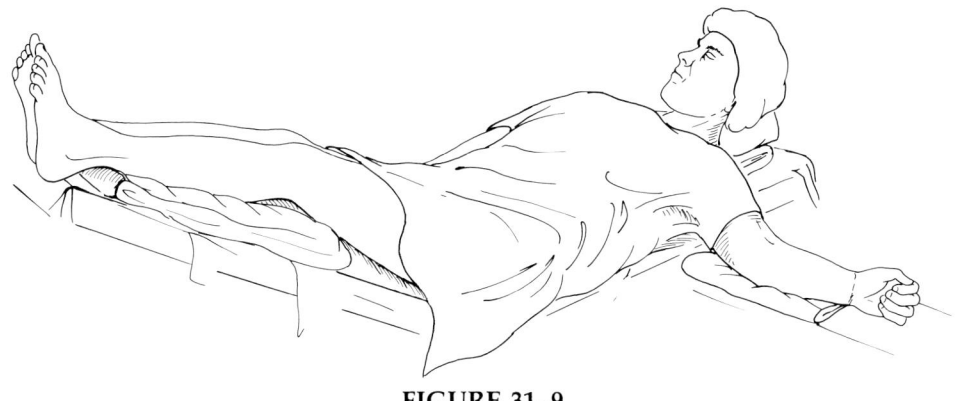

FIGURE 31–9

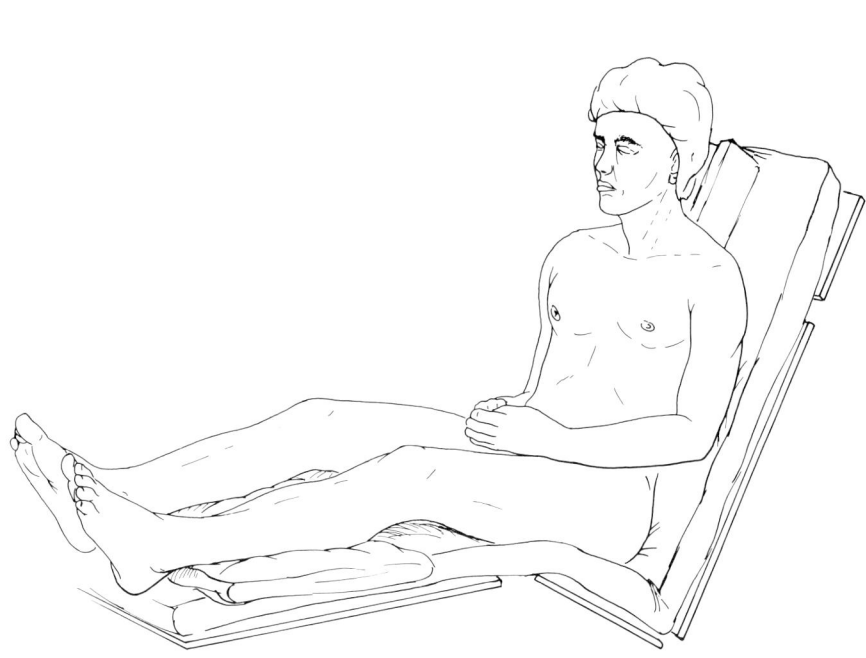

FIGURE 31–10

position and lower the foot section of the table until it is horizontal. Attach the pin fixation device to the table for the surgeon to immobilize the patient's head. Remove the head support from the surgical table. Fold the patient's arms across his waist (Fig. 31–11). Pad the elbows to protect the ulnar nerves. Wrap the legs with elastic bandages to prevent venous pooling.

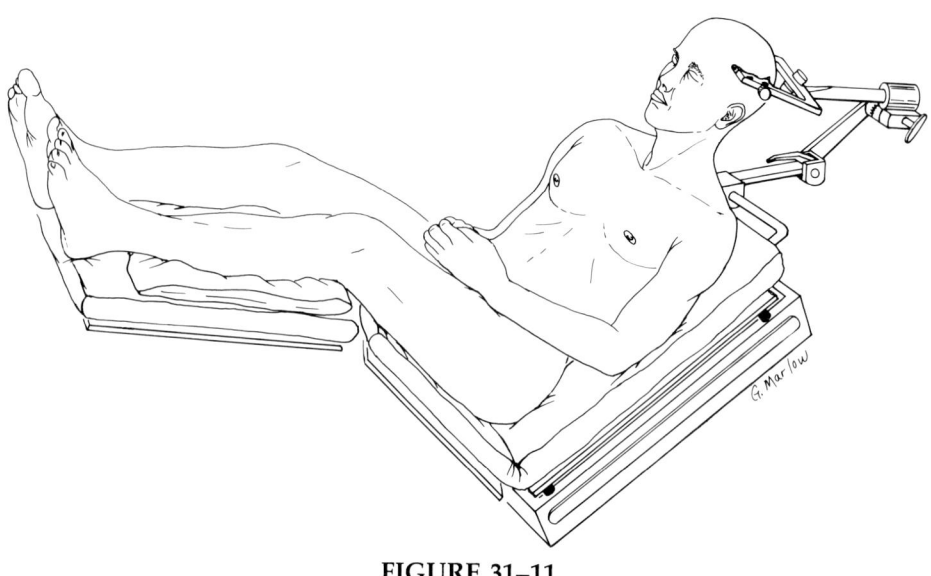

FIGURE 31–11

Because of the increased incidence of venous air emboli in the sitting position, I normally place a Doppler probe on the precordium so that venous air emboli can be heard by their characteristic sound, and position a central venous cannula at the cavoatrial junction with which to aspirate venous air emboli (see Chapter 16). In some institutions, transesophageal echocardiography is also used to detect emboli and assess their significance.

References

Anderton JM, Keen RI, Neave R: Positioning the Surgical Patient. Boston, Butterworths, 1988

Cucciara RF, Nugent M, Stewart JB, Messick JM: Air embolism in upright neurosurgical patients: Detection and localization by two-dimensional transesophageal echocardiography. Anesthesiology 60:353–355, 1984

Datta S, Alpert MH, Ostheimer GW, Brown WU, Weiss JB: Effects of maternal position on epidural anesthesia for cesarean section, acid–base status, and bupivacaine concentrations at delivery. Anesthesiology 50:205–209, 1979

Martin JT: Neuroanesthetic adjuncts for surgery in the sitting position: I. Introduction and basic equipment. Anesth Analg 49:577–587, 1970

Martin JT: Neuroanesthetic adjuncts for surgery in the sitting position: III. Intravascular electrocardiograph. Anesth Analg 49:793–805, 1970

Martin JT: Positioning in Anesthesia and Surgery. Philadelphia, WB Saunders, 1987

Sprague DH: Effects of position and uterine displacement on spinal anesthesia for cesarean section. Anesthesiology 44:164–166, 1976

Ueland K, Hansen JN: Maternal cardiovascular dynamics: II. Posture and uterine contractions. Am J Obstet Gynecol 103:1–7, 1969

Wilcox S, Vandam LD: Alas, poor Trendelenburg and his position! A critique of its uses and effectiveness. Anesth Analg 67:578, 1988

Index

Note: Page numbers in *italics* refer to illustrations.

A

Age factor, in spinal anesthesia, 180
Allen test, in arterial cannulation, 115
Alopecia, cranial, prevention of, 227
Ankle, nerve block of, *174*, 174–175
Anorectal procedure, spinal anesthesia in, 181. See also *Caudal anesthesia; Spinal anesthesia.*
Arm support, in surgical table, 225, *225*
Arterial cannulation. See *Cannulation, arterial.*
Artery(ies), brachial, cannulation of, 116, *122*, 123
　in nerve block at elbow, 159, *159*
　cannulation of, 115–123. See also *Cannulation, arterial.*
　carotid, in cervical plexus block, 214–215
　　in internal jugular vein cannulation, *78*, 78, *79*
　　in laryngeal nerve block, 7, *8*
　femoral, cannulation of, 115–116, *123*, 123
　pulmonary, catheterization of, 105–123. See also *Catheterization, pulmonary artery.*
　radial, cannulation of, 115–116, *117*
　　alternatives to, *122–131*, 123
　ulnar, in nerve block at wrist, 162–163, *163*
Arthroscopy, knee, regional anesthesia in, 172
Aspiration, gastric, glottic anesthesia and, 13, *14*
Auscultation, postintubation, pediatric, 19

B

Back support, in surgical table, 224, *224*
Bag and mask ventilation, 3–19
　adequacy of, 6
　adjunct maneuvers in, 6
　failed intubation and, 28–29
　mask fit in, 3
　oropharyngeal and nasopharyngeal airways in, 3, *4, 5, 6*
　tongue obstruction and, 3, *4, 5, 6*

"Ball-valve" obstruction, in double-lumen endobronchial tube intubation, 60
Benzodiazepine, in endoscopic intubation, 31
Bier block. See *Regional anesthesia, intravenous.*
Blood, arterial, sample of, 116
　color of, correct cannula placement and, 81, 106
Blood patch, epidural, in post-lumbar puncture headache, 183
Brachial artery, in nerve block at elbow, 159, *159*
Brachial plexus block, 145–155. See also *Nerve block, upper extremity, brachial plexus block as.*
Bronchoscope, fiberoptic, in laryngoscopy, 31–36. See also *Laryngoscopy.*
Bronchus, right, endoscopic view of, *58, 59*
Buie's position, in caudal anesthesia, 205
Bunionectomy, ankle block in, 174
Bupivacaine, in ankle block, 174
　in brachial plexus block, 146
　in caudal anesthesia, 205, 206, *206*
　in cervical plexus block, 214, 215
　in epidural anesthesia, 192
　in intercostal nerve block, 212
　in knee block, 172
　in local infiltration, 135
　in lower extremity nerve block, 167
　in lumbar epidural anesthesia, 201
　in musculocutaneous nerve block, 156
　in nerve block at elbow, 158
　in nerve block at wrist, 160
　in spinal anesthesia, 180–181, 189
　in thoracic epidural anesthesia, 202

C

Cannulation, arterial, 115–123
　Allen test in, 115
　arterial line flushing in, 116
　blood sample withdrawal in, 116
　brachial artery in, 116, *122*, 123

Cannulation *(Continued)*
　cannula insertion in, 118, *118*, 119
　dorsalis pedis in, 15, *122*, 123
　equipment in, 116
　femoral artery in, 115–116, *123*, 123
　flushing and securing of cannula in, 121, *121*
　general considerations for, 115
　guide wires in, 121
　indications for, 115
　local anesthetic injection in, 116–117, *117*
　positioning in, 116
　preparation in, 116
　radial artery in, 115–116, *117*
　　alternatives to, *122–131*, 123
　site selection in, 115–116
　transfixation technique in, 120, *120*
　central venous, 75–98
　basilic vein in, 92–94
　　"cannula-through-needle" technique in, 94–95, *94, 95*
　　equipment for, 93
　　general considerations for, 92
　　identification of, 93, *93*
　　preparation and positioning of, 93
　cannula tip location in, 75
　equipment in, 77
　femoral vein in, 95–96, *96–98*
　　equipment for, 95
　　general considerations for, 94
　　pediatric, 96, 97
　　preparation and positioning of, 96, *96*
　　procedure for, 96–97, *96–98*
　guide wire passage in, 82, *82, 83*
　history of, 75
　in pediatrics, 94, 96, 97
　indications for, 75
　intravascular electrocardiography in, 101, 102–103, *102–104*
　jugular vein in, external, 85–87, *86–89*
　　internal, 77–84
　　cannula insertion in, 84, *84*
　　equipment for, 77
　　guide passage in, 82, *83*

235

Cannulation *(Continued)*
  location of, 78, *79*
    preparation and positioning of, 78
  sites for, 75, *76*
  subclavian vein in, 89–90, *91*, *92*
    "cannula-through-needle" technique in, 90, *90–93*
    equipment for, 89
    general considerations for, 89
    preparation and positioning of, 89
    procedure for, 89–90
  intravenous, 71, *72*, *73*
Carlens tube, 54, *54*
Carotid artery, in cervical plexus block, 214–215
  in internal jugular vein cannulation, *78*, 78, *79*
  in laryngeal nerve block, 7, *8*
Cartilage, cricoid, in transtracheal anesthesia, *9*
  thyroid, in transtracheal anesthesia, *9*
Catheter, epidural, 198–100, *198–200*
Catheterization, pulmonary artery, 105–123
  catheter floating into pulmonary artery in, 111–113, *111–113*
  difficult, 113–114
  equipment in, 106
  in thermodilution cardiac output measurement, 114
  indications for, 105
  insertion sites in, 106
  introducer sheath insertion in, 107–108, *107–109*
  J-wire passage in, 106–107, *107*
  preparation in, 110, *110*
  risks of, 105
  uses for, 114
Caudal anesthesia, 192, 205–207. See also *Epidural anesthesia, caudal.*
Central venous pressure, in pulmonary artery catheterization, 111, *111*
  monitoring of, 77, *77*
Cerebrospinal fluid, aspiration of, in spinal anesthesia, 188, *188*, *189*
Cervical epidural anesthesia, indications for, 192
Cervical plexus block, 213–216
  deep, *215*, 215–216
  superficial, 213–215, *214*
Cesarean delivery, spinal anesthesia in, 181
Chest roll, for prone position, 232
Coracobrachialis muscle, in musculocutaneous nerve block, *156*, 156–157, *157*
Cricoid cartilage, in transtracheal anesthesia, *9*
Cricothyroid membrane, in cricothyroidotomy, 41–42, *42*

Cricothyroid membrane *(Continued)*
  in transtracheal anesthesia, 8, *9*
  in transtracheal jet ventilation, 38, *38*
Cricothyroidotomy, 41–44
  equipment in, 41
  general considerations for, 41
  incision in, 42, *42*, *43*
  indications for, 41
  preparation in, 41
  tube insertion in, *43*, 43–44, *44*
Croup, postextubation, pediatric, 18
Crystalloid solution, in spinal anesthesia, 183
Cuff, in pediatric intubation, 19

D

Digital nerve block, 143–144, *144*
Double-lumen endobronchial tube intubation, 53–61
  Carlens, 54, *54*
  endoscopy and, 57, 60, 69
  equipment in, 53
  in one-lung anesthesia, 55
    oxygen saturation during, 60, *61*
  indications for, 53, 53t
  insertion in, 55, *56*
  laryngoscopy and, 55, *56*
  malposition in, *59*, 59–60
  one-lung ventilation and, 60
  position check in, 57, *57*, *58*
  preparation in, 53
  right upper lobe atelectasis and, 57–58, *58*
  Robertshaw, 54, *56*
  securing tube for, 57
  types and characteristics of tubes for, 53–55, *54*

E

Elbow, nerve block at, 157–159, *158*, *159*
Electrical nerve stimulator, in regional anesthesia, 217–218, *218*
Electrocardiography, intravascular, 101–103, *102–104*
  cannula positioning in, 102–103, *102–104*
  equipment in, 101
  preparation in, 101–102, *102*
Embolism, air, venous, prevention of, 234
Endobronchial intubation, 53–61. See also *Double-lumen endobronchial tube intubation.*
Endotracheal tube, insertion of, in fiberoptic laryngoscopy, 33, *36*
  replacement of, 63–65, *64–66*
    equipment in, 63
    general considerations for, 63
    laryngoscopy in, 65
    tube changer in, 63–64, *64*
    under direct vision, 65, *65*, *66*
Ephedrine, in hypotension during epidural anesthesia, 202
  in hypotension during spinal anesthesia, 182

Epidural anesthesia, caudal, 192, 205–207
  anatomy in, 205
  continuous, 208
  equipment in, 205
  general considerations for, 205
  indications for, 192
  needle insertion in, *206*, 206–207
  pediatric, 192, 205, 208
  preparation and positioning in, 205
  test dosing in, 208
  cervical, 192
  dysfunctional, 202
  epidural space identification in, 191–192
  general considerations for, 191
  "hanging drop" technique in, 191–192
  hypotension and, 202
  "loss of resistance" technique in, 191–192, 196–197
  lumbar, 192–202
    catheter insertion and securement in, 198–200, *198–200*
    epidural space identification in, 196–197, *197*
    indications for, 192
    intravenous test dose in, 201
    local anesthetic dosing in, 201
    needle insertion in, *195*, 195–196, *196*
    onset of, 201–202
    spinal test dose in, 200, *200*
  needle in, insertion of, 195–197, *195–197*
    removal of, 199, *199*
    size of, 191
  puncture site in, 192
  spinal anesthesia vs., 191
  thoracic, 202–205, *203*, *204*
    indications for, 192
Epiglottis, in awake orotracheal intubation, 15
  pediatric, 18, *19*
Epinephrine, in ankle block, 174
  in blind nasal intubation, 22, *23*
  in caudal anesthesia, 205, 206, *206*
  in cervical plexus block, 214, 215
  in digital nerve block, 143
  in hypotension during epidural anesthesia, 202
  in hypotension during spinal anesthesia, 182
  in intercostal nerve block, 211, 212
  in knee block, 172
  in local infiltration, 135
  in lumbar epidural anesthesia, 200
  in musculocutaneous nerve block, 156
  in nerve block at elbow, 157–158
  in nerve block at wrist, 160
  in spinal anesthesia, 180–181
Esmarch bandage, in intravenous regional anesthesia, 138, *139*
  risks of, 137
Extremity, nerve block of, 145–177. See also *Nerve block, lower extremity; Nerve block, upper extremity.*

F

Femoral nerve block, 168–170, *169*
Fentanyl, in blind nasal intubation, 22, 23
 in spinal anesthesia, 182
Finger, digital nerve block of, 143–144, *144*
Foot support, in surgical table, 224, *224*
Forearm, musculocutaneous nerve block and, *156*, 156–157, *157*

G

Genitourinary procedure, lithotomy position in, 228, *228*
Glottis, endoscopic view of, *34*
 exposure of, in awake orotracheal intubation, 13, *14*, 15, *15*, 17
Glycopyrrolate, in blind nasal intubation, 22, *23*
 in endoscopic intubation, 31
Gynecologic procedure, lithotomy position for, 228, *228*

H

Headache, post-lumbar puncture, 182–183, 197
Hip, fracture of, spinal anesthesia in, 181. See also *Spinal anesthesia.*
"Horseshoe" headrest, 232, *232*
"Huber tip," in epidural needle, 191
Hypotension, during epidural anesthesia, 202
 during spinal anesthesia, 182
Hypoxemia, during one-lung anesthesia, 60, *61*

I

Infant. See also *Pediatrics.*
 intubation of, 18–19, *19*
Intubation, awake, orotracheal, 12–15, *12–15*. See also *Intubation, orotracheal.*
 bronchial, pediatric, 18–19
 endobronchial, 53–61. See also *Double-lumen endobronchial tube intubation.*
 failed, 27–29
  alternatives in, 28, *28*
  anticipation of, 27–28
  bag and mask ventilation as alternative to, 28–29
  demographics in, 27–28
  etiology of, 27–28
  general anesthesia and, 29
  general considerations for, 27
  pregnancy and, 28
 nasotracheal, 21–29
  blind, 21
   after general anesthesia, 25–26
   anesthesia of larynx and pharynx in, *14*, 22
   endoscopic vs., 21
   equipment in, 22
   laryngoscope in, 24–25, *26*
   positioning in, 24, *24*
   preparation in, 22

Intubation *(Continued)*
  sedation in, 22
  "sniffing position" in, 24, *25*
  topical nasal anesthesia in, 22, *23*
  tube insertion in, 24, *25*
 in anesthetized patient, 21
 in awake patient, 21
 indications for, 21
 orotracheal, 11–19
  awake, 12–15, *12–15*
   anesthesia of pharynx and larynx in, 13
   anesthetized vs., 12
   equipment in, 12
   glottis exposure in, 13, *14*, 15, *15*
   preparation and positioning in, 12–13, *13*
   sedation in, 13
  history of, 11
  laryngoscope blades in, curved, 11, *11*, *16*, 16–17
   straight, 11, *11*, *17*, 17–18, *18*
  pediatric, anatomic concerns in, 18–19, *19*
  "sniffing position" in, 13, *13*, 16, 17
 retrograde, 45–48
  equipment in, 45
  indications for, 45
  procedure in, 45, *46*, *47*, 47–48
 with lighted stylet, 49, *50*

J

Jet ventilation, transtracheal, 37–39
 equipment in, *37*, 37–38
 failed intubation and, 28
 procedure in, *38*, 38–39, *39*
Jugular vein, in central venous cannulation, 77–87, *78–89*. See also *Cannulation, central venous, jugular vein in.*
 in cervical plexus block, 214, *214*
 in pulmonary artery catheterization, 106

K

Kidney rest, in surgical table, 224–225, *225*
Knee, nerve block of, 172, *173*

L

Labor, epidural anesthesia during, 191, 201. See also *Epidural anesthesia.*
Laryngoscopy, double-lumen endobronchial tube intubation in, 55, *56*
 fiberoptic, 31–36
  anesthetic and vasoconstrictor in, 31
  endoscope insertion in, 33, *34*, *35*
  endotracheal tube insertion in, 33, *36*
  equipment in, 31–32
  instrument cleaning in, 33
  intravenous adjuvants in, 31
  preparation in, 32, *33*

Laryngoscopy *(Continued)*
 in blind nasotracheal intubation, 24–25, *26*
 in endotracheal tube replacement, 65
 in orotracheal intubation, after anesthesia of pharynx and larynx, 13
  curved blade in, 11, *11*, *16*, 16–17
  preparation in, 12
  straight blade in, 11, *11*, *17*, 17–18, *18*
Larynx, in awake orotracheal intubation, 13, *14*
 in nasotracheal intubation, *14*, 22
 infant, 18
 superior laryngeal nerve block of, 7, *8*
  awake orotracheal intubation and, 13
  equipment in, 7
  procedure in, 7, *8*
 transtracheal anesthesia for, 7, *8*, *9*
  awake orotracheal intubation and, 13
  equipment in, 8
  procedure in, 8, *9*
Lateral decubitus position, *230*, 230–231, *231*
Lidocaine, in arterial cannulation, 117
 in awake orotracheal intubation, 13, 14
 in basilic vein cannulation, 93
 in caudal anesthesia, 205, *206*
 in central venous cannulation, 80, 89
 in femoral vein cannulation, 96
 in intravenous cannulation, 71
 in knee block, 172
 in local infiltration, 135
 in lumbar epidural anesthesia, 193, *193*, 200, 201
 in retrograde intubation, 45
 in spinal anesthesia, 180–181, *186*, 187, 189
 in superior laryngeal nerve block, 7
 in thoracic epidural anesthesia, 203
 in transtracheal anesthesia, 8
Ligament, sacrococcygeal, in caudal anesthesia, 206, *206*
Ligamentum flavum, in epidural anesthesia, 191
 in lumbar epidural anesthesia, *195*, 195–196
 in spinal anesthesia, *186*, 187
 in thoracic epidural anesthesia, 204, *204*
Light wand, 49, *50*
Lithotomy position, 228, *229*
Lower extremity, nerve block of, 167–177. See also *Nerve block, lower extremity.*
Lumbar anesthesia, 192–202. See also *Epidural anesthesia, lumbar.*

Index

M

MacIntosh blade, 11, *11, 16,* 16–17
Magill forceps, in nasotracheal intubation, 25, *26*
Mask. See also *Bag and mask ventilation.*
 size and fit of, 3
Mayo stand, in lumbar epidural anesthesia, 193, *193*
 in spinal anesthesia, 184, *184*
Median nerve block, at elbow, 159, *159*
 at wrist, *161,* 161–162, *162*
Mepivacaine, in brachial plexus block, 146
 in lower extremity nerve block, 167
 in musculocutaneous nerve block, 156
 in nerve block at elbow, 157–158
 in nerve block at wrist, 160
Midazolam, in awake orotracheal intubation, 13
 in blind nasal intubation, 22, *23*
 in endoscopic intubation, 31
 in spinal anesthesia, 182
Miller blade, 11, *11, 17,* 17–18, *18*
Morphine, in epidural anesthesia, 192
 in thoracic epidural anesthesia, 202
Muscle, coracobrachialis, in musculocutaneous nerve block, *156,* 156–157, *157*
 sternocleidomastoid, in central venous cannulation, *78,* 78, *79*
 in cervical plexus block, 213–214, *214*
Musculocutaneous nerve block, upper extremity, *156,* 156–157, *157*
Myocardial infarction, acute, pulmonary artery catheterization and, 105

N

Nasal intubation. See *Intubation, nasotracheal.*
Nasopharyngeal airway, in bag and mask ventilation, 3, *4, 5, 6*
Nasotracheal intubation, 21–29. See also *Intubation, nasotracheal.*
Needle, epidural, 191, 195–196, *196, 197,* 199
 spinal, 179, *180*
Neonate. See also *Pediatrics.*
 tube size for, 19
Nerve block, digital, 143–144, *144*
 intercostal, 209–212
  equipment in, 209
  intercostal space marking in, 210, *210*
  needle insertion in, *210,* 210–211, *211*
  preparation and positioning in, 209–210, *210*
  skin preparation in, 210
 laryngeal, superior, 7, *8*

Nerve block *(Continued)*
 awake orotracheal intubation and, 13
 equipment in, 7
 procedure in, 7, *8*
 lower extremity, 167–177
  ankle block as, *174,* 174–175
  equipment in, 167
  femoral nerve block as, 168–170, *169*
  knee block as, 172, *173*
  lateral cutaneous nerve of thigh in, *170,* 170
  local anesthetic in, 167
  obturator nerve block as, 172, *173*
  peroneal nerve block as, *175,* 175–176, *177,* 177
  sciatic nerve block as, 167–168, *168*
  superficial peroneal nerve block as, *177,* 177
  superficial saphenous nerve block as, *177,* 177
  sural nerve block as, *176,* 176–177
  tibial nerve block as, *176,* 177
 upper extremity, 145–165, *157,* 157
  at elbow, 157–159, *158, 159*
   equipment in, 158
   median nerve block as, 159, *159*
   radial nerve block as, 159, *159*
   ulnar nerve block as, 158, *158*
  at wrist, equipment in, 160
   median nerve block as, *161,* 161–162, *162*
   radial nerve block as, 164, *164*
   ulnar nerve block as, 162–163, *163*
  brachial plexus block as, 145–155
   axillary approach in, 147, *147*
   equipment in, 146–147
   general considerations for, 145
   interscalene approach in, *154,* 154–155, *155*
   local anesthetic in, 146
    second injection of, *149,* 149–150, *150*
    test dose of, 149
   needle for, 145
    insertion of, 148, *148*
   nerve distribution and, 145, *146*
   position in, 148, *148*
   preparation in, 148, *148*
   supraclavicular approach in, 151–153
    anesthesia onset in, 153
    general considerations for, 151
    local anesthetic injection in, 153
    needle insertion in, *152,* 152–153, *153*
    positioning in, 151, *151*
    preparation in, 151, *151*
    transarterial vs. paresthesia technique in, 150
  lateral cutaneous nerve block as, *157,* 157
  musculocutaneous nerve block as, *156,* 156–157, *157*
Nerve stimulator, in regional anesthesia, 217–218, *218*
Nerves, upper extremity, *146*

Neurosurgery, sitting position in, 232–234, *233, 234*

O

Obturator nerve block, 172, *173*
One-lung anesthesia, double-lumen endobronchial tube intubation in, 55
Oropharyngeal airway, in bag and mask ventilation, 3
Orotracheal intubation, 11–19. See also *Intubation, orotracheal.*
Oxygen saturation, during one-lung anesthesia, 60, *61*

P

Paresthesias, spinal anesthesia and, 181–182
Pediatrics, arterial cannulation in, 116. See also *Cannulation, arterial.*
 caudal anesthesia in, 192, 205, 208
 central venous cannulation in, 94, 96, 97. See also *Cannulation, central venous.*
 cuff size in, 19
 dorsalis pedis cannulation in, 115, *122,* 123
 intravenous cannulation in, 71, 72, 73
 intubation in, 18–19, *19*
 orotracheal intubation in. See also *Intubation, orotracheal.*
  anatomic concerns in, 18–19, *19*
  tube selection and insertion in, 19
 postextubation croup in, 18
 tube size for, 19
Peroneal nerve block, deep, *175,* 175–176
 superficial, *177,* 177
Pharynx, in awake orotracheal intubation, 13, *14*
 in nasotracheal intubation, *14,* 22
Phenylephrine, in hypotension during spinal anesthesia, 182
Pneumothorax, emergency needle thoracentesis and, 67–68, *68*
 intercostal nerve block and, 209
 subclavian vein cannulation and, 89
Position, patient, 227–234. See also *Surgical table.*
 lateral decubitus, *230,* 230–231, *231*
 lithotomy, *228,* 229
 prone, *231,* 231–232, *232*
 sitting, 232–234, *233, 234*
 supine, *227,* 227–228, *228*
Pregnancy, failed intubation and, 28
 patient position in, 228, *228*
 spinal anesthesia in, 180
Prone position, *231,* 231–232, *232*
Pulmonary artery, catheterization of, 105–123. See also *Catheterization, pulmonary artery.*
 pressure monitoring of, in pulmonary artery catheterization, 112, *112,* 114
Pulmonary surgery, lateral decubitus position in, *230,* 230–231, *231*
Pulse oximetry, in spinal anesthesia, 182

R

Radial nerve block, at elbow, 159, *159*
  at wrist, 164, *164*
Regional anesthesia. See also names of specific types of regional anesthesia.
  anatomy in, *134*
  electrical nerve stimulator in, 217–218, *218*
  intravenous, 137–141
    anesthetic injection in, 140, *140*
    contraindications for, 137
    equipment in, 137
    Esmarch bandage in, 138, *139*
    positioning in, 138, *139*
    preparation in, 138, *139*
    tourniquet in, 138, *139*, 140–141
Renal surgery, lateral decubitus position in, *230*, 230–231, *231*
Rib, nerve block at, 209–212. See also *Nerve block, intercostal.*
Robertshaw tube, 54, *56*

S

Sacrococcygeal ligament, in caudal anesthesia, 206, *206*
Saddle block, 181. See also *Spinal anesthesia.*
Saphenous nerve block, superficial, 177, *177*
Sciatic nerve block, 167–168, *168*
Seldinger technique, in central venous cannulation, 90, 92
Sitting position, 232–234, *233*, *234*
Skin, local anesthetic injection in, *135*, 135–136
  nerve block of, for upper extremity, 157, *157*
Spinal anesthesia, 179–189
  age factor in, 180
  anesthetic injection in, *188*, 188–189, *189*
  antiseptic solution in, *184*, 184–185
  cerebrospinal fluid aspiration in, 188, *188*, *189*
  choices of, 179–180
  continuous, 189
  contraindications for, 183
  difficult, 189
  draping in, 185, *185*
  epidural anesthesia vs., 191
  equipment in, 183
  general considerations for, 179–189
  history of, 179
  hypotension during, 182
  indications for, 179
  interspace selection in, 185, 187
  local anesthetic in, 179–180
  needle insertion in, *186*, 187, *187*
  needle size in, 179, 180
  paresthesias in, 181–182
  post-lumbar puncture headache and, 182–183

Spinal anesthesia (Continued)
  preparation and positioning in, 183–185, *184*, *185*
  sedation and, 182
Sternocleidomastoid muscle, in central venous cannulation, *78*, 78, *79*
  in cervical plexus block, 213–214, *214*
Stylet, lighted, 49, *50*
Supine position, 227, *227*–228, *228*
Sural nerve block, *176*, 176–177
Surgical table, 221–225
  arm support in, 225, *225*
  electrically operated, 221, 221–222, *222*
  flexing of, 223, *223*
  foot support in, 224, *224*
  in reverse-Trendelenburg position, 223
  in Trendelenburg position, 223, *223*, 233–234
  kidney rest in, 224–225, *225*
  manually operated, 221
  patient position on, 227–234. See also *Position, patient.*
Suture, 125–130, *126–130*
  knot types for, 125
  square knot for, with both hands, 128, *128–131*, 130
  with left hand, *126*, 127, *127*

T

Tetracaine, in spinal anesthesia, 180–181
Thermodilution, cardiac output measurement by, pulmonary artery catheterization and, 114
Thigh, lateral cutaneous nerve block in, 170, *170*
Thoracentesis, needle, emergency, 67–68, *68*
Thoracic anesthesia, 202–205, *203*, *204*
  indications for, 192
Thyroid cartilage, in transtracheal anesthesia, *9*
Tibial nerve block, *176*, 177
Toe, digital nerve block of, 143–144, *144*
Tolazoline, in blind nasal intubation, 22, *23*
Topical anesthesia, nasal, in blind nasotracheal intubation, 22, *23*
Tourniquet, in intravenous cannulation, 71, *72*
  in intravenous regional anesthesia, 138, *139*, 140–141
  in pneumatic obturator and femoral nerve blocks, 167
  in spinal anesthesia, 181
Trachea, endoscopic view of, *35*, *36*
Transtracheal anesthesia, 7, *8*, *9*
  awake orotracheal intubation and, 13
  equipment in, 8
  procedure in, 8, *9*
Trendelenburg position, 223, *223*, 233–234
  in central venous cannulation, *72*, *78*, *89*

U

Ulnar nerve block, at elbow, 158, *158*
  at wrist, 162–163, *163*
Upper extremity, nerve block of, 145–165. See also *Nerve block, upper extremity.*

V

Vasoconstrictor, in blind nasal intubation, 22, *23*
  in endoscopic intubation, 31
  in nasotracheal intubation, 21
Vein(s), air embolism in, prevention of, 234
  basilic, cannulation of, 92–94. See also *Cannulation, central venous, basilic vein in.*
  cannulation of, 75–98. See also *Cannulation, central venous.*
  femoral, cannulation of, 95–97, *96–98*. See also *Cannulation, central venous, femoral vein in.*
  jugular, cannulation of, 85–87, *86–89*. See also *Cannulation, central venous, jugular vein in.*
  in cervical plexus block, 214, *214*
  in pulmonary artery catheterization, 106
  reliable locations of, intravenous cannulation and, 71, *72*, 73
  subclavian, cannulation of, 89–90, *91*, 92. See also *Cannulation, central venous, subclavian vein in.*
Ventilation, assisted, 3
  controlled, 3
  jet. See *Jet ventilation.*
  spontaneous, 3
  with bag and mask, 3–19. See also *Bag and mask ventilation.*
Ventricular pressure, right, in pulmonary artery catheterization, 111, *111*
Vocal cord, in awake orotracheal intubation, 13, *14*, 15, *17*, 17–18
  in double-lumen tube insertion, 55, *56*
  in nasotracheal intubation, 24
  pediatric, 18, *19*

W

Wrist, nerve block at, 160–164, *160–164*
  equipment in, 160
  median nerve block as, *161*, 161–162, *162*
  radial nerve block as, 164, *164*
  ulnar nerve block as, 162–163, *163*